Uncertainty and Explanation in Medicine and the Health Sciences

Olaf Dammann

Uncertainty and Explanation in Medicine and the Health Sciences

palgrave
macmillan

Olaf Dammann
Department of Public Health and Community Medicine
Tufts University School of Medicine
Boston, MA, USA

Department of Neuromedicine and Movement Science
Norwegian University of Science and Technology (NTNU)
Trondheim, Norway

Department of Philosophy
University of Johannesburg
Johannesburg, South Africa

ISBN 978-3-031-82270-4   ISBN 978-3-031-82271-1   (eBook)
https://doi.org/10.1007/978-3-031-82271-1

This Palgrave Macmillan imprint is published by the registered company Springer Nature Switzerland AG.
The registered company address is: Gewerbestrasse 11, 6330 Cham, Switzerland

If disposing of this product, please recycle the paper.

In memory of
Hans-Christian Dammann
1936–2001

PREFACE

Doubt is not a pleasant condition, but certainty is absurd
   —Voltaire

Some recent voices in the philosophy of medicine literature lament that medicine is unreliable, ineffective, to the degree that "our confidence in the effectiveness of medical intervention ought to be low" (Stegenga, 2018, p. 18). I would like to soften this verdict and defend medicine by demonstrating, first, that medicine does indeed suffer from an uncertainty that cannot be eliminated but only curbed and, second, that medicine and the health sciences use conceptual strategies such as inferences, explanations, and what I call, somewhat tongue-in-cheek, "quasi-causometers", tools to establish causation (not to prove it) in medicine and medical research.

This is an unapologetically interdisciplinary book. I have written it as a physician, epidemiologist, and philosopher with the intent to integrate methods and concepts from all three fields to analyze the ways how those working in medicine and the health sciences reduce uncertainty in medicine. Thus, the style in which the text is written is somewhere between rigorous philosophical analysis and argument on the one hand and medical research report and literature review on the other. Therefore, you will sometimes find many references to the literature and sometimes very few. Along the same lines, the chapters of Part III tend to be more "sciency" than those of Parts I and II, offering more non-philosophical detail. I hope that such inconsistencies will not affect your reading experience too much.

I am not sure I have fully succeeded in developing a novel positive account of translational health research, but I surely hope that my discussion begins to highlight some of the weaker points in the current discourse and the potential drawbacks of the lack of such discourse in the health sciences.

I have used previously published material in the following chapters. Chapter 5 is based on a handbook chapter on "Epidemiological Inferences" in A. Broadbent (Ed.), Oxford Handbook of Philosophy of Medicine. Oxford University Press, forthcoming. An earlier version of Chap. 6 was published as a chapter entitled "Explanation in Public Health" in S. Venkatapuram & A. Broadbent (Eds.), Routledge Handbook of the Philosophy of Public Health. Routledge, 2022. Chapter 8 is a revised and shortened version of Dammann, O., & Stansfield, B. K., "Neonatal Sepsis as a Cause of Retinopathy of Prematurity: An Etiological Explanation". Prog Ret Eye Res, 2023. Chapter 9 is based on Dammann, O., "Agent-Based Models as Etio-prognostic Explanations". Argumenta, 2021, and Chap. 10 is an updated version of Dammann, O., "Evidence Mapping to Justify Health Interventions". Perspect Biol Med, 2021, 64(2), 155–172.

The following acknowledgments are in order. I am grateful to Alan Leviton, Nigel Paneth, and Alex Broadbent for their comments on earlier versions of the paper that serves as the basis for Chap. 6. Special thanks to Susan Koch-Weser for directing me to the work of Paul K.J. Han and for those interesting (and fun!) conversations about health literacy and decision making. Thanks also to Lina Dammann for an illuminating discussion about uncertainty of past and future events. Gratitude to Paul Beninger for many interesting and fruitful conversations and, in particular, for pointing me to Heisenberg's 1927 paper on uncertainty. Thanks to three anonymous reviewers who offered advice on the manuscript in its very early stages and to two pre-publication reviewers (one of them Benjamin Smart) who helped improve the book in its final days of writing. And finally, much gratitude to Solveig Robinson, who read the entire manuscript and offered very helpful advice. It goes without saying that all remaining incongruities, mistakes, and follies are mine. And finally, as always, my deepest gratitude goes to my family for their love and support.

Boston, MA   Olaf Dammann

REFERENCE

Stegenga, J. (2018). *Medical nihilism*. Oxford University Press.

CONTENTS

LIST OF FIGURES

LIST OF TABLES

CHAPTER 1

Introduction

Medicine has been incredibly successful over the past two centuries. In fact, western biomedicine is often hailed as one of the greatest success stories in the history of science. It seems reasonable to propose that medical progress has contributed a great deal to the human endeavor to live better and longer lives. Among many other successful medical interventions, immunizations, antibiotics, and pain medications make it possible to prevent disease and ameliorate the associated suffering when it has already occurred. If one includes surgery and public health interventions, I don't think it is an exaggeration to say that medical progress has made an important contribution to the doubling in life expectancy worldwide over the past century, from 34 to 79 years in Europe and from 26 to 63 years in Africa.[1] Arguably, public health interventions—as simple as handwashing and as complex as global smallpox vaccination campaigns—have made similar if not greater contributions to human health over the centuries.

It seems that most people trust biomedicine and use its services on a regular basis.[2] I will call this the *conviction of medical success*. Recent papers in the areas of transplantation, immunization, and cancer therapy begin with the notion that the field at hand is a modern medical success story. For example, Bottomley, Brook, Shankar, Hester, and Issa write that "organ transplantation is a medical success story" (Bottomley et al., 2022). Barker and Markmann's historical review of human organ transplantation (Barker & Markmann, 2013) confirms that while the developmental

© The Author(s), under exclusive license to Springer Nature   1
Switzerland AG 2025
O. Dammann, *Uncertainty and Explanation in Medicine and the Health Sciences*, https://doi.org/10.1007/978-3-031-82271-1_1

period before the 1950s (skin autografts, tooth transplantations, etc.) did not bring forth much progress, it was the landmark discovery in 1912 by Georg Schöne in Paul Ehrlichs laboratory that *second* skin homografts failed even faster that the first, indicating an immune response and organ rejection. The first human-to-human kidney transplantation by Yurii Voronoy in 1933 failed spectacularly, probably due to a long delay between organ harvest and implantation, as well as a blood type mismatch. Not until the 1950s was a human kidney transplanted (by David Hume in Boston) *without* being rejected within a few days or weeks. Much of the subsequent successes in kidney transplantation are not so much due to improvements in surgical technique but due to the *immunological* work done by Peter Medawar, Rupert Billingham, and Leslie Brent in the UK and Frank Lillie and Ray Owen in the United States. Brent, Owen, and (independently) Morten Simonson discovered the key phenomenon of graft-versus-host disease (GVHD), the attack of the host's immune system by the transplanted organ. The first successful human kidney transplantation was performed in Boston by Joseph Murray, using a kidney donated by the identical twin of the recipient. Since then, chemical immunosuppression has become a mainstay of human organ transplantation. In 2019, more than 100,000 kidney, 35,000 liver, almost 9000 heart and 7000 lung, as well as 2300 pancreas and 137 small bowel transplants have been performed worldwide. For kidney transplants alone, the median survival is 12.4 years (vs. 5.4 years for those on the waiting list), and an estimated 1.4 million life years have been saved (Godfrey & Rana, 2019).

The conviction of medical success comes with an optimistic and rather hopeful attitude toward interventional innovations. Every year, as part of their outreach program, the world-renowned Cleveland clinic publishes a list of the top ten medical innovations.[3] Such positive attitude toward medical success, however, is mainly voiced by medical professionals and might not be generalizable. Still, medical success is widely hailed as the reason why we do better today than yesteryear.

Take, for example, *The New York Times Book of Medicine*, edited by Gina Kolata (2015). In it, a great collection of articles from the *NYT* bears witness to the progress medicine has made since the paper was published for the first time in September 1851. The book contains 121 articles (if I counted right) the *NYT* printed over the past 150 years on topics considered "medical". The pieces are neatly organized alphabetically by topic, ranging from AIDS and Alzheimer's, via cancer, heart disease, kidney, to mental health, transplants, and vaccines, among others. Taken together, the reprinted articles provide a breath-taking, sometimes eerie kind of time warp through the history of progress in the health sciences. Although the book highlights both exciting successes and spectacular failures, enthusiasm prevails. In her introduction, Kolata writes

> People are bigger and healthier throughout life [...] The age-adjusted risk of dying dropped 60 percent from 1935 to 2010. [...] (I)t was the result of enormous advances in medicine, a transformation so profound that it is almost hard to imagine what the world was like when The Times was first published.[4]

It looks like as if, at least according to Kolata, biomedicine is here to stay.

However, medicine is being criticized by some philosophers who argue that it does not deliver on its promises, a position that may be called *medical skepticism*. The position of medical skeptics is that medicine doesn't attain its goal: cure (Broadbent, 2018a). Alex Broadbent has raised this issue by proposing what he calls the *puzzle of ineffective medicine*, the question why many would still believe in the effectiveness of medicine although it has been far less successful than assumed (Broadbent, 2019). An even harsher judgment comes from Jacob Stegenga, whose position of *medical nihilism* holds that our confidence in the effectiveness of medicine should be low (Stegenga, 2018). Taken together, their arguments represent a *thesis of medical ineffectiveness*.

Stegenga holds that, at least in part, medical ineffectiveness can be attributed to faulty or even fraudulent research. In other words, part of the ineffectiveness of medical practice can be attributed to the underlying research. There is a kernel of truth in this position and Stegenga is not the first to lament it. For example, John Ioannidis, arguably one of the most outspoken hit-over-the-head proponents of the view that not all that glitters is gold in the health sciences, had a smash hit with his paper "Why most published research findings are false" (Ioannidis, 2005).[5] Ioannidis' work was covered by David Freedman in *The Atlantic* in 2010, who called Ioannidis "one of the world's foremost experts on the credibility of medical research" and "one of the most influential scientists alive". So, why do medics use apparently largely faulty research as the basis for their work, which renders their trade largely ineffective, and patients *still* seek medical attention in private practices and hospitals?

This is the central question Broadbent and Stegenga ask. Being seasoned philosophers of medicine, both certainly enjoy making an occasional provocative statement, but their proposal is clearly not intended to be a joke. Their books offer a whole host of observations in support of their respective arguments. Stegenga mainly blames faulty research. Broadbent says that the goal of medicine is cure and that it is just a fact that cure is rarely achieved by medical interventions. The question raised by Broadbent's puzzle is: *Why* should medicine be held in such high regard if it is indeed as ineffective as suggested? How come that medicine plays such an enormously powerful role in society and our personal lives if it really doesn't work?

"Cure" is indeed a tall order. Of note, Broadbent previously entertained a broader definition of cure as "anything that helps" in a standalone article. We can call this the "broad" definition of "cure":

> By *'cure,' I do not mean complete restoral to health as if the affliction had never afflicted. [...] I am happy to count as a cure any intervention that is reasonably effective at alleviating the ill effects of a disease, incapacity, reduced life span, and suffering.* (Broadbent, 2018b, p. 291)

However, in his 2019 book, Broadbent defends a much narrower definition, and he clearly distinguishes it from "anything that helps":

> *I suggest that* cure *be understood as an intervention that removes disease. [...] I suggest that* therapy *be understood as any intervention that alleviates the suffering or harm caused by disease but does not necessarily remove it. Defined this way, therapy might be broadly construed as to include cure (but not vice versa).* (Broadbent, 2019, p. 36)

In this book, I prefer to respond to the narrow view of cure as a more convenient point of departure. While cure might be the *ultimate* goal of medicine, it is not a proper measure for medical effectiveness, and it is not what patients can expect from a broad range of medical diagnostics, interventions, and predictions. In everyday medical work, the *immediate* goal of medical activity is to *help* by making the patient *better*, to help the patient in a situation of acute crisis, proposing mid-term solutions to reduce the impact of chronic disease and to increase their quality of life.[6] Cure may very well be the ultimate *hope* of patients, but they and those who practice medicine know that cure is rarely achieved and often unachievable. Patients do not seek medical attention because they seek cure in the long-term but because they seek immediate help. Sure, if in the long-term cure becomes possible, even better. But here and now patients want less fever, less cough, less pain and medicine can frequently deliver. In a recent editorial coauthored with my colleagues Signe Mežinska and Eugenijus Gefenas, I have called this the *auxiliary stance* of medicine,[7] defined by the practical, immediate goal of medicine to help (Dammann et al., 2022). Thus, distinguishing between the ultimate and immediate goals of medicine (cure and help, resp.) and reassigning help the role of measure of medical effectiveness would go a long way of resolving the puzzle of medical ineffectiveness. While the hope to ultimately cure may still be important as a guiding principle of surgery and medicine, a little bit of help in the short-term is enough to consider medicine a more effective endeavor than Broadbent wants to make us believe.

The idea covered in this book is simple. I argue that medicine may seem at least partially ineffective because the general expectation is that medicine can deal with *uncertainty*. I will argue that this is not true and that dealing with uncertainty is not even a task for medicine but a task for science. And since medicine is not science, it cannot deal with uncertainty. Instead, medicine relies on solid information from basic science and epidemiology. While basic bench science research provides knowledge about how a new drug works or how a disease mechanism connects an exposure like asbestos inhalation with an outcome such as malignant mesothelioma, the main branch of science that bears directly on medical action is epidemiology, the branch of science that is supposed to provide information about the causes of illness, the efficacy of new interventions, the prognosis for a patient, and so forth. But it seems to me that medicine has trouble translating scientific information into medical action. I believe this difficulty is rooted in the sheer complexity of the theoretical underpinnings of the concepts that link research information to medical practice, for example, inference, explanation, and causation.

How could it be that, if medicine doesn't work, it would give rise to what Barbara Katz Rothman calls *the biomedical empire*, "the idea of sickness as a land, a kingdom in which one holds citizenship" (Rothman, 2021, p. 69)? Rothman argues that modern biomedicine has risen to the status of a self-serving money-making system that is designed to exploit all of us and hold us hostage for its own benefit. But she clearly acknowledges that while many may agree with this perspective, most of us will also say, "Yes, but it also saved my life" (p. 7). Her book is about the argument that while "medicine saves and improves lives and does many wonderful things we can better understand what it does and why […] if we think about it as the empire, the imperial power, [Rothman is] arguing it is" (p. 9). How can something purportedly so ineffective as medicine, per medical skepticism, be so successful as to become part of a metaphor for a powerful social system, per medical imperialism?

My response is that medicine is more effective than the medical skeptics and nihilists want to make us believe. First, success has something to do with attaining a certain goal. Broadbent says that the goal of medicine is cure and that medicine is ineffective because there is no cure for many or even most diseases. Even if both statements were true, this does not yet mean that medicine is ineffective. Not reaching a goal is not equal to ineffectiveness if the expected or desired effect is not identical with said goal. While I can agree that the ultimate goal of medicine is cure, as an overarching, final goal of the entire medical endeavor, I hold that the better measure of medical success is whether medicine is capable of helping people get better. Again, I will call this position the *auxiliary stance of medicine*. From this perspective, I believe, medicine must be (and not just look) much less ineffective than Broadbent suggests, because it helps many more people get better than it cures. While one could say that this is just a moving-the-goalposts maneuver because I have changed the reference frame for the diagnosis of medical ineffectiveness by making it much easier for medicine to achieve such success, I still believe that judging medicine by its daily success in helping people get better is a much more reasonable measuring stick than judging it by whether it reaches its ultimate, lofty goal of cure. Of note, (and of importance for my position outlined below that medicine is not science), Broadbent's claim that medicine is ineffective is a claim in the sphere of *medical practice*: it relates to the effectiveness of medicine defined as the *practice of doing medicine*.

The second part of my defense of medical effectiveness has to do with Stegenga's argument that medicine should be much better than it pretends to be, but it cannot because the underlying research is bad, biased, or bogus. His perspective is not really about how medical ineffectiveness can be established (as in Broadbent's thesis) but about the reason why medicine is ineffective, e.g., by relying on faulty research. This position resonates with Ioannidis' verdict that most research results are plain false. The argument can be misinterpreted to entail that if we just did better biomedical research, we would generate better data to do better medicine which would ultimately be more useful. My response here is: hold on, not so fast! It may very well be that medicine would be better, more effective, and thereby more useful if we could just improve research data quality, minimize wrong conclusions, manage the scientific replication crisis, and so forth. But there is another thing that contributes to the impression that medicine is ineffective: it is the unlucky interaction of our misguided consistent expectation of deterministic perfection of medical explanations and the intrinsic uncertainty of the world in which we live. If we accept that much of what happens in the world, and particularly in the living world, is inherently *uncertain*, we would not be so surprised that it is simply impossible to, let me exaggerate, *always* know *exactly* why a person is sick, to find the *precise* diagnosis and treatment for *every* patient, and to predict with *certainty* what *exactly* the remaining time for a cancer patient will be. Because uncertainty is everywhere and very hard to tackle, it affects both medicine and the underlying medical research at many levels, just as it affects the weather and your chance to win the lottery.

For example, consider rosiglitazone (a.k.a., "rosi"), a drug that can be used to treat type-2 diabetes, works by sensitizing the insulin receptor. The drug had a bumpy ride after it was approved in the late 1990s—we will revisit the story in a bit more depth in Chap. 5 when we discuss explanation and inference-making in medicine. Perhaps surprisingly for some, the molecular mechanism how rosiglitazone works, i.e., by sensitizing the insulin receptor, was not fully known when the drug was approved. A few years later, a research team from Spain published the results from experiments using fetal rat fat cells (adipocytes) designed to elucidate said mechanism (Hernandez et al., 2003). Pre-treatment rosi did increase the glucose uptake by cells in the dish, but in some cells more so than in others. Thus, while there was a disposition (to borrow a term from causal power theory) among fat cells to respond to treatment with rosi with an increased glucose uptake, not all cells responded to the same degree. My inclination here would be to explain this observation by saying that in light of the very rigorously controlled conditions in the lab, the degree of glucose uptake response in fetal adipocytes is uncertain and that it is to be expected that some, but not all patients with type-2 diabetes who receive rosi, should show some improvement. At around the same time, a research team from Texas published results of experiments they conducted with 20 type-2 diabetic patients and 6 healthy controls (Miyazaki et al., 2003). The variability of the results, however, indicate that the plasma glucose level of some of the subjects who received rosi did not decrease as much as those of others, thereby indicating that the treatment was, on average, successful, but at the same time, the success was uncertain. I hold that what was seen in these research studies holds for *all* drugs: their expected effect, albeit present, remains uncertain and cannot be predicted with certainty. Later in this book (in Chap. 4) I will outline my position that the uncertainty of research results is an inherent quality of everything that goes on in our world (this is also called aleatoric uncertainty, which I will abbreviate A-uncertainty). The uncertainty of researchers and medics, however, is a cognitive state (epistemic uncertainty or E-uncertainty). In Chap. 4 I will offer details on how the two are related.

Therefore, medicine is expected to be imperfect, because medicine is uncertain as is the underlying research because the world works in uncertain ways. In fact, one could say that the entire enterprise of both medicine and medical research is tasked not only with helping each and every patient as best as we can, but it is also tasked with curbing that uncertainty as much as possible, to improve etiological knowledge, diagnostic capabilities, therapeutic options, and prognostic precision as much as possible, and not hurt too many patients in the process. However, the problem is that science can tackle uncertainty by improving its methodologies, while medicine is condemned to use those uncertain scientific results and somehow deal with it vis-à-vis the patient.

But even if medicine is more effective than Broadbent and Stegenga suggest, its residual ineffectiveness might be prominent enough to reduce the public belief in medical effectiveness appreciably. At this point, a phenomenon becomes visible that can be seen as a smoke-and-mirror strategy used by some stakeholders in the medical community to improve medicine's standing in modern society: they pretend that medicine *is* science. In the next section of this introduction and throughout the book I will defend my position that this is not in fact the case. Medicine and medical research are two very different things, and although their borders are sometimes blurry and the fields sometimes overlap, they are two very different kinds of human endeavor that I would like to keep separate, at least for the time being, in my discussion of uncertainty as a prominent source of medical ineffectiveness. My aim in this book is to offer a description of how medical and scientific experts tackle medical uncertainty, with a focus on the inferences and explanations they employ in the process. In this regard, this book offers a descriptive, not a normative account of the relationship between science and medicine.

This book has three parts. Part I provides the backdrop (Chaps. 2, 3 and 4). I explore whether medicine is effective or not (Chap. 2), outline my view that medicine is not science (Chap. 3), and offer the idea that two kinds of uncertainty (aleatoric and epistemic) at the intersection between science and medicine can help explain why medicine may appear ineffective (Chap. 4). Part II digs deeper into the concepts of inference, explanation, and causation (Chaps. 5, 6 and 7, resp.). I explicate a framework of inference-making (in epidemiology) that might contribute to some of the inferential leaps we can observe in medical practice (Chap. 5). Next, I propose an inclusive explanatory mosaicism for medicine that stands in contrast to much of philosophy of science, where explanations are often reduced to (causal-mechanical, CM) answers to "why?" questions (Chap. 6). I submit the view that while epidemiologists like to view their research as motivated by a desire to find causes, they actually *make* them by prescribing what counts as a cause and what doesn't (Chap. 7). Part III offers three examples of how the concepts outlined in previous chapters can be applied in medical and health research. The first example is a proposed etiological explanation of retinopathy of prematurity (ROP) (Chap. 8). The second is a somewhat provocative interpretation of agent-based modeling as etio-prognostic explanations (Chap. 9). The last chapter summarizes how this book can be used as a semi-formal system for evidence mapping to justify health interventions (Chap. 10).

Working from the above roadmap, here is a bit more detail about the chapters to follow.

In the first chapter I describe and discuss in a bit more detail the puzzle of medical effectiveness and how uncertainty contributes to it. My position is based on two main points. The first is that calling medicine ineffective requires a comprehensive explication of what effectiveness is. I submit that using Broadbent's goal of cure is inappropriate; although one might say that cure is the idealized final goal of medicine, most of those who work in medicine will acknowledge that seeking cure is in the most part elusive. Instead, the immediately attainable goal of medical practice is to help patients get better. This is what I call the *auxiliary stance of medicine*, its devotion to do whatever is possible to improve the single patient's health condition. The second point is that while some parts of medicine may seem ineffective, other parts are quite effective. In other words, I am saying that we are just as justified to say that medicine is effective as we are justified to say that it is ineffective; you may think of it as a glass-half-full-half-empty scenario. One of the reasons why there is effectiveness *as well* as ineffectiveness in medicine is because medicine is inherently uncertain. It is this uncertainty that, together with the misguided expectation that medicine should offer cure, gives rise to the impression that medicine is ineffective, not reaching its goal when it should and thus should not be trusted.

Chapter 3 is a brief statement that, in my view, medicine is not science. While modern biomedicine is based on modern research, it is not itself research. Medical activities are those that help patients get better, not those that generate new knowledge that supports such activities. Doing science-based medicine and doing medical science are separate activities. While some doctors are also scientists, and some scientists are also doctors, the vast majority of doctors practice medicine and most medical scientists do science. The upshot of this perspective is that medical uncertainty is rooted not only in scientific uncertainty but also in the uncertainty inherent to the translation from scientific information to medical action.

I will then offer a more thorough analysis of medical uncertainty, which is a two-pronged phenomenon (in Chap. 4). The term uncertainty can be understood in multiple ways. In our context, however, two meanings refer to two different important kinds of uncertainty. It is the *aleatoric (objective, natural) uncertainty* (henceforth A-uncertainty) inherent in the real world that leads to quite a bit of *epistemic (subjective, cognitive) uncertainty* (henceforth E-uncertainty). The first, A-uncertainty, refers to uncertainty as a characteristic or property of an event or thing; I will sometimes also call it *natural* or *objective* uncertainty. It refers to the natural wobbliness of what and how things are, and whether and when events occur. This kind of uncertainty refers to the uncertainty that Heisenberg referred to when he noted that in quantum mechanics it is impossible to locate a subatomic particle and estimate its momentum at the same moment. This, in turn, is one of the reasons why predictions of events can be (and frequently are) rather uncertain.[8]

The second meaning of the term refers to E-uncertainty, the cognitive state that results from our dealing with wobbly occurrence and prediction data. I will use the term *subjective uncertainty* interchangeably and propose a framework that locates uncertainty of facts and events in a grid defined by timepoints (past, present, future) and by four domains of medicine: etiology, diagnosis, therapy, and prognosis. I will split etiologic inquiry further into causal and mechanistic explanation. One important point of the dichotomy of uncertainty is that aleatoric (objective) uncertainty is possible only for future events, which have not yet occurred but not for past events or for past or current facts because all of the latter have already occurred, and their occurrence status is thus certain. However, we can be epistemically (subjectively) uncertain about any fact or event, past or present, and certainly future, simply based on whether we have data about them and how wobbly these are.

The chapters of Part I make the case that medical ineffectiveness and the resulting extreme response of medical nihilism are, at least in part, due to a misattribution of cure as the goal of medicine (Broadbent) and faulty research as the main, perhaps even exclusive, culprit (Stegenga). Instead, I suggest that much of the observed medical ineffectiveness can be attributed to two issues. First, medicine is not science and, therefore, results from epidemiology and the biosciences need to be made useable for medical purposes by means of inference and explanation. Second, one major difficulty for medicine and the health sciences is the natural (aleatoric) uncertainty of biological processes and, thus, the uncertainty of biomedical research results. Inference and explanation, as well as the topic of the third chapter of Part II, causometry, are concepts that are used to curb the corresponding epistemic (cognitive) uncertainty. Thus, Part II offers the conceptual pillars for tackling the issues raised in Part I.

The relationship between aleatoric and epistemic uncertainty is a transition process marked by the observation of facts, capturing it in data, and making knowledge out of those data. The inner workings of the *transitional* inference process, leading from data to information, to evidence, to knowledge, are the first topic of Chap. 5. If the observed event or fact is uncertain, data will be uncertain, and the resulting knowledge will be uncertain as well, which is precisely how I define E-uncertainty. This transition process can be seen as a kind of inference since making an inference is to make a conclusion based on evidence. It is the basis of all empirical work, where we come to conclusions based on observed data. Such inferences are made in all domains of medicine, in the form of etiologic, diagnostic, therapeutic, and prognostic inferences. The goal is to get from observation of facts to a cognitive belief state about the truth of a proposition about that fact. The main goal of drawing empirical inferences is to help us get from a state of (cognitive) uncertainty a bit closer to certainty. The state transition itself is simply the transition from one cognitive state (wobbly) to another (less wobbly). Of note, I will use the adjective "wobbly" throughout the book to refer to the uncertain-ness of events, facts, data, and cognitive responses. If you prefer more serious, technical terminology, you may consider "wobbly" an adjective that refers to the concept "WOBBLY", which is an acronym for "We Ought Better Be Looking Yonder", indicating a situation where relying solely on what seems to be the case may not be as fruitful as exploring what further inquiry might reveal.

However, this cognitive flip is not the inference itself, it is just a flip in one's belief state based on the inference, which in turn is based on evidence. The inference is the entire process that leads from the wobblier state to the less wobbly one. For example, if one thinks that it is uncertain what time of day it is based on the position of the sun in the sky (fact 1), one may want to consult a clock. If looking at my wristwatch tells me it is 12 noon (fact 2), I might infer that it is exactly midday. Before I looked, I was uncertain (belief state 1) but now I am certain what time it is (this is the flip from belief state 1 to belief state 2). Or so I think. Because if, after having checked the time on my watch, I keenly observe that the position of the sun is conspicuously off zenith (fact 1, reconsidered), I may start having doubts that my wristwatch works well. I may return to the cognitive state of uncertainty (belief state 1) and want to consult with its digital counterpart in my smartphone. If that digital clock confirms that is indeed 12 noon (fact 3), certainty returns *unless* the sun is *very much* off zenith and I start doubting the precision of my digital phone clock as well (belief state 1). At that point, I might infer that either both my clocks are off (to the exact same degree!) or my estimation of where the sun should be in the sky at noontime this time of the year is off. Knowing myself and my frequent inability to estimate the time of day based on the sun's position (fact 4), I will infer that it is more likely that I am mistaken rather than both my clocks being off and begin to trust in the certainty of it being 12 noon (belief state 2). The comparison of evidence with certain established standards does or does not allow me to draw conclusions that bring me, if not from uncertainty to certainty, then at least from uncertainty to less uncertainty, to a reduction in wobbliness. In our current context the inference is based on facts about the etiology, diagnostics, therapy, and prognosis in a specific patient's situation. These facts are, with some exceptions, naturally uncertain; the inference process will yield cognitive uncertainty that may be farther from, or closer to, the true state of affairs but still carry some risk of being uncertain. The second topic of Chap. 5 is what I call *translational inferences*, i.e., inferences that cross a gap between validity ranges. Crossing that gap is usually called making an inferential leap, of which I will discuss four examples: inference from animal to human physiology and pathophysiology, from association to causation, from population data to application in individuals, and from isolated data to complex contexts. As will become clear, inferential leaps may be possible, but they are likely to come with their own wobbliness, thereby increasing, not reducing uncertainty. Additional wobbliness is generated by the usage of results of translational inferences in *both* medicine and medical research.

The topic of Chap. 6 is explanation, and my intention is to show that multiple different kinds of explanation are used in medicine and public health. The usual distinctions in philosophy of science, such as causal versus non-causal explanations, or the frequent exclusive focus on scientific explanation with the associated question "what makes an explanation scientific?" is of secondary import in the medical context. Indeed, some of the explanations used in medicine are not scientific and might not be considered a proper topic for philosophers of science. However, they are for philosophers of medicine and epidemiology. I think that although scientific and causal explanations are undoubtedly important kinds of explanation in medicine and public health, other kinds deserve attention as well because they support medicine's immediate goal, to help people get better, and the way they do this is by reducing uncertainty.

Chapter 7, causometry, is probably the most difficult one in Part II. With its focus on one central issue in medicine and the health sciences, it explores concepts of causality and causal inference. In the final section of the chapter, I ask whether such a thing as causometry is possible. I argue that the methods used for causal inference in medicine and epidemiology, the so-called potential outcomes approach (POA) (based on counterfactual reasoning and the assumption that randomized studies yield causal results) and Hill's heuristics (based on explanatory-coherentist reasoning and the assumption that multiple, error-independent pieces of evidence support causal inference), do come close enough to causality as to represent "quasi-causometers".

In Part III I offer three chapters that describe examples of applications of the concepts covered in Part II. First, I rehearse a novel etiological explanation for retinopathy of prematurity (ROP), a devastating disorder of the retina that occurs predominantly among preterm infants. The current etiological paradigm of ROP has excessive neonatal exposure to exogenous oxygen as the main root cause; in Chap. 8 I offer an alternative etiological explanation that has neonatal infection (sepsis) as the root cause and systemic inflammation as the mechanism. The chapter ends with an application of Hill's heuristics as a quasi-causometer and the conclusion that it seems highly likely that two independent etiological pathways might lead to ROP—one with oxygen and the other with sepsis as the root cause.

The second chapter in Part II is (Chap. 9) about a research method that has become increasingly popular in population health research, agent-based models (ABMs). In ABMs, i.e., computer-based simulation models that simulate the movement through and interaction among each other of virtual agents within a two-dimensional virtual space, the occurrence and trajectory of disease in populations can be estimated based on various stochastic parameters. I argue that ABMs can be interpreted as devices that deliver etio-prognostic explanations, which take an etiological explanation, make a prediction based on it, and if confirmed, the prognostic explanation explains by having correctly predicted future events. In essence, etiological explanations explain backward in time by referring to the causes and mechanisms of event occurrences, while prognostic explanations explain forward in time by predicting future events correctly.

The last chapter of Part III and the book is an exhibit of how multiple kinds of explanatory and predictive explanation can be integrated in a joint evidence set (*JES*) made up of evidence about (A) associations between exposures and outcomes, (B) biological mechanisms, (C) confirmation of previous observations, and (D) difference-making in clinical or intervention trials. Perhaps the most important part of the underlying argument here is that if evidence can be mounted in such jointly evidential fashion, no randomization is necessary, i.e., the difference-making trials in part D do not need to be randomized-controlled trials (RCTs) because the entire, coherent evidence map provides sufficient justification for a health intervention.

Taken together, the chapters in Parts I–III provide the backdrop, concepts, and application examples of ways how medical practitioners and researchers tackle the ubiquitous uncertainties in biology and medicine. It should go without saying that if our world is truly and fundamentally indeterministic, there is no way to eliminate uncertainty. All we can do is curb its undesirable consequences such as the puzzle of medical ineffectiveness. I hope that the concepts and approaches outlined in these pages can make a small contribution toward achieving that goal.

Notes

1. https://ourworldindata.org/life-expectancy (accessed 10/07/2022).
2. The recent surge of anti-vaccination sentiment in large segments of the population is a very concerning exception. The crisis is, according to Maya Goldenberg, one of public trust rather than a war on science (Goldenberg,

2021), and much more than better science will be needed to win back that trust.

3. https://innovations.clevelandclinic.org/Summit/Top-10-Medical-Innovations.aspx (acc. 12-12-21).
4. See (Kolata, 2015, p. xiv). I will restrict my disagreement with this statement for the time being to saying that not only medicine but also public health is to be credited.
5. Of course, this paper features prominently in both Broadbent's and Stegenga's books.
6. Obviously, medicine is not the only human endeavor characterized by help. Many other helpful activities and professions are, e.g., teaching students, fighting fires, and installing traffic signs.
7. I am using the term *auxiliary* not in the sense of *additional* as it is used in everyday English but in the sense of the Latin verb *auxiliare = to help*.
8. I am thinking of predictions as cognitive-communicative acts here, where the assumption that something will happen is foretold. In the terminology I propose in Chap. 4, the target event is A-uncertain, while the act of foretelling is fraught with E-uncertainty.

REFERENCES

Barker, C. F., & Markmann, J. F. (2013). Historical overview of transplantation. *Cold Spring Harbor Perspectives in Medicine, 3*(4), a014977.

Bottomley, M. J., Brook, M. O., Shankar, S., Hester, J., & Issa, F. (2022). Towards regulatory cellular therapies in solid organ transplantation. *Trends in Immunology, 43*(1), 8–21.

Broadbent, A. (2018a). *Philosophy of medicine.* Oxford University Press.

Broadbent, A. (2018b). Prediction, understanding, and medicine. *The Journal of Medicine and Philosophy, 43*, 289–305.

Broadbent, A. (2019). *Philosophy of medicine* (p. 1). Oxford University Press.

Dammann, O., Hartnett, M. E., & Stahl, A. (2022). Retinopathy of prematurity. *Developmental Medicine & Child Neurology, 65*(5), 625–631.

Godfrey, E. L., & Rana, A. (2019). Outcomes in solid-organ transplantation: Success and stagnation. *Texas Heart Institute Journal, 46*(1), 75–76.

Goldenberg, M. (2021). *Vaccine hesitancy.* University of Pittsburg Press.

Hernandez, R., Teruel, T., & Lorenzo, M. (2003). Rosiglitazone produces insulin sensitisation by increasing expression of the insulin receptor and its tyrosine kinase activity in brown adipocytes. *Diabetologia, 46*, 1618–1628.

Ioannidis, J. P. (2005). Why most published research findings are false. *PLoS Medicine, 2*(8), e124.

Kolata, G. B. (2015). *The New York Times book of medicine.* Sterling Publishing Co..

Miyazaki, Y., He, H., Mandarino, L. J., & DeFronzo, R. A. (2003). Rosiglitazone improves downstream insulin receptor signaling in Type 2 diabetic patients. *Diabetes, 52,* 1943–1950.

Rothman, B. K. (2021). *The biomedical empire: Lessons learned from the Covid-19 pandemic.* Stanford Briefs, an imprint of Stanford University Press.

Stegenga, J. (2018). *Medical nihilism.* Oxford University Press.

PART I

Backdrop

CHAPTER 2

Medical Skepticism

INTRODUCTION

Despite its obvious successes, some think that biomedicine does not deserve the laudatory recognition it currently enjoys. In stark contrast to the conviction of medical success, philosophers of medicine have criticized medicine as largely ineffective (Broadbent, 2019), even going as far as defending a stance of "medical nihilism" (Stegenga, 2018). The reason for this distrust is their perception that medicine is largely ineffective and, thus, unsuccessful. In essence, they say that although we have antibiotics, insulin, and painkillers, we do not have a cure for cancer, for neurological diseases like Parkinson's and Alzheimer's disease, and for autoimmune disorders such as multiple sclerosis.

In his book *Philosophy of Medicine*,[1] Alex Broadbent asks two questions: what is medicine and what should we think of it? (Broadbent, 2018, p. xv). Right away after asking these questions at the beginning of the introduction, Broadbent opens with a series of statements that say it is unclear why what he calls *mainstream medicine* has made it through the millennia with apparently *increasing* popularity despite very little success in curing people of their maladies. He calls the position to focus on recent medical successes *medical whiggishness* and the opposite position *medical nihilism*, but he supports neither of the two. Instead, he suggests taking a position he calls *medical cosmopolitanism*, referring to Kwame Anthony Appiah's

O. Dammann, *Uncertainty and Explanation in Medicine and the Health Sciences*, https://doi.org/10.1007/978-3-031-82271-1_2

book *Cosmopolitanism* (Appiah, 2006), and proposes to adapt that view to medicine (181).

Before Broadbent develops this idea further, he offers a historico-conceptual overview of the varieties of medicine and then dives into two crucial points that will help him answer his first big question, what is medicine? His first point is to clarify his position about what represents the *goal* of medicine. His result is that the goal of medicine is *cure*, as opposed to, for example, pain reduction and palliative care which are things done using medical tools and in situations where cure is deemed impossible, respectively. His second point is to clarify what the *business* of medicine is.

THE PUZZLE OF MEDICAL INEFFECTIVENESS

Broadbent sees a major conundrum resulting from the tension between the conviction of medical success vis-à-vis his diagnosis of a failure of medicine which he calls the *paradox of ineffective medicine*. The paradox is the disconnect between a general strong belief in medical effectiveness although it is in fact ineffective. Broadbent asks:

> *Given that medicine is extremely unreliable at achieving its fundamental goal, namely healing the sick, why does it persist?* (Broadbent, 2019, p. 56)

Stegenga goes further by suggesting that the general ineffectiveness of medicine should lead to a general distrust in medicine. He holds that our confidence in the effectiveness of medical interventions should be low (18) and calls this view *medical nihilism*, "the view that we should have little confidence in the effectiveness of medical interventions" (Stegenga, 2018, p. 1). His proposal is based on the view that

> *The best methods that clinical scientists employ to test medical interventions [...] are, in practice, not nearly as good as they are often made out to be. As a result, we ought to be skeptical of much of the evidence generated by such methods.* (ibid.)

If this proposal sounds somewhat outrageous it is probably mainly because it flies in the face not only of witnesses of medical progress like Kolata but also of patients like you and me. Haven't we all benefited from effective modern bioscience at some point? Some philosophers of science acknowledge their gratitude even in public. For example, Donald Gillies has dedicated his book *Causality, Probability, and Medicine* to "Grazia, who has certainly benefited from scientific medicine" (Gillies, 2019).

The idea that at least some forms of medicine are ineffective is not new. For example, Broadbent offers the following quote from Oliver Wendell Holmes (1809–94):

> *Throw out opium [...] and the vapors which produce the miracle of anesthesia [...] and I firmly believe that the whole materia medica, <u>as now used</u>, could be sunk to the bottom of the sea, it would be all the better for mankind, - and all the worse for the fishes.* (Underline is italics in the original)

While Broadbent quotes from Porter (Porter, 1998, p. 680), the original quote is from an address Holmes gave to the Massachusetts Medical Society on May 30th, 1860 (Holmes, 1860, p. 37/38). The journal of that same society, the *New England Journal of Medicine*, published a brief article in 2009 (on the occasion of Holmes' 200th birthday) authored by Charles Bryan and Scott Podolsky, who mention that while Holmes mounted arguments against ineffective interventions such as bloodletting and homeopathy, he also pointed his fingers at theoretical issues that affect medical decision making, such as

> *Errors in reasoning — such as post hoc ergo propter hoc, the counting of only favorable results, or the misinterpretation of the power of suggestion — or by the seductive power of the marketplace or the pernicious fee structure whereby physicians' profits hinged on the number of drugs administered.* (Bryan & Podolsky, 2009, p. 847)

Let me veer off on a tangent for a moment, because the last notion in above quote comes eerily close to what is happening in the United States in the context of the opioid epidemic. In order to cure, medicine would need more and better knowledge coming from biomedical/pharmaceutical research. Unfortunately, the pharmaceutical industry is primarily driven by profit, while the idea to help, being the original motivation to design new drugs, takes the back seat. One most pertinent example for the resulting medical paternalism is the catastrophic story of the role of oxycodone and its producer Purdue Pharma in the opioid epidemic in the United States. The pharmaceutical company illegally stated that their drug Oxycontin (oxycodone) was less addictive than comparable medications, thereby contributing to the opioid epidemic in the United States. In 2012, a group of pain medicine experts wrote in a review article:

> *The escalating use of therapeutic opioids shows hydrocodone topping all prescriptions with 136.7 million prescriptions in 2011, with all narcotic analgesics exceeding 238 million prescriptions. It has also been illustrated that opioid analgesics are now responsible for more deaths than the number of deaths from both suicide and motor vehicle crashes, or deaths from cocaine and heroin combined.* (Manchikanti et al., 2012)

Today, more than a decade later, Purdue Pharma has successfully settled multiple law suits at the state and federal level. Corey Davis rightfully asks in the *New England Journal of Medicine*:

> *Under the settlement agreement, none of the people who made decisions that contributed to the deaths of tens of thousands of people will face criminal penalties. [Why do] pharmaceutical company executives and owners who knowingly unleashed millions of unnecessary and highly addictive pills into the market walk free? […] The answer, of course, is money.* (Davis, 2021)

Clearly, this is a formidable example of the pharmaceutical industry playing the role of the successful villain in Rothman's biomedical empire, doing harm and going unpunished. But while stories like that of the opioid catastrophe may contribute to a general lack of trust in medicine, it is not the main origin of Broadbent's medical skepticism and Stegenga's nihilism.[2]

Let us put nihilism aside for a moment and focus on skepticism. In their celebration of Holmes' life and work, Bryan and Podolsky conclude that

> *Holmes's chief relevance today derives from his legacy as a skeptic […] It is important, nonetheless, to understand Holmes as a therapeutic skeptic, not a therapeutic nihilist.* (Bryan & Podolsky, 2009, p. 846/847)

They further quote Gibian (2001) as stating that Holmes viewpoints make him a "spokesperson for an 'age of uncertainty'" (Bryan & Podolsky, 2009, p. 246). What kind of relationship pertains between skepticism and uncertainty?

Skepticism, in general, refers to a justified position of doubt. When I stand before a problem or decision, and am offered a solution, I have to make a decision to either accept it, reject it, defer the decision to a later timepoint, or not to decide at all. At least part of my considerations in such a situation is about *relative expected gains*. If I am looking to buy a new drum kit, would it be better to buy the one that sounds better or the one that is cheaper or just wait a little longer before I make those decisions? I am weighing the expected pros and cons that I envision will result from such considerations, which of course also include aspects of urgency (By when do I need the kit?) and available funds (What can I afford without hampering the feasibility of other projects?), among other things. This situation of uncertainty is one of being unsure which choice would be better than the other. I am unsure what to do because for some reason I don't feel comfortable making a decision based on simple reasoning like "brand X is better, but also more expensive than all other brands. But since you want quality and you have the money, buying brand X is the best decision". However, this scenario is not yet one of skepticism. The uncertainty rises to the level of skepticism if my position is not just one of justified hesitation based on my inability to assign greater value to one or the other expected gain, but one of genuine lack of knowledge.

Suppose I am standing at a crossroads where a recent storm seems to have blown over the signpost. I am not familiar with area, don't have a compass, or map, and no cell service. If a stranger comes along who looks reasonably trustworthy, and I ask for the road to Aberystwyth, I simply don't know whether his answer is true or not. And even if the person I ask does seem to be *really* trustworthy, I still don't know if it's true (he might be uncertain himself, or simply mistaken, or just doesn't care). In this situation, my skepticism about the truth of the given directions seems justified. I don't know the truth and perhaps even cannot know the truth until (insert your favorite truth criterion here).

Broadbent considers the therapeutic uncertainties surrounding the use of epinephrine in situations of cardio-pulmonary resuscitation without generally accepted effectiveness. Since this is an example of the availability of evidence lagging behind an intervention's use, "it might well be a cause for some skepticism, or doubt, about the effectiveness of this intervention" (p. 173) and concludes that "we might be skeptical about such medicine, but skepticism is not Nihilism, the firm belief of worthlessness" (p. 174). Thus, for Broadbent, therapeutic nihilism refers to the stance that an intervention isn't worth a dime while skepticism is doubt about the effectiveness of an intervention.

He argues further that the same also holds for prevention, the main goal of public health (ibid.). In his signature provocative style, Broadbent discusses nutrition science and concludes that "we don't really know much about how diet affects health" (p. 58). Really? We know that eating too much and too little is bad for us. We know that fruits and vegetables are better than steak and ice cream. We know which fats are better than others, why salt and sugar should be consumed in limited amounts, and that eating fugu (Japanese blowfish) can kill you if the restaurant chef doesn't really know what they are doing. I think we know a great deal about the health effects of our diets, and how one contributes to the other. In response to the potential accusation that this seems like a mere strawman argument I would respond that all I intend to say is that the notion "we don't really know much about how diet affects health" is true only if you refer to specific effects of specific nutrients on specific aspects of health. It is definitely not true when you consider the big picture knowledge we have about dietary effects on health. Still, I acknowledge that broad assertions like "eating too much is bad" can be "taken out of context [and] could (and has) been seriously misunderstood and can lead to a great deal of harm (for instance, by the many teens with eating disorders)".[3] I would certainly agree with Broadbent that we need more and better research into the details of the effects of nutrition on health, whether beneficial or detrimental, because better data are one major way to curb our uncertainty about said health effects of nutrition.

So, how do Broadbent and Stegenga arrive at the conclusion that medicine is, indeed, ineffective?

In the section on the puzzle of ineffective medicine, Broadbent says that medicine "has been ineffective in most times and in most places at delivering the cures that the people consulting it obviously want" (Broadbent, 2019, p. 55). The underlying assumption of this statement is that people who seek out medical assistance seek *cure*, which Broadbent designates as the goal of medicine in his second chapter. Broadbent seems to take it as given that people *obviously* want cure. I can certainly subscribe to the view that cure is the goal of medicine and also to his assumption that people want cure. I certainly want to be cured of the nasty cough and a fever I have had for two days, when a chest X-ray reveals that I have pneumonia. If I am lucky, the doctor thinks "pneumonia!" and will put me on an antibiotic, assuming it is bacterial pneumonia (not viral, in which case antibiotics don't work), and, at least in the United States, he will do this without obtaining a sputum test in the hope to clarify the kind of bug that is responsible for the infection. But this is a special situation, namely, one in which cure is possible *and I know it*. Knowing that a curative treatment is available justifies my *expectation* that proper treatment will probably lead to cure. Expecting cure while *knowing* that it might be elusive, as in Alzheimer's or Parkinson's disease, and so forth, is more an expression of wishful thinking than of an expectation. Calling the fact that medicine often ("in most times and in most places") fails to cure is simply unfair, setting the bar for medical effectiveness way too high. I would argue that most people, as much as they *want* cure, do not expect to be cured *if they know that cure is in fact unattainable*. They will not consider medicine ineffective because it does not *cure if this is impossible*, i.e., because it does not reach its lofty goal at all times and all places. Instead, I think that it is more likely that people would call medicine ineffective if medicine would fail to do its job, i.e., help by making them better. To be fair, this view dovetails with Broadbent's earlier, broader definition of "cure". Alas, it does not align with his later, narrower definition.

Broadbent proposes as the curative thesis the notion that cure is *both* the goal and the business of medicine (Broadbent, 2019, p. 36) and goes on to reject the latter but not the former. His argument is that if cure was the core business of medicine, those parts of medicine that fail to cure would not persist; since they do, cure is not the core business of medicine (60). He then goes on (in Chap. 4) to define the core business of medicine as understanding and prediction, which he calls the Inquiry Thesis, which "says that medicine is an inquiry into the nature and causes of health and disease, for the purpose of cure and prevention" (64). The next chapter in this book can be read as a rebuttal of the Inquiry Thesis if inquiry is taken to be *scientific* in nature. I am not alone in rejecting the idea that understanding is the business of medicine. Ben Smart has proposed to replace the Inquiry Thesis with what he calls the "Best Available Intervention Thesis", the proposal that "medicine is the sustained and organized effort to determine and prescribe the best available treatment (curative or preventative) for patients" (Smart, 2023, pp. 194:13). I do not want to offer a discussion of this proposal here. Instead, I want to point out that part of Smart's argument is that the "understanding" part of Broadbent's Inquiry Thesis is not essential to medicine. Broadbent's understanding of "understanding" is not clear, but that one interpretation is that understanding in medicine means to be able to explain and in particular to be able to provide contrastive causal explanations, e.g., "why do you have fever, rather than not?" (194:5). However, both Broadbent's Inquiry Thesis and Smart's Best Intervention Thesis respond to the question "what is the core business of medicine?", not to the question "what is the goal of medicine?", thereby leaving the curative thesis (the goal of medicine is cure) intact for me to use as an example how implausible expectations might contribute to the impression that medicine is ineffective.

IMPLAUSIBLE EXPECTATIONS

Consider the possibility that Broadbent and Stegenga might have been led astray by implausible expectations. Indeed, if medicine *were* in fact effective (e.g., by a standard different from theirs), both *puzzle* and *nihilism* just vanish into thin air. Perhaps the underlying assumption of the *puzzle* doesn't hold water. Broadbent suggests that *cure* is the goal of medicine.[4] He writes that "medicine is the sustained and organized effort to heal the sick", which he calls the curative thesis[5] (35). Whatever medicine does is oriented toward this goal, in individual patient's care and in medicine in general. Looking at medicine from this angle does indeed suggest that it doesn't reach this goal all too frequently. But what if cure is a distant, ideal goal of medicine and the immediate goal is something else, like *help*?

Cure can be viewed as a dichotomous variable. On this view, cure is either achieved or it is not, the sick are either cured or they are not, and medicine is to be considered unsuccessful in all cases where it does not provide full recovery. Alternatively, cure could be taken as a gradual improvement from sick to healthy. Here, medicine could be viewed as successful only if it brings the sick back to perfect health. However, one could use a little bit less stringent requirement and count any improvement as success. This comes closer to my view of medical success than Broadbent's.[6]

But using successful cure as an *absolute* measure of medical effectiveness would not be entirely appropriate. It might be a distal, theoretical, and perhaps even lofty goal, the light at the end of the medical tunnel, so to speak. Measured by the standard of cure, it would be hard for medicine to *ever* be judged as effective, unless one would come up with a *relative* measure of medical effectiveness, which allows for some interventions being ineffective while still allowing medicine to be considered effective *overall* or *in general*. Of course, now the difficulty arises where to put the cutoff point at which our judgment would flip from effective to ineffective. What kind of cutoff would that be, how would it be measured, on what scale, and so on. Both Broadbent and Stegenga avoid going that route. Their verdict of ineffective medicine is supported by examples of where medicine does not deliver on what Broadbent and Stegenga seem to assume is medicine's promise, i.e., cure.

I think it is not fair to judge medicine's effectiveness by its *goal*. This would be comparable to judge the effectiveness of a soccer team solely by whether they are winning *every* game. Indeed, I think that the team's effectiveness should be judged not by its successfully achieving its goal but by how well it does what it does, i.e., passing the ball precisely and cleverly, and scoring goals. Their game can be extremely effective (they score many goals) without necessarily winning, for example, if the teams they are competing against are even more effective and score more goals. Back to medicine, I think it would be fair to evaluate the effectiveness by what it does and what its effects are for patients, not by whether it achieves its goal. Broadbent calls this "what it does" medicine's *business*, and he declares *inquiry* into improved knowledge and better prediction to be that business. I disagree and will return to this proposal later when I argue that medicine is not science and that, therefore, inquiry is not its business.

Instead, I suggest that medicine's business is to achieve its immediate goal, to *help people get better*. It might be more appropriate to judge medicine's effectiveness by whether it successfully *helps* the sick feel better, suffer less. This is what I will call the *auxiliary* thesis of medicine's business. If the goal is *to help*, not necessarily *to cure*, some, if not many, medical interventions are indeed immensely successful such as pain medications, insulin replacement for diabetes, and antibiotics treatment for bacterial infections.[7] Much of surgery is also rather effective, e.g., appendectomy as a treatment for acute appendicitis. These true successes of medicine in some areas might be reason enough for many to believe in the capabilities of medicine, despite its obvious ineffectiveness in other areas of health.[8]

Think of conventional medicine in comparison to homeopathy. I think it would not be fair to call both medicine and homeopathy ineffective because both don't achieve their goal (healing), but I do think that it is fair to call medicine more effective than homeopathy because it has a better success rate in helping people feel better and suffer less. Granted, some studies find homeopathy to be at least as effective as medicine, for example, in the private practice setting when the chief complaints studied are symptoms, e.g., upper airway and ear problems (Riley et al., 2001). In more in-depth comparisons between conventional medicine and homeopathy, the latter tends to come in second (Shang et al., 2005).

This proposed shift in reference frame leaves the *puzzle of ineffectiveness* intact for Broadbent and Stegenga, but not necessarily for others. This scenario could be the case if *cure* played a much smaller role in the public's perception of what the goal of medicine is. I posit that not many people seriously expect that medicine should cure, while many, if not all, look for help and care, for medicine to make them feel better.[9] Taking the auxiliary stance explains why medicine is still here: it helps people to a degree that, on average, is sufficient to generate enough trust in medicine for it not to disappear. According to this view, *puzzle* and *nihilism* lose traction if the reference frame for medicine's effectiveness is shifted from successfully reaching its goal to doing its business successfully by providing the help patients seek.

In sum, I think that calling medicine ineffective because it does not always cure is unfair because most of us (I posit) judge by what the results of medicine's actions are for us, not by whether it achieves its goal of cure. Medicine's *business* is more immediately important for most of us than medicine's long-term goal. I shall return later to this *business* and argue in more detail, counter Broadbent, that medicines business is not inquiry toward better understanding and prediction, but simply to help.

If cure is the goal of medicine, then it is what medicine (as a human endeavor) is striving toward. I agree with Broadbent that cure is a good candidate for being the ultimate goal of medicine. But I also think that it is unfair to call medicine ineffective because it has not yet reached this lofty, overarching goal. Cure is the light at the end of the tunnel. One cannot call a bicycle ineffective because it does not bring one to the end of the tunnel in no time. While biking through the darkness, the bike brings you *forward*, and it *helps* you reach that goal. The problem is that there are tunnels without an obvious light at the end; think of the long and winding tunnels in the Swiss alps. And worse, think of long and winding tunnels where we simply don't know when we might reach the end. The bike still works and helps you getting forward, but is it fair to call it ineffective even in cases of uncertainty where the tunnel ends? Even if the tunnel doesn't end at all, as in a situation where the end of the tunnel is blocked by a landslide that needs to be successfully removed before you can reach your goal, can we really blame the bike and call it ineffective or unreliable at bringing us to our destination?

Instead, I think we should not judge medicine by whether it reaches its lofty and sometimes perhaps even elusive goal. Instead, one may want to judge medicine's success by whether it successfully does what it does as judged by the patients, i.e., *helping* people with all kinds of diseases and ailments *get better*. This brings us to Broadbent's second point, which is to clarify what the *business* of medicine is. He suggests that the two core competencies of medicine are understanding health and disease and making good predictions about them. This is what Broadbent calls the Inquiry Thesis, which posits that medicine is an inquiry into health and disease for the purpose of cure and prevention (p. 64). If you look at what medicine does from this pragmatic, non-lofty angle, medicine can persist because it at least helps us make some progress, while not always (or even not often) reaching that often elusive goal of cure. Indeed, I think that the business of medicine is not inquiry but action. Medicine is not science. The business of medicine is to *help people get better*, if possible. People don't judge medicine by how far it generally comes to its lofty goal (cure), but by how good it is at doing its business, help people get better.

I think that, at least in part, medical skepticism (and perhaps also nihilism) arises because of a misalignment between expectations and observed outcomes produced by medicine. The skeptics say that medicine is ineffective because it doesn't reach its goal (cure), but they do not explain why reaching its goal should be a measure of effectiveness. While medical interventions might be seen as ineffective vis-à-vis the expectation of *cure*, they might be viewed as less ineffective vis-à-vis the expectation of *care* (Stegenga, 36), and medical care is, I propose, generally considered *helpful* (auxiliary).[10] If we do not use the purported ultimate goal of medicine (to cure) but its arguably widely accepted immediate goal (to help) as a measure of medical effectiveness, arguments in favor of medical skepticism and perhaps also nihilism lose at least some of their force.

Reading Stegenga I initially thought of his version of nihilism applied to medicine as a suggestion not to trust medicine at all. I am grateful to one of this book's anonymous reviewers that this is not exactly what Stegenga says. Instead, he writes that "for many of our most widely used medical interventions, the best evidence available indicates that such interventions are barely effective, if at all" and that, therefore, "our confidence in the effectiveness of a medical intervention ought to be low" (Stegenga, 2018, p. 18). I understand that the reviewer wants me to soften the potential blow of Stegenga's language a little, and I am willing to do that. Still, for my central argument it doesn't really matter much if you read Stegenga as proposing to have "low confidence in medicine" or to doubt that medicine works "at all". Both versions indicate that Stegenga thinks that something is seriously wrong with medicine and that it is, as suggested by Broadbent as well, to a certain degree ineffective. In keeping with my position that the difference between having a low confidence in medicine versus no trust at all is somewhat unclear, Jonathan Fuller's view is that "[s]ometimes a low confidence is enough to justify using a drug, depending on what is to be gained or lost – it depends on how low is 'low'" (Fuller, 2020). I couldn't agree more.

PREVIEW: UNCERTAINTY

If we accept the auxiliary thesis and abandon *puzzle* and *nihilism* because we decide to accept medicine to be effective by way of being helpful, there is another issue that might contribute to the impression that medicine is less effective than advertised and contribute to medical skepticism: medicine's inherent *uncertainty*. I will go into much more detail in Chap. 4 but want to give a sneak-preview here.

No surgeon can guarantee the patient will survive the operation. No internist will tell the cancer patient that she will survive and live until old age if she only agrees to embark on a third cycle of chemotherapy. No pediatrician will swear on the grave of their stepmother that the immunization will reduce the infant's risk of infection to zero. There are always uncertainties. Not *all* smokers will develop lung disease. But some do. Not *all* individuals with HIV infection will survive for many years after receiving the diagnosis if they only slavishly adhere to their anti-retroviral therapy (ART) regimen. Life is an uncertain business and this has serious repercussions for medical practice.

There are at least two kinds of uncertainty in medicine. The first is *aleatoric uncertainty* (henceforth *A-uncertainty*), the natural uncertainty as an inherent characteristic of events. The second kind of uncertainty is *epistemic uncertainty* (*E-uncertainty*), the cognitive state of "I don't really know", which is either due to a lack of knowledge or a result of incongruities and fallacies in the knowledge generation process. In our current context, E-uncertainty arises in the communication between those who produce knowledge to be used in medicine (bioscientists, epidemiologists) and those who need to translate research results into clinical practice (the medics who interpret research results). Part of this is a lack of knowledge; for example, in the absence of etiologic information we call some diseases "idiopathic", or when we deal with what is very difficult to predict, the future.

Since the E-uncertainty arises from A-uncertainty, it should not come as a surprise that medicine seems ineffective. All human beings are different and not all medical interventions work for everyone. Certainty is rare for *anything* in life and medicine is no exception. Satisfactory explanation is difficult in medicine in the wake of A-uncertainty if precision is expected. Some have suggested that concept of uncertainty in medicine should be limited to E-uncertainty, i.e., uncertainty as a state of belief (Han, 2021). In contrast, I argue that A-uncertainty is an ingredient of all biological processes. The reliance of medicine on data about disease etiology, diagnostics, screening, therapeutic interventions, and prognosis is weakened by the A-uncertainty reflected in these data, which is due to the A-uncertainty in the underlying processes. In other words, I take uncertainty not just as some cognitive phenomenon *in* medicine but also a natural characteristic *of* medicine, which occurs in several forms and makes essential contributions to the imprecise data medical skeptics take as evidence in support of their notion that medicine is ineffective. Another aspect of this mélange of uncertainties is that misinterpretations and misunderstandings occur when scientific and particularly epidemiologic concept require translation into clinical practice, for example, when population data are used as the basis for decisions how to diagnose, treat, prognosticate for individual patients. The upshot is the *argument of uncertain medicine*, the position that medical ineffectiveness is in part due to natural A-uncertainty and the resulting E-uncertainty, and in part due to an inferential problem, when scientific data are misinterpreted, miscommunicated, or simply not well understood.

In keeping with my view of medicine as a primarily *auxiliary* enterprise, medicine is supposed to help people become and stay healthy. To achieve this goal, however, medicine needs reliable knowledge about risk factors for disease occurrence and trajectory, reliable diagnostic approaches, and therapeutic interventions. In modern medicine, this information does not rely solely and not even mainly on the individual experience of the medic but on scientific data generated in the wet lab by experimental scientists and, most important for the translation into medical practice, data generated by epidemiologists in population-based studies, and curated in the medical and health literatures in accordance with scientific inferential rules that generate etiologic, diagnostic, interventional, and prognostic explanations. These explanations justify the ways medicine conducts its business.[11] Unfortunately, the information-processing that underlies auxiliary medicine is affected by uncertainty. Of note, I think it is important to distinguish between scientific uncertainty and medical uncertainty. Sometimes, medicine is considered a scientific activity. I think this is wrong. As outlined in more detail in the next chapter, medicine is not science because it does not generate new knowledge. Medicine is helping people get better and science is the provider of data that are transformed into new knowledge to be used in medicine to help people get better.

* * *

I will not offer further discussion of medical skepticism in this book. However, I will say that medical ineffectiveness is to be expected when we expect medicine to be perfect and failsafe. Such expectations lead into the pitfalls generated by uncertainty, the topic of Chap. 4. The concepts outlined in Part II provide the means to curb uncertainty at the intersection between science and medicine, and the examples offered in Part III illustrate how these concepts can be integrated to tackle specific problems in medicine.

NOTES

1. (Broadbent, 2019). For full disclosure, Alex Broadbent was my thesis advisor at the University of Johannesburg.
2. Broadbent makes the following distinction between medical skepticism and nihilism: "Skepticism about medicine is uncertainty. Medical nihilism [...] is a strong belief in the impotence of medicine" (Broadbent, 2019, p. 158).
3. I have taken the liberty to lift the last quotation from a comment offered by an anonymous pre-publication reviewer of this book as an indication that I fully agree with this important caveat.
4. See Chap. 3 in (Broadbent, 2019).
5. In this part of his book, Broadbent appears to take "to heal" and "to cure" as synonymous.
6. But, for full disclosure, I am biased because I was trained as a physician (a long time ago) and might, thus, favor the use of a more lenient standard.
7. These are examples used by Stegenga.
8. One of Stegenga's running examples from this category is the general ineffectiveness of anti-depressant medications.
9. Stegenga alludes to this idea on p. 36.
10. Which has motivated me to call the authentic stance of doctors, nurses, and other clinicians the *auxiliary stance* and the associated theorizing *medical auxiliarianism*.
11. I will frequently refer to medicine when it might be better to refer to both medicine and public/population health. Restricting myself to medicine

will make the message clearer. Regarding public versus population health, I have referred to some important differences between them in my review of Sean Valles' book *Philosophy of Population Health* (Dammann, 2020), but none of those are of major import for my discussion in this book.

REFERENCES

Appiah, A. (2006). *Cosmopolitanism: Ethics in a world of strangers* (1st ed.). W.W. Norton & Co..

Broadbent, A. (2018). *Philosophy of medicine*. Oxford University Press.

Broadbent, A. (2019). *Philosophy of medicine* (p. 1). Oxford University Press.

Bryan, C. S., & Podolsky, S. H. (2009). Dr. Holmes at 200 — The spirit of skepticism. *New England Journal of Medicine, 361*(9), 846–847.

Dammann, O. (2020). Toward epistemic, intersectoral, and disciplinary humility for population health science. *American Journal of Public Health, 110*(4), 425–426.

Davis, C. S. (2021). The purdue pharma opioid settlement - accountability, or just the cost of doing business? *The New England Journal of Medicine, 384*(2), 97–99.

Fuller, J. (2020). Medical Nihilism by Jacob Stegenga: What is the right dose? *Studies in History and Philosophy of Science Part C: Studies in History and Philosophy of Biological and Biomedical Sciences, 81*, 101270.

Gibian, P. (2001). *Oliver Wendell Holmes and the culture of conversation*. Cambridge University Press.

Gillies, D. (2019). *Causality, probability, and medicine (1st edn)*. Routledge.

Han, P. K. J. (2021). *Uncertainty in medicine: A framework for tolerance*. Oxford University Press.

Holmes, O. W. (1860). *Currents and counter-currents in medical science. An address delivered before the Massachusetts medical society, at the annual meeting, May 30, 1860*. Ticknor and Fields.

Manchikanti, L., Helm, S., Fellows, B., Janata, J. W., Pampati, V., Grider, J. S., et al. (2012). Opioid epidemic in the United States. *Pain Physician, 15*(3 Suppl), ES9–E38.

Porter, R. (1998). *The greatest benefit to mankind: A medical history of humanity* (1st American ed.). W. W. Norton.

Riley, D., Fischer, M., Singh, B., Haidvogl, M., & Heger, M. (2001). Homeopathy and conventional medicine: An outcomes study comparing effectiveness in a primary care setting. *Journal of Alternative and Complementary Medicine, 7*(2), 149–159.

Shang, A., Huwiler-Muntener, K., Nartey, L., Juni, P., Dorig, S., Sterne, J. A., et al. (2005). Are the clinical effects of homoeopathy placebo effects? Comparative study of placebo-controlled trials of homoeopathy and allopathy. *Lancet, 366*(9487), 726–732.

Smart, B. T. H. (2023). The core business of medicine: A defence of the best available intervention thesis. *Synthese, 201*, 194.

Stegenga, J. (2018). *Medical nihilism*. Oxford University Press.

CHAPTER 3

Medicine Is Not Science

INTRODUCTION

The *New Philosophy of Medicine* is a term I like to use to distinguish philosophical work on medicine and its scientific and cultural underpinnings published after, roughly, 2010 from the work published before. This work is exemplified by, for example, Pellegrino and Thomasma's "Philosophical Basis of Medical Practice" (Pellegrino & Thomasma, 1981) and the kind of paper published in the *Journal of Medicine and Philosophy* under the editorship of Edmund Daniel Pellegrino (1920–2013) and H. Tristram Engelhardt Jr. (1941–2018). That literature revolved almost exclusively around topics like judgment, decision making, morals, and ethics, while the New Philosophy of Medicine has expanded its topical reach appreciably to include metaphysical and epistemological aspects of medicine.[1] This is the philosophical landscape this book is positioned in.

One must keep in mind that most new philosophers of medicine come from philosophy of science. Therefore, it would not be surprising if some thought of medicine *as science*, or at least as *scientific*. For instance, I earlier outlined Broadbent's view of the business of medicine as inquiry. In this chapter I want to briefly justify my position that medicine is *not* science. The upshot of this distinction is that scientific results need to be explored and digested by members of the medical community before they can be used to argue for or against diagnostic and therapeutic recommendations

© The Author(s), under exclusive license to Springer Nature Switzerland AG 2025
O. Dammann, *Uncertainty and Explanation in Medicine and the Health Sciences*, https://doi.org/10.1007/978-3-031-82271-1_3

in, e.g., medical textbooks. This requires communication across disciplinary boundaries that may contribute to misunderstandings, misinterpretations, and so forth, thereby increasing medical uncertainty.

SCIENCE IS NOT PART OF MEDICINE

It may be tempting to unify clinical care and health research under the term "medicine". For example, Raffaella Campaner appears to assume this when she writes about "the impact of pluralistic stances on the medical discourse, given its two-faceted—clinical and research—vocation" (Campaner, 2019, p. 28). What she seems to suggest is that clinical and research work are two kinds of work being done *within* medicine. If that was indeed the case, both clinical care and research were both part of medicine. However, I don't think this is true.

Of course, there is such a thing as medical research, but it is not part of medicine, while clinical care definitely is. Indeed, I believe it is exactly this "care" component that deserves to be called "medicine", not the underlying science. Scientific research provides the epistemological underpinnings needed to develop care models that work. But the production of new knowledge is neither medicine's goal nor its business. Its immediate goal is to help, to improve the health of individuals by caring for them in ways that are justified by scientific results and conclusions. The business of medicine is to implement research results and to intervene accordingly (or not) in order to achieve their respective goals. The generation of new knowledge is not part of that business.

Suggesting that medicine is a hard science is one of the smoke-and-mirror strategies used to increase consumer trust in medicine. Patients want to trust their medics, and talking and looking sciency (white lab coats!) certainly helps. But even if these superficial similarities may sometimes be interpreted as an indicator that medicine *is* science, it is not science at all. Medicine is the auxiliary activity rooted in the longstanding human tradition to help others to get better. Observational epidemiology, randomized trials, and the biosciences are scientific activities because their aim is to generate new knowledge that can be used in medicine. Medicine is an auxiliary activity that applies scientific information to help others, but it is not itself hard science. Medicine and science are completely separate activities; they do not overlap.

Let me outline this view in a bit more detail by revisiting Broadbent. He distinguishes between the goal and the business of medicine. The context of his verdict—that medicine is extremely unreliable when it comes to healing the sick—is his proposal that while cure is the goal of medicine, its business is actually *inquiry* in terms of "understanding and predicting health and disease" (p. 62). I guess that many medics would agree that this kind of inquiry is, indeed, part of their business. However, other parts are researching guidelines for diagnosis and therapy, making diagnostic and therapeutic decisions, communicating proposals for and results of diagnostic and therapeutic interventions with patients and their families, keeping up to date with the medical literature, and documenting all their decisions and actions in myriads of ways in forms, charts, and electronic health record systems. Understanding and predicting is part of this, but it is definitely not their entire business. Moreover, the understanding and prediction that *is* part of medicine's business is definitely not what I would call inquiry. Instead, I think that such understanding and prediction is the result of a medical professional's (and the medical profession's) reflections on the outcome of medical and health research. But only very little of such research, if any at all, is performed *within* medicine. While some medical and health researchers may be nurses and doctors, I would argue that the production of medical knowledge is not part of medicine, but of those applied sciences that have evolved over the centuries with just that goal, to generate knowledge that enables medical and health professionals to understand and predict health and disease. These applied sciences include fields such as anatomy, physiology, all kinds of chemistry, immunology, neuroscience, pharmacology, epidemiology, biostatistics, to name only a few. The knowledge to be applied in medicine is generated in the laboratories and offices of scientists in these fields, perhaps with the exemption of applied clinical research that is indeed performed during the daily business of medicine by medical professionals studying, for example, the effects of changes in clinical practice on clinical outcomes at the point of clinical service. But this is arguably a very small and perhaps even negligible proportion of medical and nursing research, at least in the present context, while the bulk of medical and health research is *not* conducted by doctors, but by PhDs who devote their professional lives to the generation of medical knowledge, not to its application. Therefore, I do not agree that the business of medicine is inquiry—this is the business of medical and health scientists, e.g., epidemiologists and bench bioscientists. The business of the medical professions is to *apply* the information generated by scientists to help individual patients (in medicine) and communities or other populations (in public health) by improving their health. Doing medicine simply does not include the use of scientific methods.

CALLING MEDICINE SCIENTIFIC

The strategy to talk about medicine as scientific is reflected in appellations that refer to medicine as something cool and sciency, such as "molecular medicine", "systems medicine", and "precision medicine". The National Institutes of Health (NIH), the largest federal funding source for academic biomedical research in the United States with an annual budget of more than 50 billion (sic) US dollars, includes the National Cancer Institute (NCI), which offers the following description of "molecular medicine":

> *A branch of medicine that develops ways to diagnose and treat disease by understanding the way genes, proteins, and other cellular molecules work. Molecular medicine is based on research that shows how certain genes, molecules, and cellular functions may become abnormal in diseases such as cancer.*[2]

Note that, first, NIH considers molecular medicine to be part of medicine, but it does not explicitly include molecular research under the same heading. It just notes that molecular medicine is *based on* research, which can be true for research within medicine (which I think does not exist) or outside medicine (which is where I think biomedical research is situated). Thus, the NIH definition alludes to the idea, but does not explicitly say, that molecular medicine includes genetic, molecular, cellular research, which may be considered an example of a smoke-and-mirror strategy to let medicine partake in the glory of modern bioscience, at least if you agree with me.

My own research work includes a publication titled "Whither Systems Medicine?" (Apweiler et al., 2018). The abstract states that

> *Systems medicine is the interdisciplinary approach wherein physicians and clinical investigators team up with experts from biology, biostatistics, informatics, mathematics and computational modeling to develop methods to use new and stored data to the benefit of the patient.* (Apweiler et al., 2018)

Here, the focus is not so much on molecules, but rather on data integration and modeling. However, this statement tries to keep medicine and research separate by saying that physicians and researchers collaborate in an interdisciplinary fashion. Moving on to "precision medicine", here is the definition provided by the NCI:

A form of medicine that uses information about a person's own genes or proteins to prevent, diagnose, or treat disease. In cancer, precision medicine uses specific information about a person's tumor to help make a diagnosis, plan treatment, find out how well treatment is working, or make a prognosis. Examples of precision medicine include using targeted therapies to treat specific types of cancer cells, such as HER2-positive breast cancer cells, or using tumor marker testing to help diagnose cancer. Also called personalized medicine.[3]

In this definition, precision (cancer) medicine is described as one form of medicine that uses information about the patient's own tumor to target its cells with personalized precision. In my experience, the term "personalized medicine", although not incorrect, is not much appreciated by clinicians who like to think that they have always practiced medicine in a personalized way. This position misfires because the term refers to a patient's tumor, not the person.

Of note, there is also such a thing as "precision public health". Here is one definition:

Precision public health involves the collection of more accurate population- and individual-level data on genes, exposures, behaviors, and other social/economic health determinants; enhancing public health action for improving health in subpopulations in need of recommended prevention measures; and addressing and reducing health disparities in the population by using more precision data for action.

The authors focus on the enhancement of public health activities by usage of specific kinds of data (Khoury et al., 2018, p. 580). Again, research data are described as being used in public health, but it remains open whether or not the authors see the data collection (and presumably also the analysis) component of the underlying research as part of public health or as separate from it. Just like I suggest that science is not part of medicine, I think that science is not part of public health, while its results are definitely used in public health. Still, public health and public health research are very much related, but they are still separate endeavors.

Examples of terminology that attempt to make clear that medicine is *not* science are "evidence-based medicine" (EBM) and "translational medicine". The former indicates that medicine is *based on evidence*, not generating it. The latter indicates the need to translate from "bench to bedside", i.e., from science to medicine. Still, despite all the science talk in medicine, exclamations such as "I have never seen this before in my practice!" can frequently be heard in hospital hallway conversations. What this means is that the physician thinks that, given a certain clinical problem, a similar problem has so far not occurred as part of their personal clinical experience. Early expositions of EBM poked fun at this approach by coining tongue-in-cheek variations of EBM such as "experience-based medicine" and "eminence-based-medicine".[4]

I have offered a few examples of how science-tinged names for medicine and public health are being used. Of course, I am far from suggesting that someone has introduced this terminology for the purpose of misleading patients. Still, I cannot help but sense a certain pride and perhaps even entitlement when these terms are used in medicine, just as I am confident that some, and perhaps even many, patients find the idea attractive that modern biomedicine is a thoroughly scientific endeavor and certainly a much better idea than taking the medical skeptic's or nihilist's position. Thus, I think it is fair to say that selling medicine as a scientific undertaking is a misattribution and may be devious by raising and maintaining unreasonable expectations.

My opposition to the "medicine is science" dovetails with Raffaella Campaner's recent work. The central goal of her book *Explaining Disease* (Campaner, 2022) is to elucidate the kinds of roles that explanation plays in medicine, in particular explanation of disease. In the introductory chapter, Campaner pinpoints her overarching topic, the explanation of disease with an eye toward better understanding to improve prediction and intervention in medicine. She introduces the development of philosophical theories of explanation and swiftly moves on to causal explanation in biomedicine. This clarifies Campaner's point of departure: when she says she is interested in "explaining disease" she emphasizes *causal* explanation, whose goal is to explain why disease occurs. Although causal explanation may be the most important, and perhaps the only kind of scientific explanation that provides knowledge to be used in medicine, it may also be viewed as one of multiple kinds of explanations, scientific or not, that play a role in clinical practice (see Chap. 6). Patients want causal explanations to understand why they are sick, but they also want to know what can be done and what their future will look like. In that sense, one might state that there are etiological (causal), diagnostic (detective), therapeutic (interventional), and prognostic (prospective) explanations in medicine. Of course, this is just a shift in explanatory context, a shift toward a perspective that focuses on what is being explained (explanandum), i.e., the etiology, diagnosis, therapy, or prognosis of an individual patient's course of disease. If Campaner's focus is really mainly on disease *occurrence*, her exploration of causal and mechanical explanations is completely aligned with my own, which conceptualizes etiological explanations as explanations of disease occurrence based on its causes and mechanisms (Dammann, 2020). But if her topic is to include explanations of diagnosis, therapy choice, and what the course of a case of disease is likely to be, interventional and prospective explanations would also need to be considered. One could argue that causal explanations, broadly conceived, are fundamental to all explanation and, therefore, also to diagnostic, interventional, and prognostic explanations. If we are interested in what kinds of tests are needed to make sense of a set of signs and symptoms, we ask what kind of difference in test results would be caused by the presence of a hypothesized underlying disease compared to the results to be expected in its absence. If we are interested in the kind of medication needed to get better, we ask, in essence, what intervention is most likely to cause our recovery. And if we want to know how we will be doing a few months or years down the road, we ask what changes to the disease trajectory will be caused by the intervention.

Early in the first chapter Campaner cites a brief passage from Maël Lemoine's chapter on "Explanation in medicine" in one of the abovementioned handbooks (Solomon et al., 2017) that begins with the statement, "The scientific part of medicine seeks explanations" (p. 4) and continues with a list of desiderata for how medical explanations should be conceptualized. In keeping with Lemoine's view that medicine has a scientific part, Campaner refers to "a very strict link [...] between the fact that medicine is a scientific enterprise and the elaboration of explanation in medical contexts" (ibid.) As discussed above, I don't think that medicine has a scientific part, at least not if you define medicine as what medics[5] do with and for their patients. Doctors and nurses *care* for their patients; they help them get better. However, I completely agree that medicine has scientific underpinnings, but only very few of these are generated by medics in the course of practicing medicine. The medical and health sciences that generate the knowledge used by medics are epidemiology, the laboratory sciences, psychology, sociology, and so forth. It may be that some of the individuals in these sciences are also medics, but the work they are doing is not medicine; it is scientific research. Indeed, I believe it is fair to say that most medical scientists are not medics, and their work is not part of medicine. Medicine is simply what medics do when they apply bioscientific knowledge with the aim to help others in the sphere of health and disease, without doing science themselves.

And so, I suggest keeping medicine and science separate until we have more and better arguments in support of the notion that doing medicine and doing science is the same. Campaner makes this distinction in the title of her book, which offers reflections on "medical research and clinical practice" and even more explicit when she writes that "[i]n very general terms, we can think of the *biomedical sciences* as directly and eminently involved in research and in enhancing our understanding of diseases, and of *clinical medicine* as directly involved in caring and curing" (p. 177).

* * *

After having made the case for distinguishing scientific medicine, i.e., medicine informed by science, from medical science, i.e., science that informs medicine, we now move on to one of the central points of this book, uncertainty as part of what gives rise to the appearance of medicine as ineffective. At the core of this notion is the acknowledgment of two kinds of uncertainty, aleatoric and epistemic, a distinction I will explicate in the next chapter.

NOTES

1. Key works in the *New Philosophy of Medicine* are Jeremy Howick's "Philosophy of Evidence-Based Medicine" (Howick, 2011), Miriam Solomon's "Making Medical Knowledge" (Solomon, 2015), Havi Carel's "Phenomenology of illness" (Carel, 2016), Thompson and Upshur's "Philosophy of Medicine: An Introduction" (Thompson & Upshur, 2018), Alex Broadbent's "Philosophy of Medicine" (Broadbent, 2018), and Jacob Stegenga's "Medical Nihilism" (Stegenga, 2018), and Jonathan Fuller's "The New Modern Medicine", to name only a few. The publication of three handbooks since 2016 (Broadbent, forthcoming; Schramme & Edwards, 2016; Solomon et al., 2017) bears witness to the growing interest in the field among philosophers. Part of this post-2010 turn is a growing interest among authors in causation and explanation, including Ben Smart's "Concepts and Causes in the Philosophy of Disease" (Smart, 2016), Don Gillies' "Causality, Probability, and Medicine" (Gillies, 2019), my own "Etiological Explanations" (Dammann, 2020) and Raffaella Campaner's books *Varieties of Causal Explanation in Medical Contexts* (Campaner,

2019) and *Explaining Disease: Philosophical Reflections on Medical Research and Clinical Practice* (Campaner, 2022).

2. https://www.cancer.gov/publications/dictionaries/cancer-terms/def/molecular-medicine; accessed 7 April, 2023.
3. https://www.cancer.gov/publications/dictionaries/cancer-terms/def/precision-medicine; accessed 7 April, 2023.
4. David Isaacs and Dominique Fitzgerald have suggested using a luminometer to measure the brightness of a physician's white hair to identify cases of eminence-based medicine (Isaacs & Fitzgerald, 1999).
5. I am using the term "medic" for any individual who works as a doctor, nurse, medical student, physician assistant, and so forth, i.e., anyone who works as a medical clinician with and/or for patients.

References

Apweiler, R., Beissbarth, T., Berthold, M. R., Bluthgen, N., Burmeister, Y., Dammann, O., et al. (2018). Whither systems medicine? *Experimental & Molecular Medicine, 50*(3), e453.

Broadbent, A. (2018). *Philosophy of medicine*. Oxford University Press.

Broadbent, A. (Ed.). (Forthcoming). *Oxford handbook of philosophy of medicine*.

Campaner, R. (2019). *Varieties of causal explanations in medical contexts*. Mimesis International.

Campaner, R. (2022). *Explaining disease: Philosophical reflections on medical research and clinical practice*. Springer.

Carel, H. (2016). *Phenomenology of illness* (1st ed.). Oxford University Press.

Dammann, O. (2020). *Etiological explanations: Illness causation theory*. CRC Press.

Gillies, D. (2019). *Causality, probability, and medicine (1st edn)*. Routledge.

Howick, J. (2011). *The philosophy of evidence-based medicine*. Wiley-Blackwell, BMJ Books.

Isaacs, D., & Fitzgerald, D. (1999). Seven alternatives to evidence based medicine. *BMJ, 319*(7225), 1618–1618.

Khoury, M. J., Bowen, M. S., Clyne, M., Dotson, W. D., Gwinn, M. L., Green, R. F., et al. (2018). From public health genomics to precision public health: A 20-year journey. *Genetics in Medicine, 20*(6), 574–582.

Pellegrino, E. D., & Thomasma, D. C. (1981). *A philosophical basis of medical practice: Toward a philosophy and ethic of the healing professions*. Oxford University Press.

Schramme, T., & Edwards, S. (Eds.). (2016). *Handbook of the philosophy of medicine*. Springer.

Smart, B. (2016). *Concepts and causes in the philosophy of disease*. Palgrave Macmillan.

Solomon, M. (2015). *Making medical knowledge* (1st ed.). Oxford University Press.

Solomon, M., Simon, J. R., & Kincaid, H. (2017). *The Routledge companion to philosophy of medicine*. Routledge, Taylor & Francis Group.

Stegenga, J. (2018). *Medical nihilism*. Oxford University Press.

Thompson, R. P., & Upshur, R. (2018). *Philosophy of medicine: An introduction*. Routledge, Taylor & Francis Group.

CHAPTER 4

Two Kinds of Uncertainty

Introduction

In the previous chapters I have argued that medicine might look less ineffective than the skeptics suggest if the reference point is not defined as the extent to which medicine reaches its ultimate goal, to cure, but the extent to which it does its job well and reaches its immediate goal, to help. If we can agree that effectiveness of medicine is better assessed by judging to what extent it succeeds in helping people get better, we might conclude that medicine is not so ineffective after all. But even then, medicine will seem ineffective at times. Diagnoses may be wrong, treatments do not work as intended, and prognoses do not fit what really happens to the patient.

In this chapter, I outline one of the main arguments of this book, which says that if we accept that it is true that medicine really is ineffective to a certain degree, it is not because medicine fails to cure (Broadbent), nor because medical research is bad or even fraudulent (Stegenga). Instead, medicine is at least partially ineffective because of the misguided expectation that medicine should work better than it does. This misguided expectation is due to a tendency of members of the biomedical system to ignore, downplay, or even cover up the simple fact that life, and thus medicine, is inherently uncertain.

© The Author(s), under exclusive license to Springer Nature Switzerland AG 2025
O. Dammann, *Uncertainty and Explanation in Medicine and the Health Sciences*, https://doi.org/10.1007/978-3-031-82271-1_4

At the core of the notion of uncertainty, as I see it, is my rejection for the central functional system targeted by medicine, human biology, of what some have called "Laplacian quasi-determinism", the notion that all events are causally determined without chance being a play at all. Laplacian quasi-determinism entails that event occurrence only *looks* chancy at times because we don't have enough information about the situation at hand and, therefore, do not fully grasp what is going on and cannot predict future occurrences of similar events.[1] This would be a situation in which events are not uncertain at all, but pre-determined, but our knowledge about what is going on is incomplete, leading to our uncertainty about it due to a lack of knowledge. Note that the former is about uncertainty of event occurrence (or better: the lack thereof in a deterministic world), while the latter is uncertainty as a cognitive state.

My view is that life (and perhaps the world) is inherently indeterminate. As I will expound in the next section when further explicating the distinction between aleatoric uncertainty as uncertainty *of* something (A-uncertainty) and epistemic uncertainty as uncertainty *about* something (E-uncertainty), I reject quasi-determinism in favor of a soft developmental indeterminism. In essence, I think that not much in life (except the "big trajectory" from birth to death) happens in exactly pre-determined ways. Instead, everything evolves over time, at each moment taking one of many possible trajectories of how things may evolve. The qualifier "soft" allows for some exceptions such as death and taxes, per Benjamin Franklin's quip. In medicine, we face many situations in which we are E-uncertain about something because it is A-uncertain. Interpreted this way, E-uncertainty is not just a lack of knowledge because of a lack of information but a lack of certainty because perfect certainty cannot be attained due to A-uncertainty. Certainty would be the capability of predicting an event with perfect precision, and I think that there is always some residual uncertainty because the world constantly evolves in a developmental-probabilistic, softly indeterminate way (except for death and taxes).

WHAT IS UNCERTAINTY?

Some surgeries are not successful, and the patient does not get better or even dies on the table. Anesthesia works most of the time, but some patients report they were aware of what was going on in the operating room and overheard the surgeons cracking jokes while operating.

Antibiotics usually work, but some bacterial strains have become resistant and render the antibiotic treatment ineffective. Antidepressants may or may not work well. And so on. While Stegenga's focus is on bad or faulty research as the main culprit, I propose that a major source of the apparent misalignment between expected and observed outcomes of medical interventions is *uncertainty*.

In his book *Uncertainty in Medicine*, Paul Han talks about uncertainty exclusively as a cognitive state (Han, 2021). He thinks it is impossible that all four definitions of uncertainty in the *Oxford Dictionary of English* (ODE) (p. 13) as (1) a state of mind, (2) a state of being, (3) an object, and (4) a feature of an object, can be true. I assume that his point is that for him, uncertainty is only of the first kind listed in the ODE, a state of mind, a cognitive thing. Unfortunately, Han does not state exactly *why* his uncertainty can only be a state of mind, but not any of the other three things listed in the ODE. However, he affirms that uncertainty is "ultimately a subjective, rather than an objective phenomenon, a mental state rather than a material 'thing' residing in the extra-mental world" (p.14). In essence, Han appears to be an "uncertainty monist" who thinks that there is just one thing that qualifies as uncertainty and that is a person's cognitive state with reference to aspects of a fact or the occurrence of an event. In my mind, and in keeping with the ODE, the noun *uncertainty* and the adjective *uncertain* are used in a variety of ways, and we should begin by clarifying how I will use the term before moving on to the metaphysics of uncertainty in medicine. My proposal is a call to appreciate the fourth ODE kind of uncertainty, uncertainty as a feature of something.

I suggest distinguishing between two different readings of the word "uncertainty", as a *natural property* (aleatoric or A-uncertainty), on the one hand, and uncertainty as a *belief or cognitive state* (epistemic or E-uncertainty), on the other. Thus, in contrast to Han, I propose a plurality of uncertainty, according to which there are, in my version, two kinds, aleatoric and epistemic.[2] According to this distinction, the statement "I am uncertain whether I should take an umbrella when going out for a walk" refers to my E-uncertainty, but this kind of uncertainty is rooted in the A-uncertainty of the weather. The sequence of A- and E-uncertainty is often covered by predictions such as "it is uncertain what will happen when you cut that rope" but also in the context of facts unknown as in "the exact blood sugar level of this patient at this time is uncertain". In both statements it is communicated that something (rain, blood sugar level) is uncertain and, therefore, I am uncertain, I do not know.

Thus, I will use the term uncertainty for two different things, the uncertainty of events, actions, and so on, and the uncertainty of minds. On the one hand, this view goes against Han's view, who thinks there is only one kind of uncertainty (the belief state). On the other hand, it seems to be in alignment with, for example, Merle Mishel's view, who wrote about both "uncertainty as experienced by hospital patients" (uncertainty of mind) and "events perceived as uncertain" (uncertainty of event) (Mishel, 1981, p. 259).

Perhaps the best-known account of uncertainty in philosophy of science is Heisenberg's uncertainty principle, first outlined in a letter to Pauli and later published in the *Zeitschrift für Physik* (Heisenberg, 1927).[3] The uncertainty principle holds that we cannot know both the speed and the position of a subatomic particle at any point in time. Thus, a full account of its presence is impossible (E-uncertain) because it is A-uncertain (from the perspective of quantum mechanics.) In fact, Heisenberg wrote that

> *What is wrong with the exact formulation of the causal law: "If we know the presence precisely we can infer the future" is not the inference but the premise. We cannot know the present in all its detail. All perception is a selection from many possibilities and a restriction of what is possible.* (Heisenberg, 1927, p. 197) (translation mine)

The concept of uncertainty as I am using it entails that uncertainty is not just that we cannot know the present exactly, but that the way things are, and come about, is intrinsically uncertain, independent of our beliefs about them. While the former is uncertainty as a subjective, epistemic cognitive state, the latter is uncertainty as an objective, aleatoric natural property of events. Along the same lines, Richard von Mises wrote in *Probability, Statistics and Truth*:

> *Until recently, we thought that there existed two different kinds of observations of natural phenomena, observations of a statistical character, whose exactness could not be improved beyond a certain limit, and observations on the molecular scale whose results were of a mathematically exact and deterministic character. We now recognize that no such distinction exists in nature.* (Mises, 1981 (1957), p. 217)

Distinguishing between A- and E-uncertainty makes room for the proposition of a more or less fixed relation between the two regarding the same target event. If we are uncertain whether a certain pharmacological intervention will work in a particular patient's situation, we are uncertain because the pharmaco-biological event structure, the process of the medication working in the patient's body (or not), is inherently uncertain.

This view, however, holds only for *future* events since *past* events have, trivially, already happened. They have become facts that cannot be uncertain. While this certainty of past event occurrence (or non-occurrence) is a simple objective fact, we can still be subjectively uncertain about it. For example, we know that about 66 million years ago an asteroid approximately 14 kilometers in diameter hit planet earth and left behind the Chicxulub crater, which probably initiated a global climate disaster that led to the extinction of the dinosaurs. Scientists have produced a computer model of the event and concluded that the impact generated a tsunami about 30,000 times more energetic than the 2004 tsunami in the Indian Ocean (Range et al., 2022). As interesting as this all is, and as reasonable it sounds, we cannot be certain about it, although much of it is highly likely based on corroborating evidence. However, while it is, trivially, certain that these events did or did not happen, we cannot be certain either way.

In what follows I outline my version of this dual model of uncertainty with special reference to medicine, epidemiology, and the biomedical sciences. I will argue that E-uncertainty is a mental response phenomenon in the sense of a cognitive state, as in, for example, "I am uncertain whether this patient has appendicitis" or "I am uncertain whether this chemotherapy will lead to the patient going into remission", meaning that I simply cannot talk with certainty about these current facts (appendicitis) or future events (remission). I simply do not know.

In other words, E-uncertainty is the cognitive state of not being able to talk *about* particular aspects of a target entity due to imperfect data about this aspect, i.e., the origin of E-uncertainty is the imperfect data situation at hand. E-uncertainty arises from incomplete, insufficient, or bad data. But data about facts and events arise from facts and events that are in and of themselves uncertain, such as the speed and position of Heisenberg's particles. This is what I call A-uncertainty, uncertainty as a property of events that may be associated with but is independent from E-uncertainty because the former gives rise to the latter, not the other way around. A-uncertainty is the mind-independent irregular (chancy) occurrence of events that is, I propose, at the core of the problem of medical ineffectiveness. Since A-uncertainty gives rise to data variability which in turn leads to E-uncertainty, data variability is situated at the center of the transition from A- to E-uncertainty. Our cognitive state about facts and events is based on data, their quality, validity, or incompleteness, and so forth. We must remain uncertain until we are sure that the data at hand reflect the true nature of facts and events.

The above distinction is far from novel. Indeed, it is just one of multiple ways of organizing the many aspects of uncertainty into various categories.[4] My proposed distinction probably aligns best with the distinction offered by Fox and Ülkümen, who describe A-uncertainty as "involving unknown outcomes that can differ each time one runs an experiment under similar conditions" and E-uncertainty as "involving missing knowledge concerning a fact that either is or is not true" (Fox & Ülkümen, 2011). A-uncertainty reflects the phenomenon that many events are not pre-determined and predictable. Most event occurrence does not follow mathematical laws but the rules of probability. Philosophical disposition or "powers" accounts of causation cash in by reference to A-uncertainty, basically saying that the "correlation is not causation" desideratum of causal contingency theories (causation interpreted as the difference between the probability of effect occurrence with the purported cause present and the probability in its absence) can be partially resolved by considering causal mechanisms (powers) that connect cause and effect. However, it might be that both accounts ultimately fail: contingency theories because correlation is not always causation and power theories because powers are by definition causal.[5]

At this point, two important notions need to be stressed. First, I do not hold that *all* natural facts and events are A-uncertain. Some are, some are not. Not every event is A-uncertain simply because A-uncertainty also pertains to itself. This may seem as if I am looking for a way out the backdoor of Heisenberg's "we cannot know the present" position, and I guess I am. For example, we can be certain about *facts* such as the existence of the Eiffel tower, that Pavarotti was widely considered a world-class opera singer, that most bicycles have two wheels, and so forth, since these are established facts that do not come with an A-uncertainty attached because they are already established. One can still be E-uncertain about them if one doesn't know much about the Eiffel tower, Pavarotti, and bicycles. The same is true for medical facts: we are certain that colon cancer exists, that Christian Barnard (1922–2001) did the first human-to-human heart transplant in 1967, and that smoking is associated with an increased risk for multiple cardio-pulmonary diseases. But again, these are established medical facts that cannot be A-uncertain; one can only be E-uncertain about them if one doesn't know much about colon cancer, the history of cardio-surgery, and the health risks associated with tobacco smoking. It is one of the major tasks for health data analysts to curb E-uncertainty.

Second, the story is different with uncertainty (both A- and E-) about *events*. When I say that natural events are uncertain because they are chancy, I truly mean that they are occurring randomly. This requires my commitment to an indeterministic view of the world, all the way down. Again, I agree that some events are not chancy at all, for example, the brute fact that all humans will die at some point. Also, some events do not occur randomly but due to natural laws. For example, the apple did not hover above Isaac Newton's head, but fell and hit it. This mix of certain and uncertain event is what I mean by "soft indeterminism". On this view, the world and what happens in it is an expanding event space in which some elements are certain to exist or happen, and others are not. In this book, my attention is almost exclusively directed toward those that are not.

Uncertainty in Medical Domains

Medical thinking occurs in what can be categorized as domains of medical reasoning and practice. Both A- and E-uncertainty can (and do) occur in all four domains, where different kinds of knowledge are needed to practice good medicine (Table 4.1).

Table 4.1 Example of uncertainty categorized by medical domain. Each individual item can in and of itself be uncertain (aleatoric uncertainty; A-uncertainty) and also lead to cognitive (epistemic uncertainty; E-uncertainty). Note that past events cannot be A-uncertain because they have already happened or not while they can still be E-uncertain

Time	Past	Present	Future
Domain			
Etiology			
Cause	Exposure to bacteria	Fever, cough	
Mechanism	Inflammatory response	Fever, cough	
Diagnosis		Blood test	Test positive
		X-ray	
		Oxymetrie	
Therapy		Test positive	Antibiotic
Prognosis		Antibiotic	Recovery

The first domain of medical reasoning and practice is *etiology*, where knowledge about the natural history of the disease of interest is used. On my view this includes knowledge about the causes of illness (the initial inducer) and the pathogenesis (the biological disease mechanism), which are generated by epidemiology and basic laboratory science, respectively (Dammann, 2020). The second domain is *diagnosis*, where knowledge about the kind of disease at hand is generated by medical blood tests, imaging, biopsies, and so forth. Of note, this is not novel knowledge of the scientific kind but case-specific novel knowledge about the patient. Third, *therapeutic* knowledge is crucially needed to make treatment decisions and is generated by laboratory scientists (pharmacologists) and clinical epidemiologists (performing observational studies and randomized trials). And last but not least, *prognostic* knowledge helps to forecast the development of disease in the individual patient.

E-Uncertainty in Medicine

Let's begin with E-uncertainty because it is likely the more familiar kind of uncertainty for most of us. E-uncertainty is a belief state opposite of the belief state of being certain. This is what Paul Han refers to, uncertainty attributed to the mental state of a person. In ordinary English, the noun "certainty" is frequently (perhaps even exclusively) used as a qualifier of cognitive activities, such as recalling an event or knowing something for a fact. For example, one can say that one does not recall *with certainty* whether or not it rained on a particular day last week. This statement is equivalent to saying that one is not certain whether or not it rained on a particular day last week, or to saying that one is uncertain about it. On this view, not recalling something with certainty is equivalent to being uncertain about it. It is the individual agent in the given situation, the person making the statement who is uncertain. This is uncertainty as referring to a cognitive state, a mental situation when we are not sure about the truth of a fact or whether we have a certain (no pun intended) piece of information that we are asked about.

Let us take a closer look at the scenario in Table 4.1. Uncertainty in medicine occurs in five flavors defined by the four domains of biomedical relevance, namely, as causal, mechanistic (taken together, these two are what I sometimes call etiology), diagnostic, therapeutic, and prognostic uncertainty. In each cell of Table 4.1, I have listed a fact or event relevant to one patient's possible disease that may or may not be uncertain. I have also added a simple classification of timepoints, i.e., past, present, and future. In this way, Table 4.1 offers a rather simplified illustration how the knowledge needed is generated and used in conversations with the patient.

Let's assume you are a doctor who sees a patient with a high fever and a nasty cough (at the present time). Based on common medical knowledge you hypothesize that it is likely a case of pneumonia. You order blood tests, a chest X-ray, and a measurement of blood oxygenation, all of which confirm your *diagnosis* and make it likely that this is bacterial pneumonia, while it could be also viral in origin (or both). However, medical tests are rarely 100% accurate. There are false-positives as well as false-negatives, and it is sometimes very difficult to establish the true status based on medical testing. This is a good example of how the inference about past and present events and facts rests on the *data* that are available about these facts and events, and the ways these data are interpreted. Both the available fact/event data will exhibit some variability (A-uncertainty), as will the results of the inference process (E-uncertainty). Thus, if a fact or event is naturally uncertain it might lead to, or at least contribute to, cognitive uncertainty through the data that link the two and their variability. To use a somewhat unusual and very unscientific term, the data about uncertain events and facts are often wobbly (as in "we shouldn't trust the data; we ought better be looking yonder"), and therefore, our knowledge about uncertain facts and events is wobbly as well, which is essentially my definition of E-uncertainty.

E-uncertainty of the *diagnostic* kind is simply being uncertain about wobbly data that derive from diagnostic tests. Take, for example, the suspicious shadow on a chest X-ray. The fact that the shadow is right there on the X-ray is not uncertain, because three radiologists agree on its presence. However, it is uncertain what the shadow represents; it might be an artifact without any pathological gravitas; it could be pneumonia, tuberculosis, or lung cancer, among many other things. The nature of the shadow is uncertain, which leads to cognitive diagnostic uncertainty until further evidence is collected and interpreted. Diagnostic data such as location, size, and density contribute to the generation of cognitive diagnostic uncertainty which ends when the real nature of the shadow is revealed. In our case, the diagnostic E-uncertainty is the caregivers' uncertainty about the result of the diagnostic tests, until the results come back, in this example with a positive result. The result itself depends on biological and physical aspects of how the data are generated in blood test, X-ray technology, and monitoring of systemic oxygenation. This is the natural A-uncertainty of diagnostic tests as a function of their design. The outcome of the test itself is uncertain, thus wobbly data and a wobbly cognitive state, i.e., E-uncertainty.

At this point, you can offer an *etiological* explanation to the patient, saying that they suffer from pneumonia, likely due to past exposure to bacteria origin (cause), which led to a vigorous inflammatory response in the lung (mechanism; in the past and probably still at present), which in turn causes their current symptoms.

The *etiologic* kind of E-uncertainty is uncertainty about the origin of a phenomenon at hand (fact or event), for example, the presence or new occurrence of a disease. It is uncertainty about the cause(s) and mechanism(s) of how an event came about. In Table 4.1, the past event in a patient's recent medical history is a potential exposure to bacteria and/or viruses, which may or may not have happened. Either way, there is no objective A-uncertainty of that past event because it has happened or not and so it is certain that either one of the two happened. Since this is a past event that cannot be observed directly, all we can do in the present is to do some diagnostic testing.

Mechanistic E-uncertainty is most interesting because it relates to both studies into how diseases develop (pathogenesis) and what medical interventions can be designed to interfere with such pathogenetic mechanisms for the purpose of therapeutic intervention (pharmacology). In the case of the patient in Table 4.1, the mechanism that connects the infection (past event) with the present symptoms (fever, cough) is a vigorous inflammatory response. Most patients do mount such inflammatory response to bacterial infection while others do not (A-uncertainty). The E-uncertainty of the health worker persists until they have obtained additional test results that do or don't confirm severe systemic inflammation.

Most research on mechanisms is not done in human studies but in the bioscientific laboratory. The disease mechanism is what medics call pathogenesis, the biologically plausible link between an initiator of a disease and the disease onset. Sometimes the disease mechanism concept is expanded to include the biological changes not only until disease onset but also during its further development. Of course, the bodily functions and malfunction during disease development before and after onset cannot be directly observed at the organ, cellular, and molecular level. This would be necessary to develop medical pharmaceutical interventions, but it is mostly impossible. Instead, bioscientists use simple systems such as cell cultures or animal models to design experiments that test therapeutic hypotheses.

This work is largely done by laboratories run by the pharmaceutical industry, obviously with commercial interests. However, much research into disease mechanisms is also done in not-for-profit entities, such as universities and research institutes. Regardless, the experimental paradigm also includes uncertainty. One well-known uncertainty-related problem in the biosciences is the failure of replication experiments. What works in one lab might not work in the other.[6]

Another uncertainty comes into play when in vitro (test tube and dish) results are taken to the in vivo (animal model) level. It is quite uncertain whether a successful in vivo result extends to the animal model, where many and vastly different conditions are at play. Similarly, a successful transition from animal model to application in humans is uncertain (more about this in Chap. 5 in the section on "Translational Inference"). All these natural mechanistic (pathogenetic and pharmacological) uncertainties are reflected in a prominent variability of experimental data, which in turn yields cognitive uncertainty about pathogenetic and pharmacological mechanisms, which in turn leads to what has been called "poor external validity of pre-clinical models of human disease" (Hingorani et al., 2019). Here, "poor external validity" means precisely that the fact that experimental findings in, say, a mouse model cannot be extrapolated into another model or into human biology. For example, Seok and colleagues studied this phenomenon in mice, comparing murine and human genes associated with inflammatory responses. Their main finding was that "among genes changed significantly in humans, the murine orthologs are close to random in matching their human counterparts" (Seok et al., 2013), most obviously a prominent potential source of mechanistic uncertainty. Above and beyond natural uncertainty, however, investigator-related factors may also contribute additional uncertainty. With respect to mouse models, for example, Justice and Dhillon have put it thus:

> *The usefulness of mouse models has been questioned because of irreproducibility and poor recapitulation of human conditions. Newer studies, however, point to bias in reporting results and improper data analysis as key factors that limit reproducibility and validity of preclinical mouse research.* (Justice & Dhillon, 2016)

While inflammation is a pathogenetic process, natural mechanistic uncertainty originating in the biomedical laboratory through the selection of experimental design and investigator-related factors may also render pharmacological results uncertain in similar ways.

Therapeutic E-uncertainty on the cognitive dimension refers to uncertainty about optimal therapeutic interventions that arises from research data generated by, e.g., randomized trials, where data variability reflects the natural uncertainty of therapeutic effectiveness that arises even under optimal, controlled conditions. This natural uncertainty of the therapeutic kind is based on the uncertainty of research studies in groups of individuals who may or may not respond to the intervention under investigation. In our case, the test results and the clinical presentation might give rise to the idea that antibiotics might help with the patient's recovery. Do antibiotics help everyone? They do not (A-uncertainty). And can one be certain that the treatment will help in this case? No, one cannot. This is *therapeutic* E-uncertainty.

Another example would be a randomized trial of patients with hand eczema, patients who received text message treatment adherence reminders had a 70% decrease of a hand eczema severity score after eight weeks compared to a 39% decrease among patients who did not receive such reminders (Erdil et al., 2020). It seems that text messages might be effective as a means to increase treatment adherence. However, these percentages are prone to data variability of statistical nature. In other words, another study of the same sort would likely yield rather different percentages due to the random variation of the large number of characteristics that would be different between study participants in these studies. For each individual participant, however, treatment success is uncertain. Any participant may or may not have an improved eczema severity score after eight weeks; improvement may or may not occur. It is important that on the view I am taking in this book, it is precisely this A-uncertainty of treatment success in each and every study participant that leads to the data variation we see in statistical analyses of trials. It is just not certain that everyone who received the intervention will do better, nor is it certain that everyone who did not receive the treatment will not improve.

Finally, *prognostic* E-uncertainty results on data variability from prognostic studies, which are in turn afflicted with natural prognostic uncertainty. In our example in Table 4.1, the prognostic uncertainty would be the uncertainty whether or not and how the patient will recover (A-uncertainty) and the related E-uncertainty about the prognosis, based on previously collected data. Perhaps the most common and also impactful use of prognostic is the estimation of survival prolongation after therapeutic interventions. And perhaps the most common kind of disease in which this prognostic estimation plays an important role is cancer thera- peutics. For example, it is known that in patients with early breast cancer,[7] the addition of pembrolizumab[8] to standard chemotherapy is associated with a higher percentage (65%) of a complete pathological response com- pared to standard therapy (51%) (Schmid et al., 2020, p. 810). At 36 months after randomization, 85% of pembrolizumab recipients had sur- vived without cancer-related event compared to 77% of the placebo- chemotherapy group (Schmid et al., 2022). The natural prognostic uncertainty here is the same as in etiological uncertainty above: the per- centages are averages from the two intervention groups in the trial. Being in the pembrolizumab group does not mean that an individual patient who received the drug will be among the 85% with event-free survival at 36 months. They could also be among the 15%. It could be that certain factors exist that might help determine whether some patients survive event-free to 36 months and some are not. However, it might also be that chance plays a role in determining *which ones* of the 100% of individuals will be among the 85% and which won't. Thus, based on these data, an oncologist will need to resort to saying that "in a randomized trial, 85% of pembrolizumab recipients survive event-free at 36 months compared to 77% who don't. It is, however, uncertain whether you personally will be among the 85% or the 15%". I hope that most oncologists already talk like this about uncertainty in prognostic conversations with their patients.

In sum, you cannot be certain that the fever and cough are really due to bacterial infection and lung inflammation because more than a handful other lung diseases can come with fever and a cough (*etiologic E-uncertainty*). While you order the diagnostic tests in order to reduce your *diagnostic E-uncertainty*, the testing itself is A-uncertain and can produce false results (both false-positive and false-negative). Moreover, the antibiotics may not work (*therapeutic E-uncertainty*) and/or the patient may not recover for various reasons (*prognostic E-uncertainty*).

Note that E-uncertainty can refer to one person being uncertain. Let's call this *individual* E-uncertainty. It can also refer to many or even all of us being uncertain. Let's call this *communal* E-uncertainty. For example, if I am uncertain what to eat for dinner tonight, it is *me* who does not exactly know what to have for dinner (personal uncertainty of the indi- vidual kind). In this case, nobody else can be certain what I will have for dinner (personal uncertainty of the communal kind). At the same time, the dinner and its specific culinary composition is also uncertain (factual uncertainty). In this example, both the factual uncertainty and the personal uncertainty of the individual kind result from the fact that I have not yet decided what to have for dinner. The personal uncertainty of the communal kind is a direct consequence of the former two uncertainties. But if I am uncertain when the train will arrive at the Newton Highlands station, it is technically *just me* who is uncertain (personal uncertainty of the individual kind). But this does not mean that nobody knows (personal uncertainty of the communal kind). It could be that I am on my way to the station and cannot yet see that the train is in the process of arriving at the station in a minute or two. My fellow commuters, however, can see the train coming and are thus *not* uncertain when the train will arrive.

Let us now take a closer look at what I have mentioned only in passing in this section, "A-Uncertainty in Medicine".

A-Uncertainty in Medicine

The second dimension of uncertainty relates to *A-uncertainty*, the uncertainty of effects and events. Many, if not most, facts and events happening "out there" are naturally uncertain to some degree and thus display a statistical data variability.[9] A-uncertainty comes with a statistical variability of data that leads to E-uncertainty among those who are using these data.

On this view, the presence or absence of appendicitis in a certain patient is A-uncertain independent of me being E-uncertain about it. This may seem counterintuitive since it seems either true or false that the patient's appendix is inflamed. Thus, it is either certain that it is inflamed, or it is certain that it is not. However, inflammation of the appendix is not either present or absent, there is an in-between. Inflammation is not a binary variable, but a gradual phenomenon, a process of tissue invasion by white blood cells and the accompanying production of inflammatory substances that contribute to an intricate network of tissue effects that lead to the inflammation either increasing or receding. Point being, the clear absence of appendix inflammation (no surgical intervention needed) and the clear case of acute surgical appendicitis (needs surgery now) are the extreme ends of a spectrum of inflammation intensity along which surgical appendicitis is neither present nor absent, representing a spectrum of A-uncertainty of it being present or not. While this factual A-uncertainty (located in the patient's appendix) is certainly the source of the E-uncertainty (in the physician's mind), and the latter is a result of the former. Just like the weather tomorrow is A-uncertain whether or not I am

E-uncertain about it or not, the presence or absence of appendicitis can be A-uncertain whether the surgeon feels E-uncertain about it or not. The same is true, so I argue, for the occurrence of events, mainly future events, but also some past events. It is not just the physician who is E-uncertain whether the cancer patient will live for another year or not, it really *is* A-uncertain whether they will or not. This A-uncertainty is the same whether the oncologist is E-uncertain about it or not.

Another example of A-uncertainty refers to the uncertainty associated with unknowable entities. I hold that it really *is* A-uncertain how many erythrocytes (red blood cells) there are in my blood independent of our E-uncertainty because it cannot ever be known exactly how many erythrocytes there are in my circulation. If the number cannot be known, our E-uncertainty is fixed, and we can never be certain. However, this fixed E-uncertainty is the consequence of the practical unknowability of the number of my red blood cells because we have no means of counting their exact number at any particular point in time. Although some might argue that counting them should be possible in principle if we only had the proper method available, I would respond that it is not because erythrocytes are generated and die all the time (their average lifespan is 110–120 days), so their number changes constantly. Thus, the A-uncertainty is fixed and makes the actual number in my blood vessels unknowable.

Natural A-uncertainty indicates that the existence of a fact or the occurrence of an event is uncertain. Again, the term points to a state of affairs *out there*, such as the presence or absence of a disease, or the occurrence of a medically significant event, e.g., the outcome of a surgical intervention. A-uncertainty is the natural phenomenon that some events occur randomly. When someone says "it is uncertain what the outcome of the surgery will be", they also implicitly refer to something else than their own E-uncertainty. The "it is uncertain" in this statement points to an intrinsic natural characteristic of the event in question, its "chanciness". In the case of the surgery, the outcome is A-uncertain, and *therefore* the observer is E-uncertain. In the disease status case, the exact status is A-uncertain and, therefore, we are E-uncertain. This A-uncertainty, the uncertainty of states of affairs and of event occurrence, is precisely the reason why we invented statistics to tame it because we cannot eliminate it as it is a natural property of life, an intrinsic component of how the world works.

* * *

In this chapter I have outlined the idea that, in the context of medical work, several different kinds of uncertainty may occur. I subscribe to the idea that uncertainty is not just a mental state (E-uncertainty, i.e., cognitive, subjective uncertainty about facts and events) but also a phenomenon "out there" (A-uncertainty, i.e., natural, objective uncertainty of facts and events). This is not just semantics: E- and A-uncertainty are metaphysically different kinds of uncertainty although one (E) depends on the other (A) by reference to it, both in general and in particular cases. The cognitive kind (E) is a mental state, while the natural kind (A) is a fact of life that is independent of the mental states of human observers. In medicine E-uncertainty includes uncertainty about etiological, diagnostic, and prognostic facts and events, while A-uncertainty includes uncertainty of causal, mechanistic, diagnostic, therapeutic, and prognostic facts and events.

Of note, one can be E-uncertain without A-uncertainty,[10] for example, in cases that distinguish between present and future versions of the same fact, e.g., the existence of the Louvre in Paris, France. It is not A-uncertain that the Louvre exists today because it does, but someone can still insist to be E-uncertain about it until convinced otherwise by one method or another. It is, however, clearly A-uncertain whether or not the Louvre will still exist on March 5th, 2034; we all have no other choice but being E-uncertain about that future fact until the day has arrived.

We will now move on to Part II of the book, which explicates three crucial concepts that provide the context for epistemic approaches to uncertainty in medicine: inference, explanation, and causation. The next chapter is about the bridge between A- and E-uncertainty. It is provided by data about facts and events that need to be, first, transformed into knowledge (e.g., by performing epistemic transitions using the data-information-evidence-knowledge (DIEK) algorithm) and second, to be translated into clinical action. Above and beyond the E-uncertainty generated by the natural A-uncertainty of facts and events as a source of wobbly data, the mere absence or insufficiency of data as well as inference across systems can blur the situation even further and increase E-uncertainty. This transition from A-uncertainty via wobbly data to E-uncertainty likely plays a prominent role in the anatomy of medical ineffectiveness.

NOTES

1. In this context, Paul Han refers to Einstein's "hidden variables" (Han, 2021, p. 41), a hidden layer in quantum mechanics that leads to spooky action among particles at a distance that cannot be explained. Research since the Einstein-Podolski-Rosen thought experiment was conducted in 1935 seemed to suggest that we have reason to do away with Einstein's spooks, but counterevidence has been offered (Hess & Philipp, 2001).
2. Han points out that others have used this dichotomy as well (Han, 2021, p. 36), citing the work of Walker and colleagues in the field of model-based decision support (Walker et al., 2003).
3. See Cassidy (1992, 2009) for more on Heisenberg's life and work.
4. See chapter 3 in Han (2021) for an overview of categorization schemes.
5. Patricia Cheng has offered a hybrid account (Cheng, 1997). See also Cartwright (1989) for a comprehensive philosophical analysis of the causal power concept.
6. This has led to the proposition of a "replication crisis" (Baker, 2016).
7. To be precise, these are patients with triple-negative breast cancer.
8. For the pharmacologically inclined reader, the National Cancer Institute Drug Dictionary in the United States (www.cancer.gov) defines this drug as "a humanized monoclonal immunoglobulin (g) G4 antibody directed against human cell surface receptor PD-1 (programmed death-1 or programmed cell-death-1) with potential immune checkpoint inhibitory and antineoplastic activities".
9. The exceptions are events that are naturally invariable and thus certain to occur, such that all people die at some point.
10. Thanks to Ben Smart for pointing this out.

REFERENCES

Baker, M. (2016). 1,500 scientists lift the lid on reproducibility. *Nature, 533*(7604), 452–454.

Cartwright, N. (1989). *Nature's capacities and their measurement.* Oxford University Press.

Cassidy, D. C. (1992). *Uncertainty: The life and science of Werner Heisenberg.* W.H. Freeman.

Cassidy, D. C. (2009). *Beyond uncertainty: Heisenberg, quantum physics, and the bomb.* Bellevue Literary Press.

Cheng, P. W. (1997). From covariation to causation: A causal power theory. *Psychological Review, 104*(2), 367–405.

Dammann, O. (2020). *Etiological explanations: Illness causation theory.* CRC Press.

Erdil, D., Koku Aksu, A. E., Falay Gur, T., & Gurel, M. S. (2020). Hand eczema treatment: Change behaviour with text messaging, a randomized trial. *Contact Dermatitis, 82*(3), 153–160.

Fox, C. R., & Ülkümen, G. (2011). Distinguishing two dimensions of uncertainty. In W. Brun, G. Keren, G. Kirkebøen, & H. Montgomery (Eds.), *Perspectives on thinking, judging, and decision making*. Universitetsforlaget.

Han, P. K. J. (2021). *Uncertainty in medicine: A framework for tolerance.* Oxford University Press.

Heisenberg, W. (1927). Über den anschaulichen Inhalt der quantentheoretischen Kinematik und Mechanik. *Zeitschrift für Physik, 43*(3–4), 172–198.

Hess, K., & Philipp, W. (2001). Bell's theorem and the problem of decidability between the views of Einstein and Bohr. *Proceedings of the National Academy of Sciences, 98*(25), 14228–14233.

Hingorani, A. D., Kuan, V., Finan, C., Kruger, F. A., Gaulton, A., Chopade, S., et al. (2019). Improving the odds of drug development success through human genomics: Modelling study. *Scientific Reports, 9*(1), 18911.

Justice, M. J., & Dhillon, P. (2016). Using the mouse to model human disease: Increasing validity and reproducibility. *Disease Models & Mechanisms, 9*(2), 101–103.

Mises, R. v (1981 (1957)). *Probability, statistics, and truth.* Dover.

Mishel, M. H. (1981). The measurement of uncertainty in illness. *Nursing Research, 30*(5), 258–263.

Range, M. M., Arbic, B. K., Johnson, B. C., Moore, T. C., Titov, V., Adcroft, A. J., et al. (2022). The Chicxulub impact produced a powerful global Tsunami. *AGU Advances, 3*(5). https://doi.org/10.1029/2021AV000627

Schmid, P., Cortes, J., Dent, R., Pusztai, L., McArthur, H., Kümmel, S., et al. (2022). Event-free survival with pembrolizumab in early triple-negative breast cancer. *New England Journal of Medicine, 386*(6), 556–567.

Schmid, P., Cortes, J., Pusztai, L., McArthur, H., Kümmel, S., Bergh, J., et al. (2020). Pembrolizumab for early triple-negative breast cancer. *New England Journal of Medicine, 382*(9), 810–821.

Seok, J., Warren, H. S., Cuenca, A. G., Mindrinos, M. N., Baker, H. V., Xu, W., et al. (2013). Genomic responses in mouse models poorly mimic human inflammatory diseases. *Proceedings of the National Academy of Sciences of the United States of America, 110*(9), 3507–3512.

Walker, W. E., Harremoës, P., Rotmans, J., van der Sluijs, J. P., van Asselt, M. B. A., Janssen, P., et al. (2003). Defining uncertainty: A conceptual basis for uncertainty management in model-based decision support. *Integrated Assessment, 4*(1), 5–17.

PART II

Concepts

CHAPTER 5

Inference

INTRODUCTION

In the previous chapter I have outlined the hypothesis that aleatoric (natural) uncertainty gives rise to epistemic (cognitive) uncertainty, A- and E-uncertainty, respectively. With respect to specific target entities—the entity the uncertainty is a characteristic of—the distinction between the two is straightforward: natural uncertainty is uncertainty *of* X, while cognitive uncertainty is uncertainty *about* X. For example, a patient's blood pressure at the time of admission to the emergency room is aleatorically uncertain, and the nurse is epistemically uncertain about it until she has gathered more data in order to reduce said cognitive uncertainty. The direct link between the two kinds of uncertainty is an *inferential* process, inference that links the observed to the observer, which connects the aleatoric subject matter of interest to the epistemic interest of those interested.

Returning to medical skepticism, Broadbent bases his puzzle of medical ineffectiveness on the assumption that the goal of medicine is cure and that since many diseases cannot be cured, medicine does not reach its goal and is thus ineffective. Along the same lines, Stegenga builds his case for medical nihilism on the recognition that much of the evidence medicine

Based on chapter "Epidemiological Inferences", *Oxford Handbook of Philosophy of Medicine*, A. Broadbent (ed.)

O. Dammann, *Uncertainty and Explanation in Medicine and the Health Sciences*, https://doi.org/10.1007/978-3-031-82271-1_5

relies on is faulty due to bad or even improper biomedical research. The argument I want to make in this chapter should not be viewed as a full-out rejection of the medical skeptics' positions but rather as a tweak of their stories of how medical ineffectiveness comes about.

I have already said that I disagree with Broadbent about the goal of medicine, at least partially. While he says the goal is cure, I would like to make a distinction: cure might be the long-term, distal goal of medicine, but the short-term, immediate goal is offering help. I would not disagree with his argument if cure was really what needs to be achieved to render medicine effective. I just think that if we take helpfulness as what needs to be achieved, medicine looks much better. However, medicine might still look ineffective at times, simply because it doesn't always help. I also do not fully disagree with Stegenga, who says that our confidence in medicine ought to be low. While I think that much of medicine can be trusted to help many patients (albeit not so much to cure them), I think that there is some room for a little bit of distrust. Where I do not agree with Stegenga is that bad or faulty research is a major or even the main source of said ineffectiveness.[1]

My addition to the proposal of medical skepticism—I am using this term henceforth to include nihilism for simplicity of communication[2]—is the suggestion that much of what seems to be the underlying miserable (data) situation is not necessarily due to the wrong measuring stick (Broadbent's failure to cure) or the wrong causal attribution (Stegenga's faulty research). I think that it is mainly the ubiquitous A-uncertainty of medicine that contributes to the appearance of medical ineffectiveness by generating a wobbly data situation that does not allow medicine to be the reliable, infallible health problem solver one may want it to be. The associated E-uncertainty reflects a scenario in which medicine may look ineffective where this ineffectiveness is merely a result of uncertainty and, therefore, unpredictability. My argument from uncertainty does not invalidate the verdict that medicine is sometimes ineffective; it just adds to what Stegenga and Broadbent have argued by expanding the spectrum of contributing factors.

Even if cure as the ultimate goal of medicine (qua curative thesis) is, for the purpose of estimating the effectiveness of medicine, replaced with the notion that the immediate goal of medicine, helpfulness (qua auxiliary stance), should be the arbiter of medical effectiveness (in the Broadbentian sense), I have to admit that medicine really is ineffective at times. However, I think that this ineffectiveness is to a large extent not due to bad data that are bad because they arise from bad or fraudulent research, but because the data are inherently wobbly, which, in turn, arises from the ubiquitous A-uncertainty which leads to the corresponding E-uncertainty that makes medicine look and, at least partially, be ineffective. Perhaps, if some medical wobbliness really is due to A-uncertainty it might be impossible for medicine to be much better than critics like Broadbent and Stegenga acknowledge.

The Link Between A- and E-Uncertainty

How are A-uncertainty and E-uncertainty connected? The link is provided by *data*. The data for medicine are generated in two fundamentally different ways: laboratory science focusing on the mechanism of disease occurrence and therapeutic interventions, and epidemiological research which takes care of the rest.

Whether arising from the biosciences or epidemiology, the data are what they are. They have nothing to do with our cognitive state (or at least they should not). Data are wobbly because the facts they are about are A-uncertain, which then gives rise to E-uncertainty about these, which, in medicine, can lead to etiologic (causal, mechanical), diagnostic, therapeutic, or prognostic ineffectiveness. In essence, E-uncertainty arises *by inference* from wobbly data about facts that are in and of themselves A-uncertain. It can be said that in many instances, A-uncertainty *leads* to E-uncertainty by means of wobbly data. For example, as of this writing, the location of the 2046 Winter Olympics has not yet been selected and is thus still A-uncertain. This means that we have no precise (non-wobbly) data about the location of the 2046 Winter Olympics, at least not yet. After a squabble between Sweden, Switzerland, France, and the United States for the preceding games, the French Alps will be the host in 2030, Utah in 2034, and perhaps Switzerland in 2038 and Japan in 2042. Thus, we are E-uncertain (of the communal kind) about the location of the event in '38 and '42. By the time you read this, we will probably know for certain, and the A-uncertainty with its associate E-uncertainty will disappear and be replaced by the certain fact that the winter games of 2038 and '42 will be in (fill in the blanks).

There are, however, instances of A-uncertainty without anyone being E-uncertain about it. In other words, some events can be intrinsically

A-uncertain but no one is E-uncertain about them. For example, the exact timepoint at which a certain (specific) tree in a forest will be so rotten that it breaks and falls is A-uncertain, which is not only independent of whether anyone is E-uncertain about it or not, there is also probably nobody out there who cares enough about the tree to be E-uncertain about it.

If I wait at the Boylston station in downtown Boston and the arrival time of the next D-line train to Riverside is A-uncertain, *no one* knows exactly when the train will be at my station (this is E-uncertainty of the communal kind), not even the conductor, who may have a good or even very good estimate, but she cannot *know* for certain (this is E-uncertainty of the individual sort) simply because the arrival has not occurred yet and cannot be predicted with certainty because at any point between now and the arrival something unforeseen can happen that interferes with the passage from the current position of the train to Boylston station (like, e.g., a power outage or a medical emergency among the passengers). Anything could happen to delay the train between now and then. As in this example, A-uncertainty can encompass E-uncertainty of both the individual and communal type. Indeed, one could argue that *all* (or at least most) future events are A-uncertain by definition, and so is E-uncertainty about them for everyone, i.e., both individually and communally. The same pertains to some past events although past events are certain in that they happened or not, we just cannot be sure about it. For example, we must remain E-uncertain about whether a meteor hit our blue planet at a certain timepoint while dinosaurs still roamed the earth, but the event has or has not happened and is, thus, not A-uncertain.[3] Moreover, we are also E-uncertain about whether the extinction of the dinosaurs was really due to the meteor by means of a subsequent global climate change it created that made dinosaurs' lives miserable and eventually impossible.

There are multiple ways how wobbly data can give rise to E-uncertainty in medicine. First, E-uncertainty can arise from a *lack of data* about the target event. The absence (or lack) of data results in a lack of knowledge. Many diseases of unknown origin are called "idiopathic" simply because we don't have any data about their origin. In essence, we have no idea what explains the occurrence of the disease and, thus, simply have no answer to the "why"-question that asks for an etiological explanation of the origin of the disease. In this case, causal and mechanistic uncertainties lead to E-uncertainty in the causal and mechanistic domains. A second source of E-uncertainty is *incomplete data*. Some things in medicine such as the disease mechanism or the prognosis of the course of disease are not entirely unknown but only partially known. While we know that smoking may lead to pulmonary cancer, we don't know exactly which one(s) of the 6,000 components of cigarette smoke is (are) the carcinogenic culprit. But even if we have perfect data about a target event, these data can indicate that the occurrence of similar events is inherently uncertain. Thus, data about such events, despite being perfect in the sense of being valid and reliable, will indicate just that A-uncertainty and be reflected in a resulting E-uncertainty.

Whatever the data about target events are, they provide the basis of inference processes that are used in order to cope with uncertainty. The first way this is done is the process that uses data to generate knowledge. I call this *transitional inference*, which starts with raw data, turns them into information, which can be used as evidence in support of knowledge claims (Dammann, 2018a). The second way is characterized by inferences drawn from one target system to another: from association to causation, from animal to human, from population to patient, and from simplicity to complexity. I will use the term *translational inference* to describe this way. Before we proceed, we should take a brief excursion into the research method that generates the data that connect A- and E-uncertainty.

In the remainder of this chapter, and indeed in the remainder of this book, my focus will tend to be on epidemiological research and not on the laboratory biosciences. The reason for this is my own perspective as an epidemiologist interested in explanation and causation. In the simplified framework of etiological explanations (Dammann, 2020), epidemiological research looks into the causes of disease while the biosciences zoom in on the patho-mechanism. While mechanisms play a major role in the design of pharmaceutical interventions, the application of epidemiological research results (including the results of randomized clinical trials) plays a far greater role in medicine. Thus, before we go into details of transitional and translational inferences, let me offer a brief introduction to modern epidemiology.

EPIDEMIOLOGIC EXCURSION

Epidemiology is one of the scientific disciplines that feed medicine with new knowledge. Another one is experimental laboratory science, which gathers data about the biological mechanisms of health and disease processes. The basic biosciences such as, for example, microbiology, immunology, neuroscience, or pharmacology, inter alia, provide new knowledge that is needed to understand the patho-mechanisms of disease, which in turn is needed to develop pharmaceutical interventions.

Epidemiology is a methodologically completely different approach. Having developed from a merger of medicine and population statistics, epidemiology has become the branch of the health sciences that collects data in large populations and draws various kinds of inference based on these data, needed for the development of preventive measures in public health, and for diagnosis, prognosis, and explanations in medicine. The term *epidemiology* is used not only for infectious disease research as the name seems to suggest, but for a wide variety of epidemiological subspecialties like cancer epidemiology, neuroepidemiology, perinatal epidemiology, and so on. Bioscientific work, on the other hand, is mainly, if not exclusively experimental, performed in the laboratory, using animals or simpler systems such as cell cultures, with the goal of identifying components of disease mechanisms or mechanisms of drug action. In this book, my focus is on epidemiological knowledge generated for medicine, although some of my discussion also applies to the biosciences.

Epidemiology has developed over the past centuries from medical and population statistics. The story begins in the seventeenth century with John Graunt (1620–1674), whose small booklet entitled *Natural and Political Observations Made Upon the Bills of Mortality* (Graunt, 1665) is considered one of the first clearcut examples of a study on illness occurrence patterns based on population statistics. Renowned epidemiologist Ken Rothman writes that "[w]ith this book Graunt added more to human knowledge than most of us can reasonably aspire to in a full career" and continues with a long list of firsts in Graunt's work, from the first recognition that more boys than girls are born to the first life tables to the first systematic analysis of causes of death (Rothman, 1996).[4]

From these earlier contributions has emerged what may be called *modern epidemiology*—a branch of science concerned with the design, conduct, and analysis of studies in populations (loosely defined) with the aim to provide generalizable and unbiased data about the determinants of health and disease. Modern epidemiology is the collection of methodological tools to achieve this goal. Among the major achievements of a close collaboration between modern epidemiologists and bioscientists are the development of vaccines, screening for birth defects, breast cancer diagnosis and treatment, and pinning down smoking as a major cardiovascular risk factor. Pre-modern epidemiology from Graunt to Claypon was constrained by the limited power of digital computers and some sort of methodological immaturity; modern epidemiology has emerged in the second half of the twentieth century with a unique methodological framework that is characterized by (a) a population approach, (b) a canon of recommendations for the design of bias-free and generalizable studies, (c) a strong co-operation with modern (mainly frequentist) biostatistics, and (d) a set of rules for data interpretation and inference. The result is a branch of the health sciences that has made considerable contributions to the prevention and treatment of illness. One goal (and perhaps even the *main* goal) of epidemiological research is to provide data that will help those working in preventive medicine on illness *prevention*. This is why one of the main tenets of epidemiology is its goal is to find causes of illness: if you know that a certain factor is a cause of a certain health condition, omitting or reducing an individuals' exposure to such factor should prevent the health condition under consideration.

Epidemiological research has evolved in three phases. In its earlier decades, descriptive empiricist views prevailed in epidemiological thinking, while the work has recently become predominantly prescriptive rationalist. In the 1850s, John Snow found that water from a certain set of street pumps in London was a potential cause of the cholera epidemic, and at around the same time, Ignaz Semmelweis observed in a Viennese hospital that handwashing among medical students and doctors might be a cause of reduced maternal mortality. This was epidemiology as discovery by *inference from descriptions of population patterns of illness*.

The second phase started in the early to mid-twentieth century and could be called *risk factor epidemiology*. Business was booming because many new developments in inferential statistics and study design allowed epidemiologists to move away from their traditional focus on infectious diseases and toward chronic disease research. One of the big success stories of the second phase was the research on the role of tobacco smoking in the etiology of lung cancer (Proctor, 2012). Another enormously important and successful project was initiated with the recruitment of the first patient into the Framingham Heart Study in 1948. The project is still ongoing, and data collected from three generations of inhabitants of Framingham, Massachusetts, have helped characterize cardiovascular disease and identify scores of risk factors for it (Mahmood et al., 2014).

The most recent phase of epidemiology gained traction during the later years of the second half of the twentieth century. Epidemiologists worked out methodological approaches that allowed them to design studies that avoid bias, control for confounders, detect effect modifiers, and so on.

This is what I would call *advanced analytic modern epidemiology*, tweaking the title of Ken Rothman's 1986 book ever so slightly (Rothman, 1986). Together with other trailblazing publications at around the same time, including *Epidemiologic Research* by Kleinbaum, Kupper, and Morgenstern in 1982 (Kleinbaum et al., 1982) and Miettinen's *Theoretical Epidemiology* in 1985 (Miettinen, 1985), *Modern Epidemiology* was an eye-opener for those who had always thought of epidemiology as being restricted to infectious disease research or to the description of the frequency of diseases and disorders in populations. Rothman's book helped set the stage for what has now become the focus of advanced analytic epidemiology, *causal inference.*

All modern epidemiological studies are designed to generate data from populations. I will use the term *population* for both natural populations, such as the population of the Faroe Islands (53,664 in January 2022),[5] and also for large groups of volunteers recruited by epidemiologists for the purpose of creating epidemiological *study* populations according to strict study design criteria (Pearce, 2012). Data from large numbers of individuals are generated by epidemiologists along three dimensions, each one dividing the field into two distinct kinds of epidemiology.

Descriptive epidemiology obtains population parameters such as the *prevalence* of a disease as the percentage of individuals in a population with a certain disease at a certain timepoint. *Analytic* epidemiology aims to establish mathematical relationships (associations) between risk factors (exposures) and disease or other health characteristics (outcomes). The terms *exposure* and *outcome* are used in epidemiological lingo as indicators for what statisticians call *independent* and *dependent* variables, respectively. Most analytic epidemiology is about the estimation of a statistical association between exposure and outcome variables. The exposure is the purported "risk changer" whose association with the outcome health characteristic of interest is to be estimated. The outcome variable is the variable that purportedly "depends" on the exposure status in that the outcome status is likely to change with exposure status.

Why "exposure"? This is probably a term chosen with increasing frequency over time due to the subject matter of most classic epidemiological studies such as search for the origins of cholera in London 1854 (Tulchinsky, 2018) and the extensive research by Richard Doll and Bradford Hill on the consequences of tobacco smoking (White, 1990). In both cases, the exposure really *was* an external factor that the person is exposed to, like ingestion of contaminated water from the river Thames and inhalation of cigarette smoke, resp. Note that in more recent epidemiology the term "exposure" is used for any kind of risk changer or health determinant whose relationship with a health characteristic is to be assessed, including sex, gender, race, ethnicity, genotype, etc., which are obviously not exposures in the literal sense. Still, the term "exposure" is used for these characteristics as well.

Why "outcome"? The term is probably a result of the central tenet of epidemiology, which is that epidemiology is the search for determinants or causes of disease. As in philosophy, epidemiologists think in dyads of cause and effect, where the exposure is the candidate cause and the effect is the "outcome" of that exposure.

The second dimension separates observational from interventional epidemiology. *Observational epidemiology* employs the observation of descriptive parameters and associations between exposures and outcomes as they occur in real-world population samples, without the investigators' intervention. The increase of disease incidence in one group of individuals who are exposed to a certain risk factor (E) compared to a group without that exposure (¬E) can be calculated by dividing the risk in one group by the risk in the other, yielding the *risk ratio* RR = R(E)/R(¬E), an estimate of the *relative risk* in the population the study participants are sampled from. The RR is a number between 0 and ∞, where RR=1.0 indicates no risk increase or decrease among the exposed, RR > 1.0 indicating a risk *increase*, and RR < 1.0 indicating a risk *decrease*. Because epidemiological estimates such as prevalence, incidence, and the RR come from epidemiological studies (and only rarely from entire populations) they come from groups of individuals sampled from underlying populations. One overarching kind of epidemiological inference is, therefore, from study sample data to underlying population. *Interventional* epidemiology is research in which the study participants receive an intervention (or not) and are being followed for outcome assessment. The randomized controlled trial (RCT) is the crown jewel of interventional epidemiology. Investigators create large groups by randomization, apply an intervention (typically some sort of pharmacological treatment), and wait for the outcome of interest to occur.

In the context of this chapter, a third important dimension to acknowledge is the one that distinguishes between *clinical and non-clinical* epidemiology. The former is epidemiology in the clinical setting. It can include any type of epidemiological study performed in clinical populations and it also covers the methodological aspects of diagnostic test validation. The RCT is probably the most well-known clinical study type. As the name indicates, non-clinical epidemiology generates data from populations of study volunteers that are not confined to a clinical setting.

In an earlier version of this chapter the emphasis was on epidemiological inferences (Dammann, Forthcoming). In this current version I want to highlight that all the inferences mentioned are of import to those who work in medicine as well. Of note, I do not mean to indicate that the inferences are drawn by nurses and doctors. Indeed, much of the inference-making is done by researchers, both laboratory scientists and epidemiologists, as part of their workflow, in particular at the stage of publication of their results. But again, as much as these inferences are made by researchers, they are of much import in medicine.

What is "inference"? The term "inference" refers to a cognitive process that creates, changes, or confirms a belief based on evidence that serves as premise(s) or assumptions. If that change of belief converges to what is eventually considered to be knowledge, I will refer to it as *transitional* inference (in the next section of this chapter). It specifically refers to inference-making within the process that leads from data to information, to evidence, and knowledge (DIEK)-process). If the inference-making is more about the transfer of data, information, evidence, or knowledge from one context to another, I will call it *translational* inference, the topic of the subsequent section.

Philosophers distinguish varieties of inference such as deduction, induction, and abduction, the latter sometimes also called "inference to the best explanation". A valid deductive inference makes its conclusion a necessary consequence of the premises: if the premises are true, the conclusion must be true. Induction is commonly used as a catch-all term for non-deductive inferences, or sometimes interchangeably with *enumerative* induction, which is generalizing from single or a series of observations. Abduction, or inference to the best explanation, is a non-enumerative inductive inference, selecting the hypothesis that best explains the evidence, based on the data and prior knowledge about the comparative likelihood of explanations. Medical inference is not another kind of inference on a par with these but employs the same fundamental reasoning tools.

Medical researchers will use all the kinds of inference just discussed. Mathematical calculations involve deduction; extrapolations and projections involve enumerative induction; and causal inferences require inference to the best explanation. One additional problem in medicine is not only the sheer complexity of inference that needs to be drawn for decision making, but also the degree to which data are misinterpreted and sometimes even misused to support the interests of federal agencies and the pharmaceutical industry. This can be particularly difficult and outright dangerous when apparent beneficial effects of drugs are "proven" in randomized controlled trials but negative side effects are not discovered or ignored because the trial did not follow enough participants or did not follow them long enough to detect rare side effects. Let me offer as an example the story of rosiglitazone, a drug targeting type-2 diabetes.

Rosiglitazone, sometimes abbreviated "rosi", was approved toward the end of the 1990s by the US Food and Drug Administration (FDA) based on the results from five small studies that showed efficacy but also suggested some negative effects on the patients' lipid status and heart. At least part of the pressure on the FDA to approve rosiglitazone was that another frequently used drug, troglitazone, had known hepatotoxic effect. A physician, Dr. John Buse, dared to speak out openly about his concerns that rosiglitazone might have dangerous cardiac side effects and was promptly threatened by the drug company.[6] Despite continued publication of cardiac side effects over the subsequent years, the drug's market share continued to rise until a meta-analysis published in the *New England Journal of Medicine* (the arguably most prestigious medical journal worldwide next to *The Lancet* in the UK) showed a 43% increase in heart attacks and a 64% increase in cardiac deaths (Nissen & Wolski, 2007). Naturally, sales of the drug went down appreciably. The "rosiglitazone affair" (until 2010, as told by Steven Nissen, first author of the *New England Journal* paper) reads like a cloak-and-dagger story (Nissen, 2010), including attempts by the drug company to intimidate Dr. Buse.

In response to the uncertainty about cardiovascular side effects of the otherwise effective diabetes drug, a large investigation was designed to evaluate the long-term cardiovascular effects observed in association with fluid retention (edema) in individuals treated with rosiglitazone, the "Rosiglitazone Evaluated for Cardiac Outcomes and Regulation of Glycaemia in Diabetes" (RECORD) study (Home et al., 2005). The randomized study was performed in Europe and Australasia and included more than 4000 individuals from more than 300 centers. The hope of the investigators was that the "study should provide robust data on the extent to which rosiglitazone, in combination with metformin or sulphonylurea therapy, affects CV outcomes and progression of diabetes in the long term" (Home et al., 2005). While recruitment for the RECORD study was still underway, the publication of the above-mentioned meta-analysis (Nissen & Wolski, 2007) led the RECORD study investigators to perform an unplanned interim analysis of their data. Patients receiving rosiglitazone were twice as likely to develop heart failure compared to individuals in the comparison group; still, the authors emphasized in their conclusion that "findings from this ongoing study were inconclusive regarding the effect of rosiglitazone on the overall risk of hospitalization or death from cardiovascular causes" (Home et al., 2007). The final planned results were published in *The Lancet* in 2009. Again, the investigators chose to end their data interpretation on the notion that "rosiglitazone does not increase the risk of overall cardiovascular morbidity or mortality compared with standard glucose-lowering drugs"; the study revealed that the risk for hospital admission or death due to heart failure was increased two-fold, the finding being statistically compatible with a range from 1.4-fold to 3.3-fold (Home et al., 2009).

The Center for Drug Evaluation and Research at the US Food and Drug Administration (FDA) decided in October 2007 not to take the drug off the market and, instead, required a boxed warning to indicate the risk for myocardial infarction. Another advisory committee meeting at the FDA in 2010, after the final results from the RECORD study had been published, announced more regulatory action, including the requirement from the drug sponsor of a "risk evaluation and mitigation strategy" (REMS), making sure that "the drug will be available to patients not already taking it only if they are unable to achieve glycemic control using other medications and, in consultation with their health care professional, decide not to take [other similar drugs with a different risk profile] for medical reasons" (Woodcock et al., 2010). The agency also required a comprehensive re-adjudication of the RECORD study data (re-analysis at the patient level) because questions had arisen about the validity of outcome assessments due to the study being open label, so that patients and their doctors were not blind as to the medication they were receiving and may thus have been biased in their outcome reporting due to their knowledge about previously published safety concerns.[7]

While the FDA did not go beyond these requirements to take rosiglitazone off the market, the European Medicines Agency (EMA) did.[8]

At the FDA, the results of the re-adjudication at the patient level were discussed by an expert advisory group on June 5 and 6, 2013. The statistical reviewer from the Office of Biostatistics at the FDA Center for Drug Evaluation and Research presented the data. In their conclusion they stated:

three outstanding limitations of RECORD. First, I showed that the rate of rescue medication and discontinuation from randomized treatment was higher in the rosiglitazone arm, so the interpretation of all analyses may need to consider this issue. Second, even after readjudication, a large percentage of all deaths could not be readjudicated as cardiovascular or non-cardiovascular, 38 percent on the rosiglitazone arm and 34 percent in the control arm. Finally, the trial has some design limitations, which have been discussed extensively throughout this day, such as the open label nature of RECORD, that cannot be resolved by readjudication. [...] the updated estimated hazard ratios of mortality, MACE, MI, and stroke were similar to the original reported hazard ratios, and the number of subjects with missing vital status was so small that they could not reasonably affect the estimated hazard ratio of mortality. (FDA/ CDER Report 20130605, pages 339–340)

The single most disconcerting finding of RECORD, the two-fold increased risk for hospital admission or death due to heart failure, remained unmentioned. Toward the end of the meeting, members of the public had a chance to offer their opinion and concerns. A representative of the American College of Cardiology asked for improved real-time surveillance (FDA/CDER report 20130606, p.134) and stated that "14 years since the FDA approval, [we] are still lacking conclusive evidence related to its safety" (ibid.). A representative of Public Citizen research group pointed out that 12 committee members voted to take rosiglitazone off the market in 2010 (142) and then emphasized the decision of the EMA to take rosiglitazone off the market, pointing out that "the EMA decided to protect Europeans" (152). The representative of the American Diabetes Association remained somewhat neutral, requesting the FDA to "provide guidance for drug review and approvals in the future that incorporate the diverse needs [...] and address the whole spectrum of outcomes of importance to people living with diabetes" (156/157). A member of the public with longstanding diabetes (apparently not a medical expert) stated that rosiglitazone is a most effective drug and advocated for its continued availability and use (163). In contrast, the last representative of the public—a speaker of the National Research Center for Women and Families—could not have been more explicit when they stated that "we believe that the documented safety risks would justify FDA removing this failed drug from the market entirely" (167).

After some more discussion, the committee voted on four choices: (A) removal of the REMS; (B) continuation of the REMS unchanged; (C) modification of the REMS; and (D) withdrawal of rosiglitazone from the market. The final results, after some glitches during the voting process, were 7 in favor of A, 5 B, 13 C, and one D, a result that indicates a will for change, with twice as many committee members voting in the direction of caution as member voting for removing precautionary restrictions on drug prescription. Later in 2013 the FDA removed the prescribing and dispensing restrictions for rosiglitazone but required sponsors to "ensure that health care professionals who are likely to prescribe rosiglitazone medicines are provided training based on the current state of knowledge concerning the cardiovascular risk of rosiglitazone medicines".[9] In 2015, the REMS was eliminated entirely. However, the FDA issued a non-binding guidance document in 2020, based on the deliberations at a meeting of the Endocrinologic and Metabolic Drugs Advisory Committee in the fall of 2018, which outlined the FDA's evaluation criteria of cardiovascular outcome trials, including the requirement for at least 4000 patient years of exposure to the new drug, at least 1500 patients exposed to the new drug for at least one year, and at least 500 exposed for two years, among other criteria.[10] One result of this guidance was a marked decline in industry-sponsored type 2 diabetes studies from about 200 with a start date in 2009 to half that number in 2017 (Kieffer & Robertson, 2020), which the authors interpret as a "negative industry-wide impact on investment in T2DM (type-2 diabetes mellitus; O.D.) drugs" (Kieffer & Robertson, 2020, p. 643).

My point is that it's complicated. So many factors, events, and interests play a role in medical inferences based on the interpretation of scientific results that it is very difficult at times to defend the position that scientific results can be simply translated into medical knowledge. Observational epidemiological studies reveal data about etiological risk factor constellations for specific diseases. If the perspective of an observational epidemiological study is not from risk factor to disease but from disease to longitudinal outcome, these studies can also provide prognostic data. Clinical epidemiological studies, mainly RCTs, provide data about treatment options. Diagnostic studies including screening methods are part of clinical epidemiological work as well. On the other hand, laboratory bioscience delivers pathogenetic and therapeutic data from bench experiments that are conducted on simple systems such as cell cultures or in animal models because such research cannot be done in humans for ethical reasons. Both kinds of health research have developed in parallel over the past centuries as methods for knowledge generation. Both have generated bodies of knowledge (by way of transitional inference) that can subsequently be used in medicine. However, many such inferences based on epidemiologic and bioscientific research data come with one major caveat: these data are not *directly* applicable but have to be transformed into applicable knowledge. Inferences made along the way, however, come with their own difficulties and might lead to erroneous results.

This next section continues with an outline of *epistemic transitions* as inference from data to knowledge. I use the term epistemic transition to refer to the kind of inference that is supposed to help generate knowledge from data. The main point of the section is to show that epidemiological inferences are examples of inductive inference: the inference is based on observed data, and no logical or mathematical necessity is involved.

In the subsequent section I discuss the four potential inferential leaps that strike me as common and that might contribute to the uncertainty of some explanations in medicine: inference from association to causation, from animal to human, from population data to individual patients, and from simplicity to complexity. Of note, I find it debatable whether these are, strictly speaking, kinds of inference at all. It seems to me that these are more like some kind of *interpretations*, we interpret data (information, evidence, and knowledge) from study samples as being applicable to the population the study participants have been recruited from and we use the knowledge we have generated in certain ways, but not others, to justify interventions.[11] (I will come back to the justification of interventions later in the book.) Of course, it is sometimes unclear whether these kinds of interpretation are valid. The frequently made inferences medics and medical researchers make when they go from association to causation, apply animal data to humans, apply population data to individual patients, and when they move from simplicity to complexity without further ado are examples of inference (or interpretation) that are fraught with uncertainty due to the underlying A-uncertainty of the phenomena they are about and can thus lead to E-uncertainty in all domains of medical explanation.

TRANSITIONAL INFERENCE

The first step is the process of drawing *inferences that provide a transition* from data to knowledge. Such transition is needed in all four domains of medicine to generate new knowledge. This, in turn, is needed to provide solid etiologic (causal-mechanical), diagnostic, therapeutic, and prognostic explanations (see next chapter). This important inferential process in epidemiology is the generation of knowledge (both novel knowledge for science and knowledge about the patient) from data by transformation into information and evidence to knowledge (DIEK-process). Based on prior work (Dammann, 2018a; Dammann & Smart, 2019), and a modified version of Ackoff's knowledge pyramid (Ackoff, 1989), I suggest that making epistemic transitions brings researchers from data to information, from information to evidence, and from evidence to knowledge. The process goes roughly as follows.

The natural, objective A-uncertainty of a fact or event in any of the medical domains is obviously important for the medical decision-making process. The medical agent (or agents) gathers raw *data* about the fact or event to learn more about it by, first, turning them into meaningful and shareable *information* by contextualization. The resulting information can be used as *evidence* in the process of testing hypotheses and, if consensus can be reached about its validity, as supportive of medical *knowledge*. Because we start with data and arrive at knowledge, I will use the term *epistemic transition* for the process by which medical researchers generate knowledge from data. I call this process of sequential epistemic transitions the DIEK algorithm. Let me briefly explicate the concept now; I have written about it elsewhere in more detail.[12]

Starting with Ackoff's knowledge hierarchy, which describes a cascade of epistemic transitions from data to information to knowledge to wisdom (Ackoff, 1989), I eliminate wisdom and insert evidence between information and knowledge. In that model,

- raw *data* are simply numbers, which are first generated, then put into context, which transforms them into information;
- *information* can be used as evidence if it supports a proposition by validation in comparison to a standard;
- *evidence* is information used to test (support, confirm, reject) a hypothesis;
- and if the result of such test is successful per consensus agreement among scientists and stakeholders, the proposition that is supported by the evidence at hand becomes *knowledge* (Fig. 5.1).[13]

Part of the DIEK process is making inferences based on the data, information, evidence, and knowledge it generates to allow researchers and medics to generate causal, mechanistic, diagnostic, interventional, and prognostic explanations, and to justify the development of medical

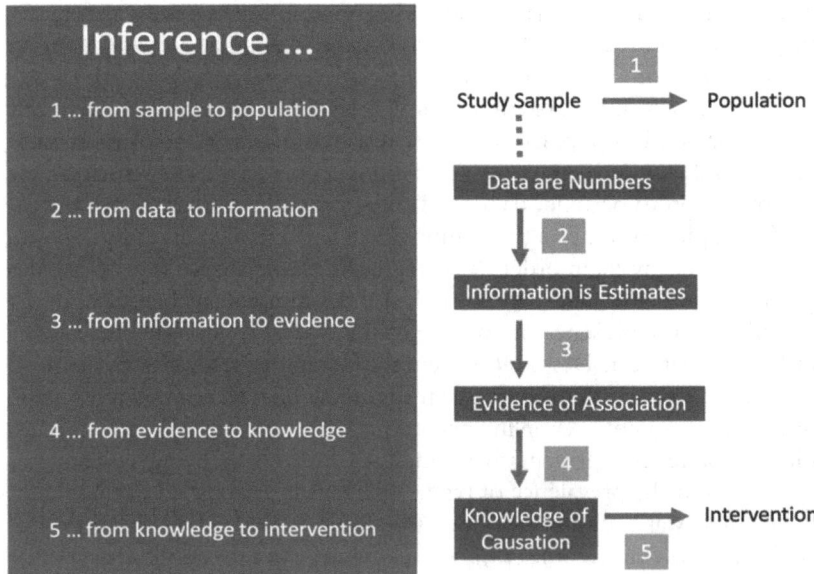

Fig. 5.1 Inferential sequence from health data to health interventions. Each inferential step is discussed in its own section in this chapter

interventions and preventive measures in public health. In what follows I will explicate this inferential process step by step, following the sequence outlined in Fig. 5.1. I will point out what kinds of internal and external constraints the scientific community has agreed upon as markers for inferential validity. It is helpful to keep in mind that all kinds of inferences drawn in the process of generating knowledge from data have the final goal in mind, i.e., to arrive at actionable knowledge for etiologic, diagnostic, therapeutic, and prognostic reasoning and to justify health interventions that come with a reasonable chance of being effective as outlined in the last chapter of this book. Again, much of my discussion emphasizes epidemiological inferences but a similar process is in principle at work when inferring from biomedical data to pathomechanistic knowledge.

Prelude: From Sample to Population

Epidemiologists generate data for the purpose of feeding them into an inferential pipeline that roughly follows the DIEK process. But before that process can begin, one major underlying assumption has to be made, i.e., the assumption that the data collected from a population *sample* reflect what is going on in the underlying population.

Indeed, very little epidemiological research is performed in entirely natural or political populations. Most research requires one or more samples from the underlying target population. For any inference from sample to population to be valid, data need to be properly derived from a proper study sample that reflects the composition of the underlying target population. For example, in order to estimate the prevalence of type 2 diabetes in France in 2008, the only entirely valid estimate can be obtained by establishing the presence or absence of the disease in all individuals living in France that year. Despite this being a Herculean task, it is not entirely impossible to do it. However, given the many financial, time, and human resource constraints, sampling techniques are used to make the process more feasible. A representative sample of individuals living in France is selected, and the prevalence of type 2 diabetes is established in these individuals and was found to be about 4% (Jaffiol, 2009). The number "4%" is raw *data* which becomes *information* when put into context, as in "the prevalence of type 2 diabetes in France in 2008 was 4%". However, the move from 4% in the study sample to 4% in all of France is an inferential leap, whose validity may be impacted by the size and composition of the study sample, by the validity of the diagnosis, which in turn depends on the validity of disease definition and clinical texting method. Let us call this *inference from sample to population* (Fig. 5.1, link #1). What would warrant such inference? While some philosophers of science, e.g., Nancy Cartwright, might say "nothing", others might say that such inference would be warranted if a similar population parameter would be the best explanation for observing the sample estimate.[14]

The inference from sample to population is, of course, closely related to what is sometimes called the "representativeness" of a study. Despite being an awfully clumsy term, it catches the problem well; it refers to how representative the sample is of the population it was drawn from and, accordingly, how close estimates are calculated based on the sample to the underlying population parameter, which remains unknown, at least until one has the time and resources to collect data from every single member of the population, which is, arguably, never the case.[15] The conceptual basics of the problem have been discussed extensively by W. Kruskal and

F. Mosteller in 1979 (Kruskal & Mosteller, 1979a, 1979b, 1979c) and indicators for representativeness are still being developed, e.g., to improve survey research (Schouten et al., 2009). In epidemiology, a related concept is "external validity" or "generalizability", which "refers to the question whether results are generalizable to persons other than the population in the original study" (Dekkers et al., 2009). Dekkers and colleagues lament how frequently external validity evaluation is disregarded in clinical trials, which they attribute to the facts that, first, randomized trials are designed to evaluate efficacy in an ideal situation, not effectiveness in a real-life setting and, second, that the concept is much more complex than its definition suggests (Dekkers et al., 2009). The authors point out that the term "external validity" is considered a misnomer by leading authors in the field (Rothman & Greenland, 1998, p. 134), because "validity" suggests that external validity can be established with exactitude, which it cannot. Philosopher Nancy Cartwright has argued cogently that all RCTs do is show for some intervention that "it-works-somewhere", while the prediction "it will work for us" is what matters most, but cannot be derived from an RCT (Cartwright, 2011). She suggests considering capacity (or power) claims about interventions, i.e., the notion that the results of an RCT might support the claim that "the treatment reliably promotes the outcome, or reliably contributes across a given range of circumstances" (Cartwright, 2011, p. 1401), while issuing the warning that it is far from simple to "to tackle, not ignore, the messy issue of 'theoretical' warrant for capacities in medical and social contexts" (ibid.).

From Data to Information

The first step in the DIEK process is about the second kind of inference which turns numbers into estimates (Fig. 5.1, link #2). Of course, this step only makes sense if the previous inferential step suggests that the data derived from the sample reflect what data drawn from the entire population would have looked like. In other words, it must be highly likely that the inference from sample to population is valid.

Once this is established, epidemiologists use data from the sample to calculate, for instance, averages or percentages that become the average (mean) of x or the percentage of y by inference. This is the process of data being put into context, by which data become information. For example, investigators gathered data from a cohort of 5219 Danish hairdressers who graduated between 1985 and 2007 (Havmose et al., 2022). They found that 45.2% had a lifetime prevalence (occurrence anytime during their lifespan) of hand eczema. In this example, 45.2% is (aggregate) *data*, which become information as soon as we infer that this data point refers to the lifetime prevalence of hand eczema among Danish hairdressers in the given sample. The inference from number to estimate is based on prior knowledge about the data generation process. We, first, know that the data used for the calculation of the percentage comes from more than 5000 Danish hairdressers and, second, that the numbers used in this calculation come from the variable "eczema anytime in life" in the given dataset, which is usually coded 0 for "no" and 1 for "yes". These two pieces of knowledge allow the investigators to infer that the 45.2% is the lifetime prevalence of hand eczema in their sample of Danish hairdressers. (Again, the inference that this percentage applies to all Danish hairdressers is the kind of inference we discussed above in the "prelude" section.)

One could argue that this process is not really *inference*, because the fact that the calculation is based on a certain variable generates a solid, deterministic relationship between the number (45.2) and the estimate (percentage of lifetime hand eczema prevalence). The number was generated by a calculation that used data from this specific variable, so the transition from data to information is not really by inference but rather by definition. I will concur that the information is based on the data alone but would still hold that one infers the *meaning* of the data based on knowledge about the ways the data were generated and that this generates information (data plus meaning). However, this meaning is not chained to the number 45.2% by definition. There could be many other variables in the same dataset that yield 45.2%, but without knowledge about the data generation process and what variables the percentages come from, the pieces of data would be indistinguishable. The inferential process is still a logical process of moving from one body of information (data (number + %) + background knowledge (data are based on variable "lifetime prevalence of hand eczema" in a sample of Danish hairdressers)) to a further conclusion, i.e., the piece of information that the percentage of lifetime hand eczema prevalence in a sample of Danish hairdressers is 45.2%. The background knowledge adds context to the data, and the result is information.

From Information to Evidence

The third kind of inference is the one from estimate to association (Fig. 5.1, #3) which utilizes the information (estimate) generated in the previous inferential step and transforms it into evidence by comparing it to a standard. Take, for example, the classic case-control study by Richard Doll and Bradford Hill in which the authors compared individuals with cancer (cases) to individuals without cancer (controls) with regard to their exposure to cigarette smoke (Doll & Hill, 1950). Among 649 male cases were 647 (99.7%) smokers while that estimate was 95.8% (622/649) among controls. Compared to each other, the two estimates suggest a (statistically significant) association between smoking and lung cancer. Information about the frequency of smoking in the two groups becomes evidence in support of the hypothesis that smoking and cancer are related. More generally speaking, the target notion that an exposure and an outcome are causally related is supported by evidence from epidemiological research that indicates such association, defined as a co-occurrence between exposure and outcome above and beyond what would be expected by chance.

Sometimes, as in the above example, the entire DIEK process is performed with valid causal inference as the main goal. Causal inference is conceptually seated at a macrolevel, while multiple kinds of microlevel sub-inferences first need to be drawn based on epidemiological data to support causal claims. At the core, the goal is to somehow infer causation from association (see next section).[16] The overarching claim that an observed association between members of a certain exposure-outcome dyad is causal is usually based on two very different kinds of qualities an epidemiologic study needs to possess that allow for two very different kinds of inference, both of which contribute to the overarching claim covered by the DIEK process in a two-step fashion. For the lack of better terms, let's distinguish *intrinsic* from *extrinsic* qualities. While intrinsic qualities are characteristics of the study at hand, extrinsic qualities are established by evaluating the study and its results compared to evidence from outside the study.[17] This section covers the first step, from information to evidence, which is supported by intrinsic qualities. The next section will cover the next step, from evidence to knowledge, based on both intrinsic and extrinsic study qualities.

Let us think of intrinsic quality as the quality of characteristics of the study itself. For example, in an observational study (the COSMOS study),

~24,000 Finnish and Swedish individuals were observed for four years regarding their weekly amount of mobile phone usage (exposure) and sleep quality (at study onset and at four years; Tettamanti et al., 2020). The underlying question was whether longer exposure to radiofrequency electromagnetic radiation is causally associated with, say, an increased risk for insomnia. According to the brief outline of relative risk calculation above, the risk of insomnia at four years among those with a high weekly duration (higher than x hours/week) of mobile phone usage (exposed) compared to individuals with a shorter duration of weekly usage (unexposed) can be calculated as the relative risk (RR), defined as the risk among the exposed divided by the risk among the unexposed. Indeed, investigators initially found a 24% increased risk for insomnia among the exposed compared to the unexposed.[18] To use this evidence in support of a valid causal inference, standard epidemiological methodology suggests to first draw on intrinsic evidence as generated by the study itself. However, to deliver such evidence, a study has to be *internally* valid.[19] This means that to be considered causal, the main study result (here: the RR = 1.24) must fulfill three key requirements: it should not be due to bias, confounding, or chance.[20]

A *bias* is any distortion of the RR estimate because of systematic or unsystematic data incongruities. For example, if study participants knew before recruitment that the study goal was to establish the association between duration of mobile phone usage and insomnia, individuals who are heavy mobile phone users *and* suffer from insomnia might be more likely to volunteer, thereby inflating the RR estimate (*selection bias*). However, this was a prospective study in which the occurrence of insomnia was established over four years after the recruitment of participants and, thus, information about insomnia could only be distorted in selection-bias-fashion if individuals with heavy mobile phone usage deliberately inflated their responses to questions about insomnia frequency.[21] This would be called *information bias*, which could be non-random (or differential) if only heavy users would inflate their answers, or random (non-differential) if the degree of inflation was the same in both groups. Selection and information bias are only two kinds of bias in a long list of currently 49 biases, collected in the "Catalog of Bias".[22] Avoidance of bias is the first requirement for internal validity.

Avoiding *confounding* is the second requirement. A confounder is what philosophers call a *common cause*. If variables A and B are statistically associated, this might not be due to a causal link between the two but due to both of them being caused by a third variable, C. For quite some time now confounding is counted among the biases; old school epidemiologists like myself, however, prefer to keep confounding separate from bias, because "bias creates an association that is not true, [while] confounding describes an association that is true, but potentially misleading".[23] Confounding can be addressed in the study design, but also in the analysis phase of the study. Other kinds of bias, such as selection and information bias, can often only be prevented by clever study design, but cannot be "controlled for", like confounding, while crunching the numbers. For an association between A and B to be considered causal, any C must be controlled for either in study design or analysis. In the COSMOS insomnia study, adjusted multivariable regression models yielded a reduction of the initial estimate of the relative risk of 1.24 (or a 24% risk increase) down to 1.09 (9% increase).[24]

The third requirement for internal validity is that the study result is *not due to chance*. To exclude that possibility, epidemiologists have developed a longstanding collaboration with biostatisticians, to the degree that part of epidemiology has morphed into a special form of biostatistics. Indeed, most modern epidemiologists have not only a good grasp on statistical methods but are experts in those statistical methods they frequently use. Such epidemio-statistical methods are applied to epidemiological study data to minimize the likelihood that the study result is due to chance. In our example from the COSMOS study, the main result was an increased risk for insomnia among the exposed (who spent more than 258 min/week on their mobile phone) compared to the unexposed (who spent less time). The estimate of the relative risk was 1.24, indicating a 24% risk increase. Could this result be due to chance? Yes, it could. Any such result could be due to chance, but statistics can be used to get a handle on that uncertainty. The calculation of a confidence interval (CI) around the point estimate (here 1.24) is standard operating procedure in risk factor analysis. This calculation gives a range of values for the RR estimate that covers the true RR in the underlying population with a certain likelihood, most frequently 95%. The 95% CI for the initial point estimate was 1.03–1.51. If there is no risk increase or decrease whatsoever, the RR would be 1.0. Thus, if the estimate *excludes* 1.0, the likelihood that the true RR is 1.0 is <5%. This threshold of 5% is the same as the threshold for a p-value to indicate statistical significance (at $p < 0.05$). If the 95% CI *includes* the 1.0 value, the result is not considered statistically significant. Indeed, the 95% CI for the adjusted RR estimate of 1.09 in the COSMOS insomnia study was 0.89–1.33, which includes 1.0, thereby indicating that the 9% risk increase did not achieve formal statistical significance and that, therefore, it cannot be said that the likelihood to observe the given risk increase of 9% (or a larger one) is less than 5%.[25] Of note, the threshold of $p < 0.05$ for deciding whether an estimate is due to chance is purely conventional, but widely adhered to in the health sciences.

Only if all three requirements for internal validity can be checked off (no bias, no confounding, no chance association) do epidemiologists even begin to use evidence as the starting point for knowledge generation.

From Evidence to Knowledge

The next inferential step is from evidence to knowledge (Fig. 5.1, link #4). Evidence is mounted in support of a hypothesis or claim. In Fig. 5.1, this is a causal hypothesis or claim, but it can also be non-causal knowledge that is inferred from the available evidence. Frequently, more than one piece of evidence is needed to support a claim. Moreover, it is often more than one kind of evidence that is required to arrive at what will be accepted as a piece of knowledge. These various pieces of evidence are put together according to rules of coherence, where a network of evidential details is woven together in a mutually supporting way. Such network is considered strongest if it includes a variety of different kinds of evidence that are error independent, i.e., where the failure of one of them does not automatically lead to the failure of others. Another item that makes an evidential network stronger is the absence, or at least paucity, of countervailing evidence. The smaller the number of pieces of evidence that contradicts the supportive evidence the better. Finally, repeated and continued confirmation of a knowledge claim, together with the absence of evidence that said knowledge claim is not solid or valid, will lead to its general acceptance.[26]

In my previous work on the data—information—evidence—knowledge transition I proposed that "knowledge consists of beliefs that 1. turn out to be predictive: predictions that are based on such beliefs turn out to be correct; 2. generate hypotheses that can be tested, and 3. that lead to interventions that are successful, 4. for a long time" (Dammann, 2018a). Thus defined, knowledge is the closest we can get in curbing E-uncertainty in medicine. Of note, we cannot curb A-uncertainty because any event has its natural A-uncertainty. But whenever we make a knowledge statement in medicine that is generally accepted as "common knowledge", we feel entitled to accept such claim as true, including the residual E-uncertainty.

For example, the statement "all bone fractures can be identified on x-ray" would not be accepted as knowledge because not all fractures can be seen on X-ray. However, the statement "bone fractures can frequently be identified on x-ray" comes closer to "common medical knowledge" but comes with the qualifier "frequently" that indicates residual A-uncertainty in terms of not all bone fractures being identifiable by X-ray, which leads to the respective E-uncertainty reflected in the belief that not all fractures can be identified on X-ray.

Obviously, the transition from evidence to knowledge is far from simple; in fact, according to the above criteria, much more is involved than just using a piece of evidence and call the claim it supports "knowledge". A comprehensive review of medical epistemology would require tackling the topic in the appropriate depth and width. With regard to medical practice, however, I think it is fair to assume that medics consider "medical knowledge" to be equivalent to "whatever the textbook says".

Postlude: From Knowledge to Intervention

After the DIEK process is finished, the knowledge gained is to be used to justify interventions (Fig. 5.1, link #5; see also Chap. 10). How do we justify health interventions? Of course, this question can be answered from multiple perspectives, for instance, by zooming in on values in health priority setting (Clark & Weale, 2012), implementability of the intervention (Klaic et al., 2022), or its acceptability (Sekhon et al., 2017). I want to focus on the kind of evidence-based knowledge that allows for the inference that the introduction of a new health intervention is justified.

Health interventions need to be supported by knowledge that builds on solid evidence as established by the last inferential step in the DIEK sequence (discussed above). While some of this knowledge is generated in epidemiology, some is provided by other branches of the health sciences. In Chap. 10 I propose a semi-formal methodological framework (multi-level evidence mapping) that helps organize and judge the available knowledge. In essence, the approach brings together the concepts of etiological explanation and explanatory-predictive coherence by offering a proposed outline for an integrated evidence map, in which knowledge about association, biology, confirmation, and difference can be documented. Perhaps high-quality evidence that is mutually supportive and non-contradictory might be a good starting point for judging the *degree* of explanatory-predictive coherence.

I have now outlined a proposed framework that conceptualizes epide-miological work as a series of goal-oriented inferences: from sample to population, from data to information, to evidence, to knowledge, to justi-fied interventions. My analysis suggests that causal inference is not the only kind of inference that epidemiologists draw. Indeed, multiple kinds of inference play important roles at multiple levels in the epidemiological workflow. Consideration of this framework (including modifications and revisions) might help identify weak spots in epidemiological reasoning.

TRANSLATIONAL INFERENCE

A second kind of E-uncertainty is due to inferential leaps that may occur while translating *from one system to another*. These are potentially faulty inferences (i) from association to causation, (ii) from animal studies to humans, (iii) from population to individual, (iv) from model simplicity to real-world complexity.

From Association to Causation

All causation as we have defined it is correlation, but the converse is not neces-sarily true, i.e. where we find correlation we cannot always predict causation.
Pearson (1900, p. 407)

Inference from correlation (or better: from association) to causation is one of the oldest inferential problems of observational research. The phil-osophical literature on causal inference in medicine and epidemiology is already large and keeps growing quickly. I will not offer a detailed analysis but only the most important facets of the debate.

The above footnote in Pearson's Grammar of Science is probably one of the most frequently rehearsed axioms in science. It is interesting that anyone would even consider the "converse" because association and cau-sation are, by definition, two very different things conceptually. While cau-sation implies a connection between two phenomena that is defined by a dependence of one on the other, a correlation (or better: association)[27] takes such dependence requirement out of the equation *by definition* such that the two phenomena are correlated such that a change in one is accom-panied by a change in the other. It is quite obvious that such correlation does not necessarily imply causation but may be generated by a common cause of both phenomena; a beloved example in perinatal epidemiology is the decline of birth rates in areas where the stork populations decline. Still, the disconnect between causation and association seems to be worthy of continuous reiteration because *somehow* humans tend to infer from one to the other. While it can certainly be argued that association is the single strongest characteristic of what we consider causation, but it is not a sufficient criterion.[28] As I will outline later in this chapter, other kinds of evidence are helpful, if not outright necessary to establish causal relationships, because they allow for causal inference based on a system of coherent, error-independent evidence.

Causal inference is inference from association to causation. Many epidemiologists see their work mainly as a response to the needs of medicine and public health and define as their main goal the identification of causal risk factors for adverse health outcomes. These risk factors are considered valuable targets for the main purpose of public health: the preservation and improvement of the health of populations by means of disease prevention and health promotion. This direct connection between epidemiology and public health has led to the notion that epidemiology is "the basic science of public health".

From the perspective of epidemiologists who want to draw causal inferences about disease occurrence, multiple problems arise. To agree what they are talking about when they talk about causation, it would be helpful to have a unified definition of causation. None exists as of today. Mervyn Susser wrote that "a cause is what makes a difference" (Susser, 1991). Rothman and colleagues think that a cause of a disease is that without which a disease would not have occurred or would have occurred at a later timepoint (Rothman et al., 2008). Leading scholar of causality in epidemiology Miguel Hernán defines causation in terms of the difference between the result observed after an intervention and the result in the absence of the intervention (Hernán, 2004). All these definitions have in common that they state what causation *does*, not what it *is*.

The two main approaches used in epidemiology for causal inference based on intrinsic and extrinsic study characteristics can be philosophically characterized as difference-making-interventionist (DMI; Vandenbroucke et al., 2016) and explanatory-coherentist (ECO; Dammann, 2018b), respectively.

The difference-making-interventionist (DMI) approach is based entirely on the *right way* to generate knowledge from data as defined by the epidemiological community. Roughly, this right way is based on counterfactual reasoning (Höfler, 2005) and the epistemological virtues of randomization, as spearheaded by C.S. Peirce and R.A. Fisher (Hall, 2007). The observed contrast in outcome between epidemiological study groups defined by exposure status, i.e., the point estimate of the association between exposure and outcome, is based on the counterfactual assumption that if the exposed had not been exposed they would have yielded the same outcome percentage/rate as the non-exposed. The true counterfactual among the exposed cannot be observed because individuals cannot be both exposed and not exposed. Thus, the non-exposed are used as the next best comparator. It is obvious that the interpretation of the counterfactual contrast between the study groups can be interpreted as causal only if no other factor (confounder) causes the outcome while the exposure is just an innocent bystander. Epidemiological methodology offers tools to reduce confounding by rendering study groups as similar to each other as possible, so that the exposure is the sole difference between them, *ceteris paribus* (Hernán & Robins, 2006, 2016; Rubin, 1974; VanderWeele, 2015). This is where randomization comes into the game, because it is considered the best possible way to achieve this goal. Indeed, in medicine, randomization is often considered the *gold standard*, because "although no study is likely on its own to prove causality, randomization reduces bias and provides a rigorous tool to examine cause-effect relationships between an intervention and outcome" (Hariton & Locascio, 2018). Indeed, many interpret the results of RCTs as direct evidence for a causal relationship between the intervention (e.g., drug versus placebo) and the outcome. On this view, at least in the eyes of most clinicians, one may view the results of an RCT as causal.[29] The question whether causation can *ever* be proven (i.e., established beyond doubt) is a discussion to have another day. Moreover, the notion that results from randomized studies guarantee causation has been met with resistance in the philosophical literature (Cartwright, 2010; Rocca & Anjum, 2020; Worrall, 2007). Still, randomization is considered the litmus test for causal inference in the DMI world: "Causal inference from large observational databases (big data) can be viewed as an attempt to emulate a randomized experiment—the target experiment or target trial—that would answer the question of interest" (Hernán & Robins, 2016). Simply put, target-trial emulation consists in collecting and arranging the data in ways that emulate the design of a randomized study so that it yields results that can be interpreted as estimates of a causal effect.[30]

The ECO approach posits that it is impossible to extract solid causal information from an individual epidemiological study simply because causation is not in the data just as sandcastles are not in the sand—they must be built. As Nancy Cartwright put it: "no causes in, no causes out" (Cartwright, 1989). My interpretation of this notion is that we cannot get causal information out of a data model if we don't already have causal information about the data covered by that model. If we do not have the background knowledge that smoking causes lung cancer, we cannot say that an association between smoking and lung cancer in an observational (non-randomized) epidemiological study reflects that causal relationship. If one is looking at the results of a single epidemiological study, the ECO approach consists in putting the study results into perspective by way of comparison to extrinsic criteria. In other words, it requires the presence of evidence from outside sources that supports the causal hypothesis, not from the study itself.

The classic procedure for this is the one proposed by Sir Austin Bradford Hill (Hill, 1965), who suggested a list of nine questions the answers to which can jointly support a causal hypothesis if answered in the affirmative.[31] Is the association between exposure and outcome strong? Is the relationship biologically plausible? Is there corroborating evidence from relationships between similar exposures and outcomes? And so on. The Hill "viewpoints" (as Hill called them) have been used widely in the epidemiological and philosophical literature. Space constraints prevent a full discussion of this literature here. Suffice it to say that despite originating from the debate about smoking and lung cancer in the 1950s and 1960s, Hill's viewpoints are still being used in medical research, and one can land papers about such research in respectable biomedical journals (Awadh et al., 2017; Frank et al., 2016). The point of the ECO approach is to refrain from causal inference solely based on observational data organized in the currently most widely used way as sanctioned by the DMI, which in turn relies heavily, if not entirely, on the assumption that results from randomized experiments must be causal. Instead, it is suggested to put results of observational studies in perspective by building a coherent story with support from multiple angles using different kinds of evidence (Dammann, 2018b).

Whichever method for causal inference is used, the most frequent goal in medicine is to develop interventions that work. Such interventions are best based on solid knowledge, which comes from randomized clinical trials, or from observational data analyzed like a target trial, or from a coherent body of multiple kinds of evidence, each one suggesting cogently why the planned should work. This is inference from association to causation based on the transition from evidence to knowledge.

The next section is about a second sort of translational inference, which is more pertinent to the context of basic laboratory science into the patho-genetic mechanisms of disease and, thus, pharmacological intervention than to epidemiologic research: the inference from animal experiment to application in humans.

Inference from Animal Experiment to Human Application

Inferring the mechanism of a certain disease from evidence generated in animal experiments can create uncertainty about the understanding of the patho-mechanism in humans if the physiology of animals and humans do not align. In general, inferring from animals to the human system can be valid to a certain extent, but the correspondence is often not 100%. This inferential leap adds uncertainty to the E-uncertainty based on A-uncertain animal data.

The idea of the scientific laboratory experiment goes back hundreds of years. In essence, laboratory research rests on the idea that one can test a hypothesis by trying it out. The idea is that if we believe that doing X will result in Y in a certain defined context Q, the best way to find out if that is true is by *doing it*. For example, if the question is whether throwing a rock (X) at a window will shatter it (Y) in the pleasant sunny climate of North Carolina (Q), the first thing would be to go to North Carolina, find a window and a suitable stone, and go for it. In some such instances the glass will shatter (thin glass, big rock), but in other instances it won't. The irregularity of such results will awaken the interest of every scientist and lead to the next experimental level at which the experimental conditions are modified. This can be done in different ways. For example, to find out whether changing the size of the rock or the thickness of the glass will lead to more or less success one would do just that: different stone, different glass, and so forth. But the original question (does X lead to Y in Q?) can be modified in many other ways. For example, does X *always* lead to Y in Q? What other things than Y does X lead to in Q? Does X lead to Y in contexts other than Q? And so on. All these modified questions can be answered by conducting experiments in various ways, and, importantly, repeatedly so that investigators can observe whether any result of an exper-iment is a one-off or whether it reflects a regularity to the degree that the experimental evidence can be generalized. The only alternative is to base knowledge on previous experience (indeed, a surprisingly common way of justifying medical decisions), on anecdotal evidence, or on "evidence" of thin air. As physicist and philosopher of science Mano Singham observed, people like and sometimes even prefer pseudo-scientific evidence; however, knowledge based on scientific experiments is more reliable because it is generated by consensus generated by experts based on an agreed-upon methods and vetted in a complex process of discussion, peer review, and publication (Singham, 2020, p. 3). My main point here is that the experimental approach is thought of as the chief method in science because it is the only genuine scientific method to test hypotheses. It is thought of as yielding more reliable data than simple observational evidence and as yielding more solid results than anecdotal evidence because of the social process of "making knowledge" by community assessment.

For these reasons, the biomedical research community relies heavily, if not exclusively, on experimental bench research. From the perspective of medical domains in which explanations are sought, biomedical laboratory research is mainly in charge of elucidating pathogenetic and therapeutic evidence. It is obvious why biomedical researchers use the laboratory approach to pathogenetic and therapeutic evidence: both are mechanistic realms, areas of biology where the action is inside the body of the patient. And while scientists need *some* way to try out their ideas, using the human body is prohibited by ethical standards. As an *Ersatz* for the human body investigators therefore use experimental systems that are easily manipulated and ethically feasible.

Of course, this situation creates all kinds of problems, ethical, practical, but also theoretical. To generate knowledge about detailed (e.g., molecular, genetic) mechanisms, biologists resort to individual cells and cell cultures (simple systems) or to small animal models from the roundworm *C. elegans* to zebrafish to small rodents like mice and rats. Sometimes, researchers use even larger animals, up to the primate level for their studies. For obvious reasons, not all agree that this is ethically a problem-free zone. The practical problems are also not negligible. First, running an animal research laboratory is no simple job. From simple animal care to complicated experimental setup, from the food and drink restrictions inside the laboratory space to extensive biohazard regulations, a biomedical laboratory is an extremely complicated environment. Of most interest in our context, however, is the theoretical problem of inferring from animal to human biology. Although it seems plausible that mouse lungs, guts, and perhaps even brains work by the same underlying principles as their human counterparts, Pandora Pound and their colleagues from the Reviewing Animal Trials Systematically (RATS) Group asked a bit provocatively, "Where is the evidence that animal research benefits humans?" (Pound et al., 2004). They reject justifications of animal research and ask for more transparent and systematic evaluation of animal research that is supposed to have import for humans. In a literature search on systematic reviews on animal studies and their contribution to clinical medicine, they identified six reviews on calcium channel blockers for stroke, low-level laser therapy for wound healing, fluid resuscitation for bleeding, thrombolysis for stroke, stress and coronary heart disease, and endothelin receptor blockade in heart failure (Pound et al., 2004). One important finding was that clinical trials in some of these areas were initiated despite evidence from animal experiments that the intervention could be harmful, obviously suggesting that clinical researchers considered the animal work irrelevant. Moreover, they identified multiple methodological problems at the level of experimental designs. Their conclusion is important for the uncertainty theme of this book:

> Even if animal experiments provide valid results and sufficiently precise estimates of treatment effects to discount the effects of chance, the extent to which the results can reasonably be generalised to humans remains open to question. Perhaps it was because of this uncertainty that the data from animal studies were disregarded in the above cases. (Pound et al., 2004, p. 516)

The above-referenced paper was published in 2004. More recently, and with emphasis on mental illness, an area of research that adds yet another level of inferential complexity to the story, psychology professor Espen Sjøberg concludes that

> Animal models can be very useful for investigating the mechanisms behind a human condition. This new knowledge can help improve our understanding and treatment of this condition, but the researcher must not assume that the observed animal behaviour also applies to humans. Ultimately, animal models only provide solid evidence for the animal used, and indicative evidence of human behaviour. (Sjoberg, 2017, p. 10)

Sjøberg also offers some suggestions how to avoid logical fallacies in animal experiments, including, but not limited to, being aware of one's own limitations (arguably very difficult for the eager competitive bioscientist), develop an a priori hypothesis and analysis plan (this should go without saying in a serious research lab), double blind the experiment (meaning that the investigator should be blind to the original hypothesis and the identity of the experimental groups), avoid anthropomorphizing (and making assumptions about the inner workings of animals), and avoid the file drawer effect by trying to publish negative results despite the pushback to be expected from some journal editors.

Taken together, caution is indicated when inferring from experimental animal to human, and this caution should probably be even more pronounced when inferring from simple systems (like cell studies) to humans. Finally, even in these simple systems, biological mechanisms sometimes appear to differ between the animal species from which cells are harvested. For example, Lam and colleagues have documented appreciable differences between cells harvested from mice and rats in their inflammatory response to pro-inflammatory stimuli (Lam et al., 2017). The details of these differences are not important here. What is important is the caveat hanging over inferences from experimental animal to humans when it comes to studies of specific biological mechanisms that are studied to improve our understanding of pathogenesis or pharmacological issues relevant to human health and disease.

From Population Data to Individual Application

Another problematic inference is from epidemiological data to individual cases in medicine. Epidemiology is the main provider of data for medical usage. These data come from large studies with many participants and thus reflect average measures (actually, estimates) of the association between a certain risk factor and a certain disease. If individuals exposed to risk factor X are (on average) twice as likely to develop disease Y compared to individuals not so exposed, in an epidemiological study this would result in a relative risk (RR) of 2, indicating a two-fold risk, e.g., 20%, among those with the risk factor compared to those without, e.g., 10%. Such information about risk and relative risk is often used in medicine when consulting patients. Obviously, however, the above percentages are based on *many* individuals and cannot be applied to a single person. The inference from population to person is less than straightforward. We can go from observed frequencies such as percents (ranging from 0 to 100%) to likelihoods (ranging from 0 to 1) when referring to populations, but how can we go from likelihoods in populations to likelihoods in individuals?

The immediate goal of medicine from the perspective of the auxiliary stance is to help, and this help is offered mainly to individual patients. Thus, the "target entity" of medicine is the person who comes with a complaint, needs to be properly diagnosed, deserves an explanation how their status of ill health came about, wants a treatment plan to be developed, and receives information about their prognosis given this treatment versus alternative treatment strategies. The medic (including nurses, doctors, physician assistants, and so on) needs data that allow them to provide such initial help with the intermediate goal of improving the patient's condition, so they feel and function better. Medics perform these tasks by using data to outline etiological explanations (C), explore the disease mechanism (M), make diagnoses (D), decide on treatment strategies (T), and provide prognostic information (P). These "CMDTP" data come with a certain amount of variability, from biomedical research that may be fraught with artificial uncertainty due to bad/fraudulent research, and also with natural uncertainty due to the chanciness of facts and events.

As previously mentioned, the main research technique to provide CMDTP data is modern epidemiology. Epidemiologic research works with the concept of a "study" which refers to the proper design, implementation, and analysis of health information from large groups of individuals. The underlying idea is that using information from many individuals has advantages over the collection of data from individual or only a few. For example, the observation that Kristi, a hairdresser in Trondheim, has developed skin eczema over the years offers weaker evidence in the support of the inference that it is something about Kristi's job as a hairdresser that may have led to her skin eczema than evidence gathered from multiple epidemiological studies that the incidence of hand eczema in hairdressers (about 21%) is four times that found in office workers (5%) (Jamil et al., 2022). Why is that? Note that the inference we want to make was that is a proposition that mixes a single-person perspective (Kristi's job, her eczema) with a more generalized notion about the risks of working as a hairdresser and skin eczema in general. The simple observation that Kristi is a hairdresser *and* suffers from hand eczema is not enough to generalize an association or even causal relationship between being a hairdresser and contracting hand eczema *in general*. Why not? Simply because it might be a co-occurrence by chance. If *many* hairdressers have hand eczema, the inference would be stronger. As mentioned above, it turns out that roughly one-fifth of hairdressers have hand eczema. This would not yet support the hypothesis that hairdressers are at increased risk for hand eczema, because it could turn out that one-fifth of the entire population, say, every person in the world regions covered by the meta-analysis quoted above, turns out to have hand eczema. Indeed, it might be that the prevalence of hand eczema in the entire population is *higher* than 21%, which would indicate that the risk for hand eczema in hairdressers is *lower* than in the general population, which would be evidence against the hypothesis that being a hairdresser plays a role in the etiology of Kristi's hand eczema. This is why a proper comparison group is always important. In our example, such a comparison group would be the office workers with their 5% prevalence of hand eczema. The comparison of 21% versus 5% is what supports the *general notion* that being a hairdresser (compared to being an office worker) is associated with an increased risk of developing hand eczema. The simplest epidemiological measure for the strength of the association would be a relative risk (RR) of 4.2, calculated as 21% divided by 5%.

However, the inferential leap becomes apparent when we consider that the original proposition was that "it is something about *Kristi's job* as a hairdresser that may have led to *her skin eczema*", the emphasis being on Kristi's job and Kristi's hand eczema. All potential technical difficulties of how the research studies and meta-analysis were conducted and analyzed aside, what exactly is that it allows for the application of the epidemiological population data expressed in percents and a calculated RR to Kristi, who is obviously a single person. Percents are averages of variables that are coded as 0 or 1, here: hand eczema being present is coded as 1, its absence is coded as 0. Thus, if 21 out of 100 individuals have hand eczema, they are coded 1, the other 79 as zero. The average is 21 * 1 + 79 * 0 / 100 = 21, expressed as 21 per hundred = 21%. Kristi, however, is an individual with hand eczema and there are no 99 other Kristis with or without hand eczema so one can calculate an average and apply the concept of percents to the population of 100 Kristis. But worse, Kristi is only one Kristi, so percents cannot be applied to her *at all*. This is an inferential incongruity of vast importance in medicine. None of the information from population studies can be applied to individual patients without putting the inference into proper perspective, by telling Kristi that her being a hairdresser *might* have contributed to her hand eczema because hand eczema is about four times more common in hairdressers like her than in office workers. To be completely honest, the medic would need to tell Kristi that there is *no way* of knowing for certain that something about her being a hairdresser did actually cause her hand eczema. The acknowledgment of this uncertainty vis-à-vis a patient who is probably not happy with such response is part of what authentic medicine should do, and not avoid such pain points of conversation by employing defensive strategies such as omitting these kinds of caveat or hiding behind medical jargon.

What is it then that makes the epidemiological RR concept so popular in medicine, where it is used a lot for etiological inference, and in the law, where it is used to determine whether it is "more likely than not" that the murder was committed by the gardener?

The basic problem here is the concept of risk, which introduces a second inferential incongruity. The term risk is used in multiple ways, and its meaning in individuals and populations is slightly different. The inferential incongruity is that information about the population risk (of hand eczema) cannot be used to estimate individual risk (of hand eczema). A strong version of this incongruity says that population risk and individual risk are entirely different things and thus incompatible. *Population risk*, interpreted as risk in populations, is the likelihood of occurrence of a certain disease in populations. This likelihood is, again, a prospective, hence unmeasurable entity. However, it can be estimated in epidemiological studies by observing the population in question over time and establishing the incidence of the disease. This can be done by counting the number of newly occurring cases of the disease and dividing it by the sum of all time units each person contributes to the study. This incidence rate (IR) is the best estimate of the risk of the disease in a population; a simpler, but less appreciated one is the prevalence of disease in the population, i.e., the number of individuals with the disease divided but the number of members of the population at a certain timepoint or over a time interval. The estimate calculation, however, can only be done at the end of the study, when the numbers are in. Thus, the risk estimate is a retrospective entity, not a prospective one as is population risk. Of course, once we have a solid risk estimate (I will leave aside at this point how solidity would be defined) we will use it prospectively. We would infer from a population risk estimate of 21% hand eczema in hairdressers in Norway that we can expect the same percentage of hand eczema to occur in an independent population of hairdressers in, say, Sweden. In other words, we would translate the 21% (retrospective) prevalence in Norway into an expected prevalence of 21% in Sweden, which we then translate into a risk of 0.21 likelihood (prospective). Notice that this inference from retrospective estimate, e.g., counted and calculated percents, to prospective likelihood, i.e., population risk, might be yet another inferential incongruity. Still, many years of frequentist statistics based on estimates etc. suggest that this inference cannot be too misleading.

Statistics is indeed a most frequently used method in epidemiology, and it is the epidemiologists' not-so-secret weapon against invalid inference from chance occurrences that contribute to the natural event uncertainty of such estimates in populations. This uncertainty is due to the fact that we live in a proba-deterministic (aka, deter-probabilistic) world where the percentage of hand eczema will vary among populations. It might be that its prevalence in Sweden is higher or lower than in Norway. To be honest, the estimate of 21.4% comes from three studies and reflects a pooled incidence rate, not a percentage. (I have, incorrectly, transferred the IR into a percentage to make the text easier to follow.) The pooled IRs come with a 95% confidence interval (CI) ranging from 15.3 to 27.4. This range covers the "true" IR in the underlying population with a likelihood of 95%. The variability of these data results from the natural uncertainty of the occurrence of hand eczema in various populations. Statistical approaches such as the calculation of pooled estimates and confidence intervals have been invented to get a handle on this uncertainty.[32]

Let us now move from population risk to individual or *personal risk*. A good start is to mention that with a few exceptions, medicine has a uniquely individualistic concept of health. In other words, I think that more often than not, medical thinking revolves around the health of individuals rather than the health of populations. Arguably, we think about *ourselves* as individuals, not as members of a certain community when it comes to health issues including health risks.

The perception of *personal risk* is something like a justified expectation that one may become sick from a disease, or have an accident, or experience a certain loss, and so on. In general, personal risk can be thought of as a situation where an individual sees herself vis-à-vis a particular danger, a threat. Let's call being in such situation *being at risk*. In this sense, we are always at risk of *something*, anything that may be harmful or at least unwelcome. On this view, individual risk is a mental concept. We think about being at risk; we perceive a possibility of contracting a disease. As soon as we own something we think about being at risk of losing it; as soon as we have achieved something we fear that it might be taken away. Health is just such a thing.

Viewed the other way around, our health is threatened by illness, accidents, etc. At any point, we *might* develop a health condition (unless it is a disease that you have only once, such as certain infectious diseases that leave the person immune to a second episode). If one drives down the turnpike in a car, one is at risk of getting involved in an accident. Let us call such circumscribed situation that specifies the circumstances in which a specific risk factor might lead to an undesirable outcome a *risk scenario.* Risk scenarios can be very general, such as the one that holds that we all are at risk of developing cancer at some point in our lives.[33] Some other scenarios are more specific, such as being at risk of developing rabies when you wake up at night in the summer with a juvenile lost bat circling the light fixture attached to your bedroom ceiling. You may or may not have been bitten by the animal (their teeth are so small it wouldn't even wake you up). You also may or may not encounter a bat that carries rabies, so you may or may not be at risk of rabies yourself.

The many kinds of individual risk scenarios are based on prior conditions (personal, social, or environmental factors) and on future events (such as being bitten by a bat), which differ for every person. Therefore, every person has a slightly different personal risk scenario for the same disease; my risk of developing breast cancer is *by definition* different from yours simply because I am me, not you. We can think of risk as a personalized expectation of an individual about her future health condition. This expectation may be more or less justified based on prior knowledge, and individuals may not even be aware of it. Being at risk is being in a specific situation that represents an instantiation of a specific risk scenario, defined as a unique combination of endogenous and exogenous circumstances a person finds herself in that mold this person's realm of possible future events. Everyone is in one such situation; most of us are in many such situations. Risk is everywhere.

Personal risk is a qualitative thing, not a quantitative measure. It is a mental state, a cognitive position, that makes us think that something awful can happen. As soon as one starts talking about quantifiers such as "high" or "low" risk or about a "21% risk of contracting hand eczema when becoming a hairdresser", we refer to a different, population kind of risk that is only estimable based on data from populations. Strictly speaking, such population risk estimates do not apply to individuals per se. The only way is to apply it to *individuals as members of groups* of individuals who are situated in roughly the same risk scenario. On this view, one could have told Kristi when she started her apprenticeship as a hairdresser that based on epidemiological research the likelihood among hairdressers of developing hand eczema is 0.21, and 0.05 among office workers and that the risk of hairdressers is thus four times that of office workers. Still, the numerical values of those likelihoods have no quantitative meaning for Kristi as a person, only for hairdressers in general.

At the personal level, risk is a likelihood that is different from likelihoods in populations. In fact, risk at the personal level, interpreted as a probability, is probably better characterized as something like a subjective degree of belief, not a stable frequency of events in the long run. Therefore, statements such as "Tom has a 50% chance of contracting the measles over the next 5 years" are meaningless because the frequentist view does not apply to individuals, unless there is a way to capture degrees of belief in percentages.

Might there be a way to apply population risk to individuals directly, without invoking the "member of group" detour? Jonathan Fuller has tackled this question head on and comes to the conclusion that at least a partial solution to the problem is possible by interpreting individual probabilities as representing "our rational credence conditional on the evidence (and on several assumptions)" (Fuller, 2022, p. 1128). He calls this "epistemic interpretation of individual patient probabilities". He argues that epidemiologic evidence comes in the form of population-based risk estimates based on averages calculated for the population at hand. In many instances, the evidence comes from clinical trials and is then processed using the evidence-based medicine (EBM) framework, which considers meta-analyses of multiple such trials in the form of systematic reviews the best evidence medicine can have. Fuller considers this problematic, because the EBM framework interprets patients' risk ontically as a propensity (1121) and suggests an epistemic reinterpretation as "credences, in which epidemiological evidence is instead seen as informing medical uncertainty" (ibid.). Fuller correctly states that epidemiological data yield estimates such as absolute risk (AR, derived from the population as the population proportion that have developed the disease of interest after a predefined observation period) and absolute risk reduction (ARR, the absolute difference between AR in those with a certain risk factor and those without). These estimates have meaning at the population level, but not for individual patients. The population estimates are interpretable as indicating population probabilities based on frequentist data. Still, says Fuller, using such measures in reference to single patients is ubiquitous in EBM, and, for that matter, in medical care generally. This inferential leap is rooted, per Fuller, in the interpretation of a patient's risk as a probability. What's problematic is that just that patient's risk is not defined in any other way than by inference from just those population-based estimates like AR and ARR.

To dig deeper, Fuller goes on to ask what probabilities are in the first place and refers to Hacking (Hacking, 2001) and Gillies (2000), who distinguish between belief-type and frequency-type, and between subjective and objective probabilities, respectively. In our current context of uncertainty in medicine, it seems that E-uncertainty arises in the realm of belief-type, subjective interpretations of probability, while A-uncertainty is aligned with frequency-type, objective, data-related uncertainty.

Fuller holds that the most plausible ontic interpretation of an individual patient's risk is as a propensity, a physical tendency toward a particular outcome, like fried potatoes have a propensity to turn black after a while if you leave the pan on the burner unattended. But he does not consider the propensity view applicable to patient outcome context, simply because he thinks that most medical outcomes are not *that* chancy. Fuller outlines why epidemiological measures do not actually provide propensities and some other cogent reasons that pave the way for his rejecting the ontic propensity interpretation. Instead, he thinks that single patient risk is better interpreted as something not mind-independent like a propensity, but as a degree of belief (credence), which is one sort of available epistemic interpretations.[34] For our current context, Fuller pulls it all together by bringing uncertainty into the game when he writes:

> Medical evidence is often seen as having some bearing on medical uncertainty, hopefully reducing it by providing new information but sometimes increasing it by challenging existing thinking. Credences are a ready and useful way of representing uncertainty. Epidemiological evidence informs uncertainty by grounding our credences in frequencies. (Fuller, 2022, p. 1126)[35]

It would be interesting to explore exactly *how* epidemiology helps grounding credences in frequencies. For the time being I believe that population risk estimates (population probabilities) *have no meaning for individuals* and thus cannot be used without further ado when thinking about or talking to individual patients. Part of the problem is that risk is an inherently prospective concept. It is the likelihood that something will happen to people (both alone and as member of a population). Because risk is a prospective concept it cannot be directly observed, neither in populations nor in individuals, until it "happens". In individuals, the risk idea vanishes, because the disease of interest (e.g., hand eczema) has occurred, and the person is not at risk anymore. All one can do is estimate risks and relative risks in populations, but once the study is done, there is no population risk (likelihood) anymore. All there is are estimates like prevalence percents or IRs. But percents and rates over time are not probabilities; they are percents and rates. Again, such incongruities need to be considered and should be included in patient conversations and in research considerations. No simple task, but a necessary part of practicing authentic medicine.

The story becomes even trickier because the etiological question in Kristi's case is, did Kristi contract hand eczema *because* of her work as a hairdresser? This would potentially be the case if Kristie were a hairdresser (as she is) *and* suffers from hand eczema (as she does) *and* if something about being a hairdresser causes hand eczema. The first two items can be confirmed by getting a social history from Kristi and a dermatologist's diagnosis of hand eczema. The third part, however, needs to be supported by biomedical research data, where the causal information comes from epidemiology and the mechanistic information comes from laboratory studies.

Causal inference is the holy grail of epidemiology and the biosciences. While the biomedical scientist would be interested in the question whether a certain substance used by hairdressers *can* cause hand eczema, the epidemiologist would want to find out whether such substance *does* cause it. Note that the epidemiologist can only find out whether some substance is causal at the population level, simply because population research is what epidemiologists do. They cannot speak to the issue whether said substance actually did cause Kristi's hand eczema. That inference from epidemiological data to individuals, however, is exactly where the incongruity I have discussed is at work, the incongruity between population data and their application in individual cases as well as the related incongruity between different meanings of risk (likelihood of disease) in persons and in individuals.

From Simplified Research to Complex Real World

The fourth inferential leap is the one from simplicity to complexity. It is related to, but not at all the same as the leap from animal to human discussed above. It is the opposite of drawing simple inferences from complex data, where sophisticated statistical methods have to be applied to identify simple signals in, e.g., multilevel population health data (Park et al., 2018). The inferential leap I want to raise awareness about is the one that works the other way around, from simple to complex.

Most medical interventions are tested in randomized controlled trials (RCTs). The efficacy of a drug in the artificial research setting of the RCT is not necessarily mirrored by the efficiency of the drug in real-world scenarios.[36] This scenario may lead to a situation in which medication choice and estimated efficiency of the drug become uncertain as well, simply because data gathered under ideal but artificial circumstances do not necessarily align well with data collected in not-so-ideal, but more natural circumstances.

As described above, laboratory research is sometimes done with the intent to keep the experimental setting as simple as possible with the goal of minimizing the possibility that extraneous variables affect the results of the experiment. This happens when, for example, researchers isolate individual cells or groups of cells of the same cell type from an experimental animal and perform experiments in which under identical conditions one set of cells is treated with a certain stimulus, while the other (control) cells receive a sham treatment. In such an experimental setting, the "identical conditions" assumption is supposed to minimize the possibility that influences other than the stimulus are responsible for any difference, however defined, between the two experimental groups after the intervention has been performed that could be interpreted as resulting from the stimulation.

A situation in which experimental simplicity and results from such settings is used to infer mechanistic insight for a much more complex scenario is cancer research. For example, molecular studies in cell lines of renal cancer cells are interpreted as evidence that a certain molecule X "might function as a cancer-promoting factor and possible new therapeutic target for renal cell carcinoma" (Lou et al., 2023). Granted, the authors of this research paper use cautious language by saying they *might* have identified a potential cancer-promoting factor, but they still must somehow believe that the evidence they found about the presence and function of molecule X in a simple system (cancer cell lines) has some sort of meaning for the much more complex system of renal cell carcinoma, otherwise they would not even consider the possibility.

This sort of inference from simple to complex is clear evidence for the prevailing reductionist way of thinking in modern biomedicine. According to this view, complex processes and mechanisms are composed of simpler elements that can be identified and assigned causal-mechanical function. The view postulates that a whole is composed of pieces that, if identified, explain the structure and/or function of the whole. This is, indeed, a rather mechanistic view of the biological world and does not account for phenomena such as nonlinearity, chaos, tipping points, and emergence (Corradini & O'Connor, 2010; Northrop, 2011).

The tendency to think simple in the daunting presence of complexity is ubiquitous in modern biomedicine. For example, genetics is a discipline of biology in which simple Mendelian patterns of inheritance were the major paradigm for the longest time. Indeed, some geneticists still seem to think of *all* diseases as essentially caused by genetic mechanisms (personal observation). However, the recognition that not all disease etiology is that simple gives rise to statements like this one:

> *common diseases are highly heterogenous, with a small proportion of cases having relatively simple etiology (sic) dominated by a single genetic mutation, while the vast majority of cases are caused by the combined effect of multiple genetic and environmental factors each contributing a minor influence.*
> (Sham & Cherny, 2011, p. 2)

I might be wrong but I sense that the authors of the above quotation, despite their insight of disease complexity and their response by writing for a book on complex disease analysis (Zeggini & Morris, 2011), still think that genes play the primary role in the etiological disease drama of most diseases, and that environmental factors are secondary. I hold that it is more likely that disease etiology is not either genetic or environmental but *always* both.[37]

Lauren Ross has offered an analysis of explanation in the context of complex psychiatric diseases (Ross, 2023). She refers to common claims that psychiatric diseases are frequently considered causally complex without much further explication what this notion means. Ross outlines four causal "architectures", two at the token level (mono- and multicausal) and two at the type level (causal homogeneity and heterogeneity). Within each level, complexity increases from mono- to multicausal and from homo- to heterogeneity. She identifies three main challenges for explaining the disease of the multicausal model. First, scientists need to identify all the causes, which becomes increasingly difficult over time because the pool of unidentified causes becomes smaller and smaller. Second, Ross notes that scientists do not just need a list of causes, but also a "coherent story about how all of these factors work together to produce the disease" (8). I could not agree more since this is, in fact, the mechanistic component of "etiological explanations", which I define as a "plausible description of a set of causes and pathogenetic mechanisms in whose presence illness occurs consistently more frequently than in their absence" (Dammann, 2020, p. 40). Third, multicausality comes with the unfortunate downside that scientists don't like it because it gets too complicated for those who study disease in the lab. More explanatory challenges come with Ross' second dichotomy, causal homogeneity versus heterogeneity. While the former characterizes the kind of disease or disorder that always has the same set of causes across all instances, the latter allows for multiple different sets of causes in multiple different instances of disease.[38] This distinction also does not come without explanatory problems, Ross writes. First, no single set of causes identified in one instant can explain all occurrences, simply because there are other sets in other instances. The second challenge is an interesting question: why do different sets of causes lead to similar effects? Finally, Ross offers an additional challenge, posed by the fact that some diseases are *defined* by their causal structure, which one needs to know to correctly identify instances of such diseases. This results in a catch-22 situation, where one cannot study the causes of a disease because one would first need to know its causes.

Ross' analysis makes one thing eminently clear about the explanation of disease: it's complicated. Inferring from simple experimental settings to the complexity of real-life disease causation might be possible, but requires much careful consideration of challenges, for example, those reviewed by Ross.

*   *   *

This chapter has offered an analysis of two kinds of inference I consider important when thinking through the architecture of epidemiological and bioscientific approaches to uncertainty in medicine, i.e., transitional and translational inference. While the former specifies the inferential steps from data to information to evidence to knowledge, the latter refers to inferential leaps from one thought system to another, i.e., from association to causation, from animal to human, from population to individual, and from simple to complex. All these inferences (of both types) are philosophically richer than my brief account suggests. I am aware that I am merely scratching the surface in many ways, but I hope that my outline can serve as a point of departure for further consideration.

The next chapter will cover the concept of explanation in medicine and epidemiology. I submit that explanation is a major strategy to tackle medical uncertainty, especially if not restricted to causal explanation as is often done in philosophy of science. In essence, I propose that a broad variety of explanations are used to curb medical uncertainty.

NOTES

1. It also seems that Stegenga's "master argument" using Bayes' theorem (p.176) suggests a formal relationship between the confidence we have in medical interventions given the available evidence ($P(H|E)$) on the one hand and, on the other, the probabilities that the evidence we have given the intervention works ($P(E|H)$) and the two individual probabilities that the evidence is true ($P(E)$) and the intervention works ($P(H)$). Devanesan has offered a counterargument based on the fact that "the complexity and heterogeneity of medicine is so vexing" and, thus, makes it unlikely that Stegenga's "master argument" can be generalized in a helpful way (Devanesan, 2020, 101189, p. 7). Upshur and Goldenberg think that Stegenga's "cynical conclusions rest on an untenable notion of the nature of the facts" (Upshur & Goldenberg, 2020, p. 75) and that "there is an evolving plasticity to facts and evidence and an enduring and perhaps increasing amount of uncertainty" (Upshur & Goldenberg, 2020, p. 81), a recognition that dovetails beautifully with my argument put forth in this book.
2. Broadbent differentiates between medical skepticism as a kind of E-uncertainty about medicine and medical nihilism as a "strong belief in the impotence of medicine" (Broadbent, 2019, p. 158).
3. I am grateful to Lina Dammann for an enlightening discussion about the uncertainty of future versus past events.
4. For more detailed historical perspectives on pioneers of epidemiology see work on Percival Pott (Young, 2005), James Lind (Baron, 2009), William Farr (Halliday, 2016), John Snow (Snowise, 2021), Ignaz Semmelweis (Loudon, 2013), and (to finally break through this line-up of male pioneers) Janet Lane Claypon (Morabia, 2010)
5. https://hagstova.fo/en/population/population/population (accessed 3/7/2022)
6. See United States Senate Finance Committee Report at https://www.finance.senate.gov/imo/media/doc/prb111507a.pdf.
7. The results of the re-evaluation of the RECORD trial were published in (Mahaffey et al. (2013).

8. https://www.ema.europa.eu/en/news/european-medicines-agency-recommends-suspension-avandia-avandamet-avaglim. A clinical expert in the matter, Dr. Bernard Cheung, summarized his views on the controversy in 2014, misinterpreting a 28% increased risk for heart attacks with a p-value of 0.4 as "not an overwhelming result" (data are from an updated meta-analysis by Nissen and Wolski (Nissen & Wolski, 2010)), and lamenting the fact that a re-introduction of the drug to the European market is unlikely because it would not be "economically worthwhile" for the drug company (Cheung, 2014).
9. https://www.fda.gov/drugs/drug-safety-and-availability/fda-drug-safety-communication-fda-requires-removal-some-prescribing-and-dispensing-restrictions
10. https://www.fda.gov/regulatory-information/search-fda-guidance-documents/type-2-diabetes-mellitus-evaluating-safety-new-drugs-improving-glycemic-control-guidance-industry
11. See Cartwright (2012) for a lucid discussion of the problems associated with the external validity of randomized trials and effectiveness predictions.
12. See Dammann (2018a) for a more detailed but still concise description.
13. It is not my goal to embark on a philosophical analysis of the concepts of data, information, evidence, and knowledge. I will simply use these terms as they are used in epidemiology and medicine.
14. Thanks to Alex Broadbent for pointing this out to me.
15. I am using the term "parameter" in the statistical sense; it refers to population values as opposed to sample statistics.
16. Frequently in this context, association is called "correlation". I am avoiding this term here to avoid confusion: the term is not only used in a general sense (meaning "statistical association") but also the name for a particular kind of statistical approach, i.e., correlation analysis.
17. This is not to be confused with internal and external study validity, which are related, but different concepts.
18. The investigators in this study used a statistical method that yields odds ratios (ORs) as an estimate of the relative risk.
19. *External* validity, on the other hand, refers to how well study results can be generalized, i.e., extrapolated from the study sample to other populations (see Section "Epidemiologic Excursion"). Note that looking at external validity makes sense only if a study is internally valid.
20. Current textbook epidemiology includes confounding among the biases as "confounding bias". It will become clear why I prefer to keep the concepts separate.
21. This is an example of the Hawthorne effect—people who know they are observed behave differently from when not.

22. See https://catalogofbias.org/
23. From a slide presentation authored by Dr. Nigel Paneth, available at http://www.pitt.edu/~super7/18011-19001/18951.ppt
24. The main confounders investigators adjusted for were age, sex, country, sleep outcome at baseline, current smoking, alcohol consumption, body mass index, educational level, weekly headache, mental and physical health score (SF-12), and diagnosis of depression. Data were also weighted to account for relative exposure to lower (3G) versus higher (2G) radiofrequency.
25. For an entertaining discussion *Why 5%?* see (Gauvreau & Pagano, 1994)
26. For a more formal explication of knowledge generation by evidence see Conee and Feldman (2004) and McCain (2014).
27. The term "correlation" is often used rather loosely in philosophy, meaning that two variables "go together". In statistics, however, this would be called an "association", while the term correlation is reserved for associations between two continuous variables, such as age and body height.
28. It is also not a necessary condition because one can have data that suggest no correlation while there is one; consider causal relationships that follow a quadratic equation where data are available only at both ends of a hyperbolic curve but not in between.
29. Randomization is, by definition, never an intrinsic feature of observational (non-randomized) studies. Therefore, I have not listed it as one of the requirements for internal validity used for the assessment of observational studies.
30. Miguel Hernán has offered an interesting plain-language defense of the target-trial emulation approach in one of the world's most prestigious medical journals (Hernán, 2021).
31. I have previously written about Hill's heuristics in chapter 4.5 of Dammann and Smart (2019) and in more detail in chapter 8 of Dammann (2020).
32. The concept of statistical significance has been developed for similar reasons. I will not go into this topic, not just because it is of only marginal importance for our discussion, but also because a large number of statisticians and other scientists have suggested to abandon the concept because it is frequently misused (Amrhein et al., 2019). They have also suggested to use the term "compatibility interval" instead of "confidence interval" because confidence is a mental state, not a numerical entity. The interval denotes the "true" values the point estimate would be compatible with.
33. Note that I used the verb "develop" in the last sentence: the usage of this verb in everyday conversations and in medical lingo, to describe a situation in which a previously healthy person *becomes* ill. I think it might be worthwhile to ponder the question whether developmental thinking might be a way to describe disease occurrence.

34. Fuller refers to Gillies (2000) for an overview of this issue.
35. Fuller does not go into much detail about how it can be justified to set credences to epidemiologic estimates, but refers to his own previous work (Fuller & Flores, 2015) and to principles discussed in Lewis (1980) and Hacking (2001).
36. It is interesting that most publications on "real-world evidence" is based on data from electronic health records, which arguably do not represent real-world scenarios but hospital or healthcare system scenarios.
37. During the time I took an epidemiology class with Ken Rothman in the early 1990s, an oncologist stated on National Public Radio that cancer is 75% genetic and 25% environmental. Rothman's comment was that this notion is wrong because *all* diseases are 100% genetic and 100% environmental.
38. This seems to be what Rothman has described in his sufficient-component cause model (Rothman, 1976).

REFERENCES

Ackoff, R. L. (1989). From data to wisdom. *Journal of Applied Systems Analysis, 16*, 3–9.

Amrhein, V., Greenland, S., & McShane, B. (2019). Scientists rise up against statistical significance. *Nature, 567*(7748), 305–307.

Awadh, A., Chughtai, A. A., Dyda, A., Sheikh, M., Heslop, D. J., & MacIntyre, C. R. (2017). Does Zika virus cause microcephaly - Applying the Bradford Hill viewpoints. *PLoS Currents, 9*.

Baron, J. H. (2009). Sailors' scurvy before and after James Lind - a reassessment. *Nutrition Reviews, 67*(6), 315–332.

Broadbent, A. (2019). *Philosophy of medicine* (p. 1). Oxford University Press.

Cartwright, N. (1989). *Nature's capacities and their measurement.* Oxford University Press.

Cartwright, N. (2010). What are randomised controlled trials good for? *Philosophical Studies: An International Journal for Philosophy in the Analytic Tradition, 147*(1), 59–70.

Cartwright, N. (2011). A philosopher's view of the long road from RCTs to effectiveness. *The Lancet, 377*(9775), 1400–1401.

Cartwright, N. (2012). Will this policy work for you? predicting effectiveness better: How philosophy helps. *Philosophy of Science, 79*(5), 973–989.

Cheung, B. M. Y. (2014). Behind the rosiglitazone controversy. *Expert Review of Clinical Pharmacology, 3*, 723–725.

Clark, S., & Weale, A. (2012). Social values in health priority setting: A conceptual framework. *Journal of Health Organization and Management, 26*(3), 293–316.

Conee, E. B., & Feldman, R. (2004). *Evidentialism: Essays in epistemology*. Oxford University Press.

Corradini, A., & O'Connor, T. (2010). *Emergence in science and philosophy*. Routledge.

Dammann, O. (2018a). Data, information, evidence, and knowledge: A proposal for health informatics and data science. *Online Journal of Public Health Informatics, 10*(3), e224.

Dammann, O. (2018b). Hill's heuristics and explanatory coherentism in epidemiology. *American Journal of Epidemiology, 187*(1), 1–6.

Dammann, O. (2020). *Etiological explanations: Illness causation theory*. CRC Press.

Dammann, O. (Forthcoming). Epidemiological inferences. In A. Broadbent (Ed.), *Oxford handbook of philosophy of medicine*. Oxford University Press.

Dammann, O., & Smart, B. (2019). *Causation in population health informatics and data science*. Springer.

Dekkers, O. M., Elm, E. v., Algra, A., Romijn, J. A., & Vandenbroucke, J. P. (2009). How to assess the external validity of therapeutic trials: A conceptual approach. *International Journal of Epidemiology, 39*(1), 89–94.

Devanesan, A. (2020). Medical nihilism: The limits of a decontextualised critique of medicine. *Studies in History and Philosophy of Biological and Biomedical Sciences, 79*, 101189.

Doll, R., & Hill, A. B. (1950). Smoking and carcinoma of the lung. *BMJ, 2*(4682), 739–748.

Frank, C., Faber, M., & Stark, K. (2016). Causal or not: Applying the Bradford Hill aspects of evidence to the association between Zika virus and microcephaly. *EMBO Molecular Medicine, 8*(4), 305–307.

Fuller, J. (2022). Epidemiological evidence: Use at your 'own risk'? *Philosophy of Science, 87*(5), 1119–1129.

Fuller, J., & Flores, L. J. (2015). The Risk GP Model: The standard model of prediction in medicine. *Studies in History and Philosophy of Biological and Biomedical Sciences, 54*, 49–61.

Gauvreau, K., & Pagano, M. (1994). Why 5%? *Nutrition, 10*(1), 93–94.

Gillies, D. (2000). *Philosophical theories of probability*. Routledge.

Graunt, J. (1665). *Natural and political observations mentioned in a following index, and made upon the bills of mortality* (3rd edn). Printed by John Martyn, and James Allestry.

Hacking, I. (2001). *An introduction to probability and inductive logic*. Cambridge University Press.

Hall, N. S. (2007). R. A. Fisher and his advocacy of randomization. *Journal of the History of Biology, 40*(2), 295–325.

Halliday, S. (2016). William Farr: Campaigning statistician. *Journal of Medical Biography, 8*(4), 220–227.

Hariton, E., & Locascio, J. J. (2018). Randomised controlled trials - the gold standard for effectiveness research. *BJOG: An International Journal of Obstetrics & Gynaecology, 125*(13), 1716–1716.

Havmose, M., Thyssen, J. P., Zachariae, C., & Johansen, J. D. (2022). Long-term follow-up of hand eczema in hairdressers: A prospective cohort study of Danish hairdressers graduating from 1985 to 2007. *Journal of the European Academy of Dermatology and Venereology, 36*(2), 263–270.

Hernán, M. A. (2004). A definition of causal effect for epidemiological research. *Journal of Epidemiology and Community Health, 58*(4), 265–271.

Hernán, M. A. (2021). Methods of public health research — Strengthening causal inference from observational data. *New England Journal of Medicine, 385*(15), 1345–1348.

Hernán, M. A., & Robins, J. M. (2006). Estimating causal effects from epidemiologic data. *Journal of Epidemiology and Community Health, 60*, 578–586.

Hernán, M. A., & Robins, J. M. (2016). Using big data to emulate a target trial when a randomized trial is not available. *American Journal of Epidemiology, 183*(8), 758–764.

Hill, A. B. (1965). The environment and disease: Association or causation? *Proceedings of the Royal Society of Medicine, 58*, 295–300.

Höfler, M. (2005). Causal inference based on counterfactuals. *BMC Medical Research Methodology, 5*(1), 28.

Home, P. D., Pocock, S. J., Beck-Nielsen, H., Gomis, R., Hanefeld, M., Dargie, H., Komajda, M., Gubb, J., Biswas, N., & Jones, N. P. (2005). Rosiglitazone Evaluated for Cardiac Outcomes and Regulation of Glycaemia in Diabetes (RECORD): Study design and protocol. *Diabetologia, 48*, 1726–1735.

Home, P. D., Pocock, S. J., Beck-Nielsen, H., Curtis, P. S., Gomis, R., Hanefeld, M., Jones, N. P., Komajda, M., McMurray, J. J. V., & RECORD Study Team. (2009). Rosiglitazone evaluated for cardiovascular outcomes in oral agent combination therapy for type 2 diabetes (RECORD): A multicentre, randomised, open-label trial. *Lancet, 373*, 2125–2135.

Home, P. D., Pocock, S. J., Beck-Nielsen, H., Gomis, R., Hanefeld, M., Jones, N. P., Komajda, M., McMurray, J. J. V., & RECORD Study Group. (2007). Rosiglitazone evaluated for cardiovascular outcomes--an interim analysis. *The New England Journal of Medicine, 357*, 28–38.

Jaffiol, C. (2009). Current management of type 2 diabetes in France. *Bulletin de l'Académie Nationale de Médecine, 193*(7), 1645–1661.

Jamil, W., Svensson, A., Josefson, A., Lindberg, M., & Von Kobyletzki, L. (2022). Incidence rate of hand eczema in different occupations: A systematic review and meta-analysis. *Acta Dermato-Venereologica, 102*, adv00681.

Kieffer, C. M., & Robertson, A. S. (2020). Impact of FDA-required cardiovascular outcome trials on type 2 diabetes clinical study initiation from 2008 to 2017. *Therapeutic Innovation & Regulatory Science, 54*, 640–644.

Klaic, M., Kapp, S., Hudson, P., Chapman, W., Denehy, L., Story, D., et al. (2022). Implementability of healthcare interventions: An overview of reviews and development of a conceptual framework. *Implementation Science, 17*(1), 10.

Kleinbaum, D. G., Kupper, L. L., & Morgenstern, H. (1982). *Epidemiologic research: Principles and quantitative methods.* Lifetime Learning Publications.

Kruskal, W., & Mosteller, F. (1979a). Representative sampling, I: Non-scientific literature. *International Statistical Review/Revue Internationale de Statistique, 47*(1), 13–24.

Kruskal, W., & Mosteller, F. (1979b). Representative sampling, II: Scientific literature, excluding statistics. *International Statistical Review/Revue Internationale de Statistique, 47*(2), 111–127.

Kruskal, W., & Mosteller, F. (1979c). Representative sampling, III: The current statistical literature. *International Statistical Review/Revue Internationale de Statistique, 47*(3), 245–265.

Lam, D., Lively, S., & Schlichter, L. C. (2017). Responses of rat and mouse primary microglia to pro- and anti-inflammatory stimuli: Molecular profiles, K+ channels and migration. *Journal of Neuroinflammation, 14*(1), 166.

Lewis, D. (1980). A subjectivist's guide to objective chance. In R. C. Jeffrey (Ed.), *Studies in inductive logic and probability* (Vol. II, pp. 263–293). University of California Press.

Lou, J., Liu, X., Fan, X., Xu, X., Wang, Z., & Wang, L. (2023). Lncrna FEZf1–as1 negatively regulates ETNK1 to promote malignant progression of renal cell carcinoma. *Journal Of Medical Biochemistry, 42*(2), 232–238.

Loudon, I. (2013). Ignaz Phillip Semmelweis' studies of death in childbirth. *Journal of the Royal Society of Medicine, 106*(11), 461–463.

Mahaffey, K. W., Hafley, G., Dickerson, S., Burns, S., Tourt-Uhlig, S., White, J., Newby, L. K., Komajda, M., McMurray, J., Bigelow, R., Home, P. D., & Lopes, R. D. (2013). Results of a reevaluation of cardiovascular outcomes in the RECORD trial. *American Heart Journal, 166*(240–249), e241.

Mahmood, S. S., Levy, D., Vasan, R. S., & Wang, T. J. (2014). The Framingham Heart Study and the epidemiology of cardiovascular disease: A historical perspective. *Lancet, 383*(9921), 999–1008.

McCain, K. (2014). *Evidentialism and epistemic justification* (1st ed.). Routledge, Taylor & Francis Group.

Miettinen, O. S. (1985). *Theoretical epidemiology.* John Wiley & Sons.

Morabia, A. (2010). Janet Lane-Claypon--interphase epitome. *Epidemiology, 21*(4), 573–576.

Nissen, S. E. (2010). The rise and fall of rosiglitazone. *European Heart Journal, 31,* 773–776.

Nissen, S. E., & Wolski, K. (2007). Effect of rosiglitazone on the risk of myocardial infarction and death from cardiovascular causes. *The New England Journal of Medicine, 356,* 2457–2471.

Nissen, S. E., & Wolski, K. (2010). Rosiglitazone revisited: An updated meta-analysis of risk for myocardial infarction and cardiovascular mortality. *Archives of Internal Medicine, 170,* 1191–1201.

Northrop, R. B. (2011). *Introduction to complexity and complex systems.* Taylor & Francis.

Park, S. Y., Staicu, A.-M., Xiao, L., & Crainiceanu, C. M. (2018). Simple fixed-effects inference for complex functional models. *Biostatistics, 19*(2), 137–152.

Pearce, N. (2012). Classification of epidemiological study designs. *International Journal of Epidemiology, 41*(2), 393–397.

Pearson, K. (1900). *The grammar of science* (2nd ed.). A. and C. Black.

Pound, P., Ebrahim, S., Sandercock, P., Bracken, M. B., Roberts, I., & Reviewing Animal Trials Systematically, G. (2004). Where is the evidence that animal research benefits humans? *BMJ, 328*(7438), 514–517.

Proctor, R. N. (2012). The history of the discovery of the cigarette-lung cancer link: Evidentiary traditions, corporate denial, global toll. *Tobacco Control, 21*(2), 87–91.

Rocca, E., & Anjum, R. L. (2020). Causal evidence and dispositions in medicine and public health. *International Journal of Environmental Research and Public Health, 17*(6), 1813.

Ross, L. (2023). Explanation in contexts of causal complexity: Lessons from psychiatric genetics. In William C. Bausman, Janella K. Baxter & Oliver M. Lean (eds.), *From Biological Practice to Scientific Metaphysics.* Minneapolis: University of Minnesota Press.

Rothman, K. J. (1976). Causes. *American Journal of Epidemiology, 104,* 87–92.

Rothman, K. J. (1986). *Modern epidemiology.* Little, Brown & Company.

Rothman, K. J. (1996). Lessons from John Graunt. *Lancet, 347*(8993), 37–39.

Rothman, K. J., & Greenland, S. (1998). *Modern epidemiology* (2nd ed.). Lippincott-Raven.

Rothman, K. J., Greenland, S., Poole, C., & Lash, T. L. (2008). Causation and causal inference. In K. J. Rothman, S. Greenland, & T. L. Lash (Eds.), *Modern epidemiology* (3rd ed., pp. 5–31). Lippincott Williams & Wilkins.

Rubin, D. B. (1974). Estimating causal effects of treatments in randomized and nonrandomized studies. *Journal of Educational Psychology, 66*(5), 688–701.

Schouten, B., Cobben, F., & Bethlehem, J. (2009). Indicators for the representativeness of survey response. *Survey Methodology, 35*(1), 101–113.

Sekhon, M., Cartwright, M., & Francis, J. J. (2017). Acceptability of healthcare interventions: An overview of reviews and development of a theoretical framework. *BMC Health Services Research, 17*(1), 88.

Sham, P. C., & Cherny, S. S. (2011). Genetic architecture of complex diseases. In E. Zeggini & A. Morris (Eds.), *Analysis of complex disease association studies* (pp. 1–13). Academic Press.

Singham, M. (2020). *The great paradox of science: Why its conclusions can be relied upon even though they cannot be proven.* Oxford University Press.

Sjoberg, E. A. (2017). Logical fallacies in animal model research. *Behavioral and Brain Functions, 13*(1), Article no. 3.

Snowise, N. G. (2021). Memorials to John Snow - Pioneer in anaesthesia and epidemiology. *Journal of Medical Biography, 31*(1), 47–50. https://doi.org/10.1177/09677720211013807

Susser, M. (1991). What is a cause and how do we know one? A grammar for pragmatic epidemiology. *American Journal of Epidemiology, 133*, 635–648.

Tettamanti, G., Auvinen, A., Åkerstedt, T., Kojo, K., Ahlbom, A., Heinävaara, S., et al. (2020). Long-term effect of mobile phone use on sleep quality: Results from the cohort study of mobile phone use and health (COSMOS). *Environment International, 140*, 105687.

Tulchinsky, T. H. (2018). John snow, cholera, the broad street pump; Waterborne diseases then and now. In *Case studies in public health* (pp. 77–99). Elsevier.

Upshur, R., & Goldenberg, M. J. (2020). Countering medical nihilism by reconnecting facts and values. *Studies in History and Philosophy of Science, 84*, 75–83.

Vandenbroucke, J. P., Broadbent, A., & Pearce, N. (2016). Causality and causal inference in epidemiology: The need for a pluralistic approach. *International Journal of Epidemiology, 45*(6), 1776–1786.

VanderWeele, T. J. (2015). *Explanation in causal inference: Methods for mediation and interaction.* Oxford University Press.

White, C. (1990). Research on smoking and lung cancer: A landmark in the history of chronic disease epidemiology. *The Yale Journal of Biology and Medicine, 63*(1), 29–46.

Woodcock, J., Sharfstein, J. M., & Hamburg, M. (2010). Regulatory action on rosiglitazone by the U.S. food and drug administration. *New England Journal of Medicine, 363*, 1489–1491.

Worrall, J. (2007). Why there's no cause to randomize. *British Journal for the Philosophy of Science, 58*(3), 451–488.

Young, R. H. (2005). A brief history of the pathology of the gonads. *Modern Pathology, 18*(Suppl 2), S3–S17.

Zeggini, E., & Morris, A. P. (2011). *Analysis of complex disease association studies: A practical guide* (1st ed.). Academic Press/Elsevier.

CHAPTER 6

Explanation

INTRODUCTION

In the previous chapters, we have discussed the puzzle of medical ineffectiveness and some of the ways aleatoric (A-) and epistemic (E-) uncertainty in medicine contribute to this problem. One way of dealing with uncertainty in medicine is to focus on the strategies of transitional and translational inference, i.e., the inferential techniques that help with the transition from data to knowledge and from one conceptual system to another, respectively. In this chapter, we will turn our attention toward *explanation*, the ways medics and medical researchers try to tackle uncertainty in a productive fashion.

How can E-uncertainty be reduced if E-uncertainty about X is derived by translational inference from A-uncertainty of X? Would not the A-uncertainty need to be reduced first? I submit that A-uncertainty is intrinsic to something and cannot be changed. If the world is always wobbly, will not any data about it always be wobbly, so our cognitive state about it will always be wobbly as well? Moreover, is uncertainty not a dichotomy, either present or absent?

Based on chapter "Explanation in Public Health" in *Routledge Handbook of Philosophy of Public Health*, Venkatapuram and Broadbent (eds.).

O. Dammann, *Uncertainty and Explanation in Medicine and the Health Sciences*, https://doi.org/10.1007/978-3-031-82271-1_6

Let me begin by addressing the notion that uncertainty is dichotomous. Sometimes, we tend to think of things as dichotomous while they are not. Things that are *named* in a dichotomous way may seem to *be* dichotomous although they are not. For example, honesty and dishonesty seem to be two alternative things while they are really two areas with some overlapping gray space that has a bit of both. Tractable and intractable are similarly wobbly terms that aren't two specific things but two broad realms of tractability with fuzzy boundaries. Along these lines, I think it is fair to say that certainty and uncertainty are neither completely mutually exclusive nor exhaustive in describing elements of the realm of things that we may call certain or uncertain. In keeping with this notion, I believe that uncertainty comes in degrees. Many events are naturally uncertain in the sense of being *very* uncertain, like the exact position and momentum of Heisenberg's particles at any single point in time, other things are *sort of* uncertain like the timing of earthquakes, and other things are completely certain, like the fact that all humans will die at some point. Arguably, the most interesting cases are the aleatoric *sort of* uncertain ones, and one way of dealing with the associated epistemic *sort of* uncertainty is explaining it away, thereby reducing E-uncertainty.

What do I mean by "explaining uncertainty away"? As alluded to above, I think that uncertainty is not a dichotomous thing and can thus occur at different levels. I think it can be reduced by offering explanations that provide answers to questions like why, how, when, where does what occur? In medicine such questions are posed by patients every day and explanations are provided every day by medical professionals. Similar questions are asked by medics and biomedical researchers and are answered (by those same researchers) in the form of study results. In fact, I think this is what explanations are supposed to do: they reduce (or in some unfortunate situations increase) uncertainty. Changing the uncertainty level of something (aleatoric) and someone (epistemic) is how explanation is conceptualized in this book.

In the remainder of this chapter, I will take an explanatory mosaicist approach, because I don't think that only what is accepted as a scientific explanation is worthy of the medical philosophers' attention. I will begin by outlining the distinction between explanations that describe and clarify (D-C explanations) and explanations that provide answers to why- and how-questions (etiological explanations). I propose that it will be beneficial to understand how researchers and practitioners of medicine explain their actions in the health workflow, from problem assessment via goal definition and intervention to evaluation. This workflow is essentially the same in all four domains of medicine (etiology, diagnostics, therapeutics, and prognosis). Further, I will discuss the types and subtypes of explanation used in medical and public health research and practice: scientific, justificatory, methodological, and prospective. In doing this, I take the discussion far beyond the usual focus in philosophy of science as answers to "why?"-questions. The chapter ends with a few comments on my proposal.

Much of this chapter does not read as if it is about explanation *in medicine*. However, my general conceptual discussion of explanation will make it clear how different kinds of explanation may work in medicine, which will help us get a better grasp on how uncertainty is reduced in medicine. The upshot of the chapter will be that explaining medical uncertainty away requires not just scientific or causal explanations, the main kinds of explanation dealt with in philosophy of science, but also non-causal and perhaps even non-scientific kinds of explanations as well.

EXPLANATION: WHAT'S IN A NAME?

What are we talking about when we talk about *explanation*? Of course, there are multiple definitions of the term, both in general and philosophical usage. In everyday language, explanation often means to describe or to clarify. Philosophers of science make distinctions between kinds of explanation as being scientific versus non-scientific, causal versus non-causal, or answers to why- versus answers to non-why-questions.

For example, the Merriam-Webster Thesaurus states that, in general, explanation is "a statement that makes something clear", and the Encyclopedia Britannica defines the philosophical concept of explanation as a "set of statements that makes intelligible the existence or occurrence of an object, event, or state of affairs".[1] Wikipedia, probably the most commonly used archive of common knowledge, says:

> *An explanation is a set of* statements *usually constructed to* describe *a set of facts which clarifies the causes,* context, *and* consequences *of those facts. This description may establish* rules *or* laws, *and may clarify the existing rules or laws in relation to any objects, or phenomena examined. (Italics mine)*[2]

This definition states that explanations do two things: they describe and clarify. Let's call such explanations *descriptive-clarificatory* (D-C) explanations. Accordingly, the first important explanatory function of D-C explanations is to *describe*, that is, to provide a description of elements of a fact or event. It may seem a bit far-fetched to distinguish the descriptive from the clarificatory component of an explanation because one could say that in some way or another *all* descriptions are potentially clarifying. At the same time, all clarificatory explanations might be seen as providing a description of the explanandum (the target phenomenon to be explained).

The statement "2 = 1 + 1" is both one possible description of what "2" is (the sum of two 1's) and at the same time also one possible clarification for someone who does not yet know that 2 is the sum of 1 + 1. The D-C kind of explanation seeks to offer information about a fact or event and to clarify it, providing a more or less detailed narrative about something so that it can be better understood. This is sometimes also called an *explication*. A narrative about the cellular structure of the liver clarifies what liver tissue looks like in terms of its cellular tissue composition. Thus, a knowledge increase is part of the goal of clarificatory explanations, but if the explanation is not made by someone to someone else, it does not need to increase anyone's knowledge to be clarificatory. It can just sit somewhere, e.g., in a textbook, and merely have the potential to clarify and still be a clarificatory explanation that is just not yet doing its explanatory job, but certainly could if someone opened the book and read the explanation. Arguably, such a D-C explanation remains one even when it is read by someone who already knows everything about liver histology. It suffices to just be a narrative about something that has the potential to make this something intelligible, or at least more intelligible, for someone who doesn't know much about it. Any narrative that potentially clarifies something does the clarifying by telling a story that describes the thing to be clarified.

But are there descriptive explanations that are *not* clarificatory as well? For example, in response to the question "what is the sun?" one might respond "the sun is a huge ball of burning matter that is located at the center of our solar system and it is so big that its gravity keeps the planets spinning around it in its grip", which is a description *and* a clarification. The response "the sun is a hot, bright spot that can sometimes be seen in the sky" is also a description and a clarification since it clarifies that the sun is hot, bright, and sometimes visible in the sky. However, the clarificatory strength and, therefore, value of the second explanation can be seen as inferior to the first one. Still both explanations describe and clarify. I am not yet sure that description and clarification are two characteristics of one and the same thing, which would be the case if all descriptive explanations would also have the potential to clarify and if all clarificatory explanations had the potential to describe.

In the philosophical literature, however, the meaning of the term "explanation" is frequently restricted to *scientific* explanation (Skow, 2015). While there does not seem to be consensus on exactly how scientific explanation should be defined, there appears to be at least some agreement that many scientific explanations can be characterized as answers to *why*-questions that explain *why* certain propositions are true and events occur. On this view, a scientific explanation is a narrative about the causal history of an event or fact (Lewis, 1986; Lipton, 1991; Salmon, 1984). Such causal history provides a narrative of how something comes about. In our simple $1 + 1 = 2$ example equation, the sum 2 comes about *because* one adds $1 + 1$. The addition is the mechanism that causes the sum, given that the elements of the addition do in fact add up to 2. The result 2 exists also independently of the addition of two 1's because it can be the result of many other additions (like $1.9 + 0.1$ or $1.1 + 0.9$, and so on). However, feeding 0.3 and 1.9 into the addition does not produce the result of 2. Instead, the result would be 2.2. Thus, the result of the addition is explained by both the elements of the addition and the addition mechanism. In our example $1 + 1 = 2$, 2 is the result of the addition and the addition, therefore, part of an explanation of *why* the result is 2. Another part of the explanation is the numeric value of the number 1 and the mathematical convention that adding two 1s gives you one 2.

A causal explanation can also serve as a descriptive and a clarifying explanation. Causal explanations like "children tend to grow because you feed them" can function as answers to Why-questions like "why do children tend to grow?", while also describing what tends to happen when you feed your child and clarifying what might happen if you don't. Why can descriptive and clarificatory explanations not necessarily work as causal explanations?

It may be the case that all causal explanations are also descriptive and clarificatory, but not all descriptive and clarificatory explanations are causal. When I describe pneumonia as a disease that comes with general malaise, fever, breathing difficulties, abnormal auscultatory lung sounds and abnormal chest X-ray results, I offer a descriptive explanation of the clinical presentation and some possible diagnostic findings, which is also a clarificatory explanation for those who don't yet know exactly what pneumonia is. However, the explanation does not offer any causal information, i.e., an explanation how pneumonia develops as a disease in a previously healthy individual. Thus, an etiological explanation of pneumonia serves a descriptive and clarificatory role by outlining what constitutes pneumonia but part of that potentially clarificatory description is a description of *why* and *how* pneumonia occurs.[3]

Although the predominant view in philosophy of science of what a scientific explanation is and does appears to refer to explanation that provides answers to why-questions, consulting with a philosophical dictionary reveals the following definition:

> *[Explanation is] an act of making something intelligible or understandable, as when we explain an event by showing why or how it occurred.* (Audi, 1999, p. 298)

Interestingly, the first part of this definition seems to refer to D-C explanations, while the second refers to etiological explanations as an example for D-C explanations. In the remainder of the entry, the author distinguishes between causal explanations that answer why-questions from explanations that refer to the process that delineates the process how the fact or event came about, thus offering an answer to how-questions. I am referring to etiological explanations as doing both, by referring to both causes and mechanisms of event occurrence by way of giving a causal and a mechanical explanation, respectively. However, I admit that the distinction gets a bit blurry if one thinks of answers of how-questions (mechanical or causal process questions) as answers that would also qualify as answers to why-questions (causal questions). Instead of neatly distinguishing between reference to the cause (bacterial infection) as an answer to the why-question about a case of pneumonia and to the mechanism (pulmonary inflammation) as an answer to the how-question, it would probably be fair to consider either answer as a proper answer to both questions *in everyday medical conversations.* Although bacteria are the cause and inflammation is the mechanism, the patient who asks "Why do I have pneumonia?" might be content with an answer that refers to either bacteria or inflammation, i.e., either "Because you have a bacterial infection of the lung" or "Because you have a massive inflammatory response in your lung" might count. Similarly, the question "How did this happen?" would be answered by "bacteria infected your lung" and "you developed a massive inflammatory response in your lung". My point is that in everyday medical communication, causes and mechanisms are not always, and perhaps not even often, kept separate, while philosophers tend to do this to keep the explanatorial architecture straight.

Going back to an everyday-life-dictionary, the American Heritage Dictionary entry dovetails well with the distinction between the explanatory functions of D-C versus etiologic explanations. It refers to explanation as "the act of explaining", which is in turn defined as

1. To make plain or comprehensible. 2. To define; expound [...] 3. To offer reasons for or cause of; justify [...].[4]

These three (sub)definitions of "explaining" are nested in the sense that the first two refer to D-C explanations and cover the third, which refers to etiological explanations, just as Audi does in the previous quote above.

I will not offer a deep dive into models of explanation in this chapter but want to at least cover some of the discourse about scientific explanation in the philosophical literature in the next section. If medicine is supposed to be science-based, and if medical explanations are supposed to reduce uncertainty in medicine, shouldn't all explanations used in medicine be scientific? I will then move on to offer a very broad and inclusive (mosaicist) view of explanation as it is used in medicine, where both D-C explanations and etiological explanations are ubiquitous. Most importantly, my survey of explanations used in medicine and population health includes but is not restricted to why-question-responses. Activities like data interpretation, decision making, planning, and policy development involve explanations that are non-scientific and are part of medicine's business as well. Most of these activities are based on scientific evidence, but they also require types of explanation that are not answers to why-questions. The main reason not to restrict myself to the usual pattern of how explanation is generally discussed in the philosophical literature is that I am interested in explanation in medical *practice* in which other types of explanation play important roles.

EXPLANATION EXPLAINED

In this section I propose a very broad and inclusive conceptualization of explanation in medicine, namely, the view that an explanation is any auxiliary response (as in "helpful", not just "accessorial") to questions asked to increase understanding and the scope of action. According to this view, all D-C explanations (including etiologic explanations) are explanations *because* they lead to an actual or potential increase in understanding by providing descriptive and clarifying answers.

I deliberately do not restrict myself to scientific explanations. Scientific explanation has to do with *understanding*. In the preface of his *Scientific Explanation and the Causal Structure of the World* (1984, p. ix), Wesley Salmon wrote that "we secure scientific understanding by providing scientific explanations". The link between explanation and understanding is an oft-cited one. For example, Henk de Regt focuses on explanatory understanding, "the understanding of why a phenomenon occurs that results from a scientific explanation of that phenomenon" (de Regt, 2017, footnote on p. 2), while excluding "objectual understanding, understanding-how, and understanding-that" (ibid.). De Regt's explanatory understanding seems identical with Salmon's scientific understanding since both refer to scientific explanation as its source. However, de Regt appears to restrict scientific explanation to the explanation why a phenomenon occurs, which is a subset of the set of all explanations, while Salmon seems to apply the term "scientific explanation" to all "understanding of events and phenomena" (Salmon 1997, pp. 79–91; cited by De Regt:2). I explicitly do *not* follow Henk de Regt because I do not want to be restricted to scientific explanations as answers to why-questions. Instead, I believe that explanations in the form of answers to how-, what-, where-questions are asked by scientists and non-scientists, both within the practice of science and outside. The remainder of this section delves a bit deeper into these kinds of distinctions between scientific and non-scientific explanations, causal and non-causal explanations, and explanations as answers to why-questions, and so on. Although this expedition into the murky waters of explanation can be somewhat mind-bending at times, I do believe it is important to consider such intricacies as a basis of the general notion that explanation is a chief approach to the curbing of uncertainty in medicine.

Scientific Explanation

Even a superficial survey of the literature reveals that the terms *explanation* and *scientific explanation* are sometimes used interchangeably. It is not clear, however, whether this is a consequence of focus in philosophy of science, where scientific explanations play a central role because they are scientific explanations, or a serious proposal to conceptualize both as being the same kind of thing. The following quote from a prominent philosophy of science handbook suggests just that to drop the modifier "scientific" from "scientific explanation":

> *'Scientific explanation' is the traditional name for a topic that philosophers of science are supposed to have something to say about. But it is a bad name for that topic. For one thing, theories of scientific explanation don't have an activity that is exclusive to scientists as their subject matter. Nonscientists do it, too, all the time; they just have less specialized knowledge to use and direct their attention to less complicated phenomena. This suggests that we drop the adjective 'scientific' and call the topic 'explanation.'* (Skow, 2016)

This proposal would suggest that scientific explanation and explanations are one and the same. On this view, all explanations are scientific, which makes sense only if one thinks of any explanatory activity as scientific or of any goal of explanation as a scientific goal. It also suggests that anything that does *not* qualify as an explanation cannot be a scientific explanation, which makes sense based on the logic of statements such as "if Riley is not a dog, she cannot be a Dachshund". Also, Skow seems to interpret "scientific" as a modifier that means "being done exclusively by scientists". This, in turn, suggests that the activity of explaining is somehow restricted to scientists and, in generalized form, that something is not scientific if it is not done by scientists. This would mean that if a non-scientist, for example, a philosopher, gives an explanation it cannot be scientific, thus not be an explanation at all (because according to Skow explanation and scientific explanation are the same). I am not sure I'm prepared to subscribe to this exclusive view. In fact, I am not sure that "being done by scientists" is a good definition of "scientific". I would agree if Skow actually means that any explanation is a scientific explanation because any explanation can be used in a scientific context, by scientists or non-scientists, to make a scientific argument and *therefore* count as a scientific explanation. This comes close to my own view of scientific explanation, which I will further expound below.

At any rate, philosophers of science often explicitly restrict their discussions of explanation to scientific explanations. What makes an explanation scientific? What is added by the modifier "scientific" to the term "explanation"? In the philosophy of science literature, the two main forms of scientific explanation are unificationist (UN) and causal-mechanical (CM) models of explanation. I will mention UN only in passing and offer a more extensive discussion of the CM account.

The UN was proposed by Friedman (1974) and Kitcher (1989). It attempts to provide "a unified account of a range of different phenomena" (Woodward, 2017). Focusing on Kitcher's version, I read him as saying that we need to explain many phenomena to understand nature and if we can find a stringent pattern of explanatory arguments that can help explain a wide range of phenomena, we are on the right track to finding a unificationist explanation. In his piece *The Importance of Scientific Understanding* Salmon distinguishes between the UN and CM by saying that the latter provides help opening black boxes while the former helps forming a world view (Weltanschauung) (Salmon, 1997, p. 83).

CM explanations are a hybrid of *causal explanations*, which explain *why* an event or phenomenon occurs, and *mechanical explanations*, which explain *how* it occurs. Explanations of the CM sort explain why and how an event occurs; it does not tell us what the event is, or when it occurred, or where, and so forth. The CM model arises predominantly from Wesley Salmon's work (1984), who thought of CM explanations as what Wright called *etiological explanations* (Wright, 1976). I very much appreciate this terminology because it dovetails with the usage of "etiology" in medicine as the causal story why and how a disease occurs, which is why I have used that approach in my previous work as a model for explanations of illness occurrence (Dammann, 2017, 2020, 2021b).

To qualify as a scientific explanation, Salmon holds that an explanation needs to (i) refer to natural phenomena and (ii) be an answer to a why-question. Salmon's first point is in reference to natural phenomena, which requires a precise definition of what Salmon means by "natural phenomenon". Unfortunately, he does not provide one, but even without further instruction from Salmon himself, I think it is fair to assume that he intends to refer to physical, chemical, and biological phenomena as they occur in nature. If that is true, explaining the link between thunder and lightning or the etiology of breast cancer would be a scientific explanation, while an explanation of the mechanisms at work in a clock, car, or rocket would not. While these mechanisms can be reduced to physical phenomena, they are not natural phenomena, since clocks, cars, and rockets are not natural things but artifacts. Perhaps we should strip the above assumption of its "as they occur in nature" modifier and stick with "physical, chemical, and biological phenomena" only. This would include the engineering sciences among the sciences that use scientific explanations, which seems right. And this, in turn, would mean that non-scientific explanations are explanations outside physics, chemistry, biology, and engineering, excluding psychology, sociology, semiotics, mathematics as non-scientific, which does *not* seem right at least to those who think of these as fields of scientific inquiry. Luckily, Salmon only *seems* to restrict his characterization of scientific explanations to explanations of *natural* phenomena. Indeed, he states that

> [t]he main purpose of the present book is to examine the nature of scientific explanation [and] issues to be considered apply not only to modern physics but rather to the whole range of scientific disciplines from archaeology to zoology, including a great many that occupy alphabetically intermediate positions. (Salmon, 1984, p. 9)

According to this, we may feel comfortable applying Salmon's discussion, including his notion of scientific explanation, to all scientific disciplines. However, Salmon's focus on scientific *disciplines*, whether some or all, clearly indicates that he considers explanations scientific if they are used in the context of one or more scientific disciplines. According to this context-defined view, as opposed to Skow's explainer-defined view, any explanation that is used exclusively outside of the realm of science does not qualify as scientific. One way to specify this a bit further would be to say that Salmon's account appears to define scientific explanation as being used in the business of scientific practice (including the practice of scientific theory; again, this is what I think would be most helpful; v.i.). Another possible interpretation is that an explanation is scientific if it explains something scientific. It is not the context but content what distinguishes between scientific and non-scientific explanations. Salmon's account is not so much about who does the explaining, like Skow's scientists (let us call this the explainer view). It is also not about the context in which the explaining is done, i.e., in science (let's call this the context view). Instead, it is about what is being explained, i.e., the explanandum (content view). Of course, both context and content view leave much room for interpretation what makes the context or content of an explanation scientific.

Answers to Why-Questions

Salmon's second requirement is that scientific explanations ought to be answers to why-questions. He claims that "[i]t is crucially important to distinguish *scientific* explanations from such other types. [...] A request for a scientific explanation [...] can always be reasonably posed by means of a why-question" (ibid., p. 10; italics Salmon's). What he means is explanations that explain why and how a phenomenon occurs, a.k.a. etiological explanations. For example, Salmon distinguishes between explanations and *descriptions* by reference to the Port-Royal Logic (Arnauld & Nicole, f.p. 1964) and quotes the passage: "Our minds are not satisfied unless they know not only *that* a thing is but *why* it is" (PRL, 1964, p. 33 per (Salmon, 1984, p. 4)). Our non-scientific spatial, procedural, and temporal D-C explanations would count as explaining *that*, not as explaining *why*. What exactly is it that renders why-answers scientific while non-why-answers are non-scientific?

Woodward and Ross hold that scientific explanations can be distinguished from non-scientific explanations because they are "explanations of *why* things happen" (ibid.; the authors' italics). They suggest that one contrast entailed in the notion "scientific explanation" is the "contrast between those 'explanations' that are characteristic of 'science' and those explanations that are not" (Woodward & Ross, 2021, p. 3). Of course, we now need to ask what Woodward and Ross mean by "characteristic of 'science'". This is obviously not a trivial question, and Woodward and Ross seem to follow Salmon and the Port-Royal Logic by distinguishing explanatory from "merely descriptive" accounts, but they swiftly acknowledge that different accounts of explanation define such contrast in different ways. Interestingly, Woodward and Ross give an example of what they think all accounts of scientific explanation they discuss would agree *not* to be explanatory but merely descriptive, namely, "an account of the appearance of a particular species of bird of the sort found in a bird guidebook" (ibid., p. 4). They argue that such an account is, "however accurate, not an explanation of anything of interest to biologists". This introduces another way to distinguish between scientific and non-scientific explanation (next to explainer, content, and context views), i.e., by *concern*. But how do we know what is of interest to biologists and that descriptions of birds in bird guidebooks are *not* of interest to them? In all likelihood, Woodward and Ross do not mean to propose this distinction by concern as a valid criterion, simply because any explanation that explains *something* of interest to *some* biologists would count as a scientific explanation, such as an explanation of baseball rules to a biologist's grandchild, or of the peculiar location of the motor in a biologist's mid-engine car, and even the description of a capercaillie in the British Book of Birds if its biologist reader feels it is incorrect.

It is also sometimes said that explanations *in general* (not just those with the modifier "scientific" attached) are generally answers to why-questions. Of course, this would rid us of the option to use being an answer to a why-question to distinguish scientific from non-scientific explanations. For example, Skow (2016) holds that philosophical theories of explanation are simply not intended to cover what- and where-questions, but only "cases where someone explains *why* something is the case" (Skow's italics). Similarly, Bas van Fraassen (1980) refers to why-questions in Chap. 6 of his *Scientific Image*, stating that "[a]n explanation is an answer to a why-question. So, a theory of explanations must be a theory of why-questions" (van Fraassen, 1980, p. 134). Of note, van Fraassen does not say that "scientific explanations are answers to" but that "explanation is an answer to". Either he refers to *all* explanations including scientific explanations, or he *says* explanation, but *means* scientific explanation, as could be inferred from the broader topic of his book. In either case, van Fraassen's notion definitely includes scientific explanations. He does not, however, say explicitly that he thinks of all explanations as scientific.

If it is true that both explanations in general and scientific explanations are answers to why-questions, scientific explanations are either a proper subset of explanations in general, or the two sets are identical. In the first case, all scientific explanations would be explanations, but there are also non-scientific explanations. Unfortunately, the why-question distinction between scientific and non-scientific explanations doesn't work here because the non-scientific explanations would also be a proper subset of all explanations and therefore also be answers to why-questions. The second case of explanation/scientific explanation identity would mean there are no other explanations than scientific ones and Salmon's explanations of words, stories, and ways to get to a party could not be counted as explanations at all unless they are considered scientific for other reasons yet to be identified. The other two set-theoretical options don't need to be considered at all because (1) scientific explanations intersecting with explanations would leave at least some scientific explanations behind as non-explanations, which is a direct contradiction, and (2) being a completely separate non-overlapping set of explanations would be nonsensical since it would render all scientific explanations something that is not an explanation. In either case, the contradiction precludes the why-distinction. The only way out of this dilemma would be to assume that van Fraassen does indeed intend his why-distinction to hold for scientific explanations.

It seems reasonable to adopt the view that while all scientific explanations are answers to why-question, not all answers to why-questions are scientific explanations. In the philosophical literature, the opinion that *some* explanations are not scientific explanations abounds (examples above). In other words, the set of scientific explanations is considered a proper and non-identical subset of all answers to why-questions. Salmon briefly acknowledges this (Salmon, 1984, p. 10), giving as examples questions that ask for motivational reasons (like, e.g., "Why did you go to the drugstore today?" or "Why did God single out Job", and so on).

Non-scientific Explanations

Rejecting Skowian equivalence suggests that at least some philosophers think that there is such a thing as a non-scientific explanation. To support the notion that there is such a thing as a non-scientific explanation, one would need to show that there are explanations that still qualify as explanations while being non-scientific. This would be possible if, while all scientific explanations are explanations, not all explanations are scientific explanations. Of course, all of this does not align well with Skow's equivalence view. Nevertheless, eminent philosopher of explanation Wesley Salmon offers ordinary-life examples of non-scientific explanations, referring to explanations of words, stories, and directions to a party (Salmon, 1984, p. 10).

Intuition suggests that we use the term explanation for scientific explanations *and* for non-scientific ones as well. This becomes evident in the use of the term in ordinary-life situations, such as an explanation of my motivation not to have my hair cut for a few months (just because I can) or the explanation provided by the instruction booklet of how my new miter saw works (very well indeed, despite being battery driven). In fact, there are some philosophers who define "explanation" *very* broadly. For example, in his "critical notice" on van Fraassen's *Scientific Image*, Martin E. Gerwin writes that he defines "explanation as a set of true statements, one of which describes the phenomenon to be explained" (Gerwin, 1985, p. 363), which resonates with our D-C explanations above. For example, if you ask me "Where can I find the F.A.O. Schwartz bear in Boston", I provide an explanation in the form of an answer to a where-question by telling you to go to 800 Washington Street and take a look around. The explanation explains *where* you can find the bear. Let us call this a *spatial* explanation. And if you ask me how to get there and I recommend taking the orange line of the T (short for MBTA, the local public transportation agency in the Massachusetts Bay area, also a play on words referencing the "T(ea) Party" in Boston 1773) to the Tufts Medical Center stop, I provide another explanation that specifies *how* to get there. Let's call this a *procedural* explanation. If you ask further since when the bear has been where it is now, I provide an explanation that tells you since when it has been there by responding: "Since 2004". This could be classified as a *temporal* explanation. These types of explanation seem to be in keeping with the Wikipedia (D-C) definition quoted above.

I think that most of these explanations would be considered non-scientific by most philosophers. One may think of them as D-C explanations because they describe and clarify, but the capability to clarify is probably not sufficient to make a D-C explanation a scientific one. Why not? Although they are true in the sense of being factually correct and although they provide useful information, perhaps even increase the knowledge of the explainee, or at least update some of her beliefs, most would not call these scientific, simply because they do not serve the scientific purpose of increasing the understanding of phenomena that have not been understood before *by anyone*. On this view, an explanation that helps me understand how electricity works would not qualify as a scientific explanation while the explanation that helped us understand *for the first time* how electricity works would, although the utterance that communicates the explanation could be the same in both cases. This would be a functional account of scientific explanation that focuses on the function of the explanation regarding increase of *novel* understanding.

Let us take another look at the relationship between scientific explanations and answers to why-questions. The proposal seems to be that if an explanation is supposed to be a scientific one it needs to be a response to a why-question. If Salmon and Van Fraassen got it right and scientific explanations are answers to why-questions, responses to non-why-questions would not qualify as scientific explanations. A non-why-question may be defined as a question that does not ask "why?" and that cannot be rephrased as a why-question. Take, for example, the response "Water consists of two hydrogen and one oxygen atom" to the question "What is water?" This question cannot be sensibly rephrased as a why-question. Rephrasing it as "Why is water liquid?", "translucent?", and "wet?", etc., would not be a valid rephrasing. Thus, according to Salmon and Van Fraassen's why-question criterion, the H_2O-explanation would not count as a scientific explanation. At least to me, this is somewhat counterintuitive, considering that it does in fact explain the structure of water in scientific (physical-chemical) terms and that the information conferred by it may indeed be helpful in, or even necessary for, the conduct of certain scientific experiments and the understanding of certain scientific contexts. Therefore, I think it is permissible to say that the H_2O-explanation is in fact a scientific explanation, even though it cannot be rephrased as an answer to a why-question. This would now open the door for at least some answers to non-why-questions to be included among the members of the set of scientific explanations. While I agree that some answers to why-questions will not count as scientific explanations, I also think there is reason to think of at least some non-why-questions as being scientific. On this view, some of my earlier examples for spatial, procedural, and temporal questions would qualify as asking for a scientific explanation although they cannot be rephrased as a why-question. This allows for an account of scientific explanation as providing a response to why-questions or to non-why-questions of scientific concern, of content, or in scientific contexts. Let us call this the set of "scientific explanations defined in the broadest sense" view, henceforth abbreviated the "broad view".

Since it still seems difficult to pinpoint exactly what makes a scientific explanation scientific, let us take a look at what might make an explanation non-scientific. I already stated that I think that not being about a natural phenomenon or not being rephrasable as an answer to a why-question appears not to suffice. If that is true, what other criteria does an explanation need to fulfill in order not to count as a scientific explanation? I have argued above that the H_2O-explanation is a scientific explanation because it explains the explanandum in scientific terms (using the content view) and can be useful in scientific settings (context view). If that is true, one criterion, albeit arguably trivial, for a non-scientific explanation is that it has *nothing* to do with any scientific context, content, or concern. Is this where Salmon's Job and drugstore examples come in? Arguably, explanations of why God selected Job and why my neighbor went to the drugstore have, prima facie, nothing to do with science. However, could the former not become important in the science and theology discourse, and the latter in motivational psychology? We would need to define what kinds of activities we would grant the status of science and, accordingly, what kinds of activities would be considered scientific, so that explanations used in the context of such activities would be scientific, while explanations outside these activities would not. One (again, arguably trivial) way out would be to say that in some way or another *any and all* explanations could be useful in some scientific activity, however defined. Being potentially helpful in a scientific context seems too permissive a characterization of scientific explanations, simply because it would render *all* explanations potentially scientific.

Even for me as a sympathizer with the broad view, this seems to be too easy a way out. Intuitively speaking, there should be a context in which an explanation cannot be considered scientific in any way. Otherwise, all explanations would be scientific explanations. Luckily, in the spirit of good old falsificationism, we need only one black swan to show that not all swans are white. We need to show that there is indeed an explanation that cannot be scientific in any way to demonstrate that not all explanations are scientific in the broad sense.

To do this, it seems reasonable to search for the black non-scientific swan in the big pond of explanations. As an extreme example, astrology might be one. The explanation "Because you were born under the sign of Libra" to the question "Why do I like harmony, gentleness, and the outdoors?" will certainly not be considered a scientific question, despite being an answer to a why-question. Indeed, one could design a scientific study that compares a large group of Libras with a similarly large group of non-Libras regarding their personality types and being-outdoor-preferences as judged by questionnaires applied interview-style by interviewers who do not know the interviewee. In such a study, the accuracy of the explanation would be explored in what could reasonably be called a scientific setting. Ergo, the outdoors-because-Libra explanation would qualify as scientific under the broad view. However, we can respond with the simple move of rejecting the broad view as too broad and adopt another one, the "scientific as in the *practice of*" view, henceforth called the *narrow* view. On this view, an explanation is considered scientific only if it is used *for the purpose of doing science*, not if a priest explains why chemically speaking the water in the baptism font does not differ much from tap water (content) or if a molecular biologist explains why he failed to order the correct antibody for the experiment (context). This would, for example, render the above H_2O-explanation scientific if and only if it is used for the purpose of doing science, but not if it is used to explain what water consists of in a high-school chemistry class setting. Similarly, on the narrow view, the Libra-explanation would count as scientific in our Libra-study outlined above, as it is part of the scientific question to be answered by that study, i.e., "do

Libras appreciate harmony, gentleness, and the outdoors, while non-Libras don't". However, it would not count as scientific if it occurred during a friendly chat about astrological explanations between two scientists during a department holiday party. Obviously, this narrow view would lead to cases of the same explanation being scientific in one situation but non-scientific in others. Other narrow views, such as being scientific only if given by a scientist (explainer view), also don't seem right because scientific explanations should still be scientific if given by physicians or nurses.

It seems that we still have not found an acceptable mark for all scientific explanations among all explanations, apparently at least in part because we cannot (yet) properly distinguish between scientific and non-scientific explanation. However, at least for the time being, it seems that intuition suggests that there are both scientific and non-scientific explanations, although it is a bit tricky to find a suitable demarcation line between the two. Let us look a bit more into the idea that answers to why-questions are causal and, thus, scientific explanations.

Causal Explanation

Some authors have suggested that all explanations should be thought of as *causal* explanations. Salmon writes that

> [E]xplanation is a two-tiered affair. At the most basic level, it is necessary, to subsume the event-to-be-explained under an appropriate set of statistical relevance relations [...]. At the second level, [...] the statistical relevance relations that are invoked at the first level must be explained in terms of causal relations. (Salmon, 1984, p. 22) (Salmon's italics)

In other words, an explanation explains by providing an account of the *causal origin* of the event or phenomenon to be explained. Salmon's is not the only causal account of explanation. David Lewis also wrote that "to explain an event is to provide some information about its causal history" (Lewis, 1986, p. 217). He characterizes the act of explaining something to someone else in terms of the *transmission of information* (218) and holds that "[a] why-question [...] is a request for explanatory information" (229). However, as Dellsén observes, "since Salmon (1984) and Lewis (1986), not many philosophers have defended the view that *all* explanations are causal explanations" (Dellsén, 2016, p. 377). Bird lists no less than six kinds of theories of explanation, causal theories being one of them, and although he acknowledges that there may be some overlap, he asserts that "causal explanation is not a nomic explanation" (Bird, 1998, p. 62). Thus, it seems fair to say that not all would agree that all explanation is causal explanation.

Now, is all *scientific* explanation causal? For example, in his *Causal Explanation* Lewis rejects the idea that "there is such a thing as a non-causal explanation of particular events" (Lewis, 1986, p. 221). If indeed all explanations are causal, and if scientific explanations are a proper subset of all explanations, there cannot be such a thing as a non-causal scientific explanation. A recent discourse about non-causal explanation in philosophy of science suggests otherwise.[5] I do not want to rehash this discourse here for reasons of space and scope, but suffice it to say that this literature strongly suggests that there is such a thing as a non-causal explanation and that, relying on Lange, "non-causal explanations have long been recognized in both mathematics and science" (Lange, 2017, p. xii). I suspect that part of the reason for the increased interest in non-causal explanation is that some philosophers of science are unhappy about the ubiquitous brain stem reflex among members of their discipline who equate explanation with scientific explanation with causal explanation. In their introduction to the multi-author book *Explanation Beyond Causation*, Alexander Reutlinger and Juha Saatsi state their motivation for editing the book by pointing toward the *pragmatic* question, "what exactly scientists are doing and aiming to achieve when they explain something" (Reutlinger & Saatsi, 2018, p. 1). They stress that until roughly 2010, causal-mechanical explanations have been considered the paradigm of scientific explanation, but that since then, work on non-causal explanation of empirical phenomena has been on the rise. I will not go into much detail about their excellent collection of chapters on non-causal explanation, nor do I see the need to discuss single author works in the field such as Marc Lange's *Because Without Cause* (Lange, 2017). Suffice it to say that, apparently, in philosophical discourse about explanation, the main focus is on scientific explanation, and that providing a scientific explanation is considered basically the same as telling a story about why (and how) a phenomenon occurred. Thus, what is new in this literature is that some non-causal explanations seem to explain empirical phenomena, in other words, the occurrence of events out in the observable real world. Some examples of non-causal explanation in science are mathematical explanations (the focus of Lange's book). Reutlinger and Saatsi give a fun toy example, asking what explains the fact that 23 strawberries cannot be distributed equally among 3 philosophers (4). But is the answer to the 23 strawberries question really a non-causal explanation? Is the question not asking what gives rise to the impossibility to divide 23 by 3 without remainder, and is this "what gives rise to" not equivalent to a why-question, answers to which are frequently thought of as causal (or causal-mechanical)? Could one not say that the rules of arithmetic are the cause and our tendency to follow rules is the mechanism? Together this would represent a full causal-mechanical (etiologic) explanation of how the fact came about. Moreover, the fact that the required explanation isn't really required to explain an event but a fact does not distinguish between causal and non-causal explanations. Facts are generated by events at some point, which can be explained by a causal-mechanical explanation; in this sense, it is possible to give a causal-mechanical explanation not only for events but also for facts. What explains the fact that I see the backside of a big urban hospital when I look out of my office window? A story about how the two buildings involved were built at some point in downtown Boston (on land taken from the local Chinatown community[6] and before then from the Massachusett tribes) and that I am sitting in one looking at the other would, arguably, count as a cause, and some story involving matter and light, my retina and visual cortex would count as a mechanism. Lange refers to examples like the 23 strawberries question as distinctively mathematical explanations, which he distinguishes from "ordinary scientific explanations that use mathematics" (Lange, 2017, p. 9) by reference to the fact that their explanandum is *necessary*.[7]

What is the relationship between causal explanations and answers to why-questions? If causal questions are *always* asked with sentences starting on "Why", then being a causal explanation and an answer to a why-question is one and the same. However, if it is possible to ask a causal question without invoking "why", then the two are somehow different. For example, in Salmon's causal-mechanical model of explanation, which amalgamates causes and mechanisms into causal-mechanical processes, the causal component might be an answer to a why-question, but the mechanical component answers a how-question as well.

Another example comes from David-Hillel Ruben, who asks "Are all singular explanations causal explanations?" (Ruben, 1990, p. 209). Like other philosophers who meander between "explanation" and "scientific explanation", Ruben admits that "throughout the book I have moved rather freely between "explanation" and "causal explanation". Thus, if

Ruben can toggle between explanation and causal explanation without harm, and if all scientific explanations are indeed causal explanations, at least to some extent the meandering could be among all three entities. It would not matter whether we talk about explanations, scientific explanations, or causal explanations: everything we say could be meant to hold interchangeably for all three entities.

This seems highly unlikely. Still, the relationship between the concepts of explanation, scientific explanation, and causal explanation is far from clear, which is mainly due to a certain blurriness of their boundaries as per our above discussion. Indeed, Woodward and Ross (2021) write that "[t]he boundaries of the category 'scientific explanation' are far from clear" (ibid., p. 13) In particular, I am interested in their set-theoretical relationships based on how they are supposed to do their explanatory work. Do they overlap, forming intersections, and to what extent? Is one a proper subset of another one? From our preliminary and superficial discussion above, it seems that the answer is that explanation, scientific explanation, and causal explanation are different things while there is room for the possibility that they overlap, although the inter-conceptual demarcation lines remain unclear at times. Still, it seems right to say that explanations *include* scientific explanations, some of which are causal explanations while others are not, leaving some room for explanations that are both non-scientific and non-causal.

This gives rise to the possibility that there might be some kind of non-causal, non-why type of explanation that may *still be relevant to science* and which, therefore, may potentially be worthy of philosophers of science's attention. In particular, I am interested in clarifying whether there really is a good reason to exclude answers to *how-, what-, where-, who-, when-*questions, and so forth, from the pool of *scientific* explanations, for example, just because they cannot be rephrased as a why-question?

FOUR TYPES OF EXPLANATION

What are the things that call for an explanation in medicine? I have previously suggested a workflow-based framework for explanation in public health (Dammann, 2022) that I believe can serve as a blueprint for explanation in medicine as well. What types of explanation are used to do the explaining and what are their functions in medical and population health practice? In what follows, I will be flexible regarding the distinction between *public health* and *population health* but will attempt to be mindful of potential differences when it comes to issues of explanation. In broad terms, I suggest thinking of *public health* as the institutionalized effort to protect the public's health and of *population health* as the health of populations, pragmatically defined by some as groups with >1 member (Keyes & Galea, 2016).

The simple four-step schema depicted in Fig. 6.1 illustrates the sequence of tasks for medical and population health practitioners. It begins (somewhat arbitrarily since one could jump into the cycle at any point) with a health *assessment* of patient or population and continues with a work plan, a *definition* of goals. If an *intervention* is deemed necessary and appropriate it is implemented, followed by an *evaluation* of success. Again, these four consecutive steps do not differ much between medicine and population health.

The kinds of explanation used in medicine vary according to what is being explained (explanandum), what kind of information is used to do the explaining (explanans), and for what purpose the explanation is given.

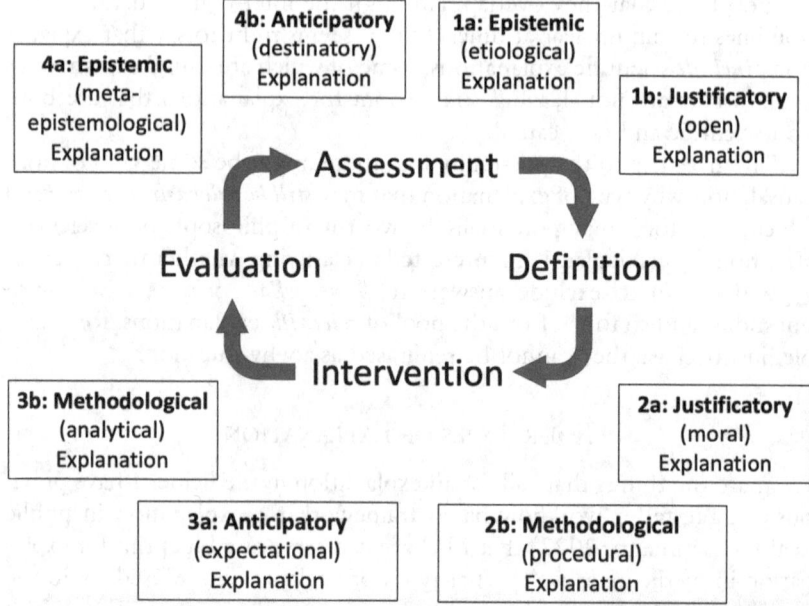

Fig. 6.1 Workflow-based framework for explanation in medicine and public health

In what follows, I propose to distinguish four kinds of explanation that are used for four different purposes: to generate knowledge (*epistemic* explanation),[8] to explain the rationale for the action (*justificatory* explanation), to clarify data design and analysis (*methodological* explanation), and to plan further steps (*anticipatory* explanation)[9] (Table 6.1). I do not mean to suggest that this list exhausts all possible kinds of explanation used in medicine and public health, just those that I find most helpful in understanding the explanatory work done in the context of the health workflow cycle.

The following subsections briefly touch on each of the four *kinds* of explanation, i.e., epistemic, justificatory, methodological, and anticipatory. Note that I propose two *types* for each kind, which results in eight types of explanation (as outlined in Fig. 6.1 and Table 6.1) that are part of the transition from each of the four activities in the healthwork cycle. My examples will be mainly from population health, but similar examples can be given for medicine as well.

Epistemic Explanation

One of the main ways to collect the necessary evidence for public health is surveillance. Public health surveillance is defined as "the ongoing,

Table 6.1 Characteristics of kinds and types of explanation in medicine and population health

Kind	Type	Explanandum	Explanans	No. in Fig. 6.1
Epistemic	Etiological	Occurrence	Causal-mechanical origin	1a
	Meta-epistemological	Knowledge gain	Description of knowledge gained	4a
Justificatory	Open	Reason for action	Justification of action	1b
	Moral	Obligation to act	Moral justification	2a
Methodological	Procedural	Intervention method	Means of intervention	2b
	Analytical	Success measurement	Means of measurement	3b
Anticipatory	Expectational	Expected results	Clarify expected outcome	3a
	Destinatory	What's next?	Description of plan	4b

systematic collection, analysis, and interpretation of health data, essential to the planning, implementation and evaluation of public health practice, closely integrated with the dissemination of these data to those who need to know and linked to prevention and control" (Hall et al., 2012).

The Centers for Disease Control and Prevention (CDC) in the United States consider surveillance "the cornerstone of public health practice" (Richards et al., 2014). Surveillance provides data that help "detect and monitor diseases, injuries, and conditions; assess the impact of interventions; and assist in the management of large-scale disease incidents" (Richards et al., 2014, p. 472). For the detection of *occurrence*, a target condition is defined, and surveillance staff and technology tools are prepared to detect the occurrence of that target condition to an extent higher than expected. Data are accumulated over a defined time period and compared to expected occurrence numbers. For example, if an infectious disease occurs more frequently than expected in a certain area over a certain period of time, this would be considered an outbreak.

However, this evidence is not provided by surveillance alone. Another important source of data is epidemiologic research, the branch of the health sciences that is charged with the design, conduct, and analysis of population-based studies to understand the distribution and determinants of health and disease in populations (Rothman et al., 2021). Contrary to popular belief, fueled by its prominent role in the media during the COVID-19 pandemic, epidemiology is not just the science of epidemics. Infectious disease epidemiology is only one branch among many in modern epidemiology. Epidemiologists study the occurrence (prevalence, incidence) of practically *any* health phenomenon in populations under the heading *descriptive epidemiology* and the statistical association (often mislabeled "correlation") between purportedly causal risk factors (exposures) and any kind of illness (outcome) using *analytical epidemiology* methods. Modern epidemiological theory started with predominantly methodological considerations in the 1970s (MacMahon & Pugh, 1970) and 1980s (Kleinbaum et al., 1982; Miettinen, 1985; Rothman, 1986) and has reached new heights with Nancy Krieger's ecosocial theory of health (Krieger, 2001; Krieger, 2011), Miguel A. Hernán and James M. Robins' framework for causal inference (Hernán & Robins, 2020), and Tyler VanderWeele's explanatory approach (VanderWeele, 2015).

For VanderWeele, an explanation is putting a phenomenon "with a particular context so that the phenomenon is better understood" (VanderWeele, 2015, p. 7), which dovetails with the Merriam-Webster definition of explanation referred to above. His main topic is epidemiological modelling tools for the analysis of mediation, which he briefly defines as "the phenomenon whereby a cause affects its intermediate and the change in the intermediate goes on to affect the outcome" (VanderWeele, 2015, p. 7), and interaction, which "relate[s] to when, and for whom, a cause affects a particular outcome" (VanderWeele, 2015, p. 9). On this view, a *mediator* is just that an intermediate factor that provides the link between cause and effect. *Interaction*, on the other hand, is a somewhat more complex concept but more important for population health science. In much simplified terms, interaction is a phenomenon of "mixed effects", which results in different magnitudes of influence of cause C on effect E in strata defined by the presence or absence of a third factor F. In other words, the CE relationship R_{CE} among individuals with F differs appreciably from R_{CE} among individuals without F. Stated formally: $(R_{CE}|F) \neq (R_{CE} |\neg F)$. In public health, the importance of this phenomenon is obvious because one needs to know whether the effect of some intervention should be expected to be different in one subpopulation with F compared to one without F. Identifying factor F in this scenario would obviously have enormous impact on whether and how the intervention would be implemented. The same holds for clinical (medical) contexts as well, illustrating the general import of clinical epidemiological methods and findings as a basis for medical action. For example, Paul M. Ridker and colleagues conducted a randomized trial of low-dose aspirin in almost 40,000 women aged 45 or older and followed them for 10 years and registered the occurrence of cardiovascular events and stroke (Ridker et al., 2005). While the intervention was associated with a risk reduction for myocardial infarction by 34% among women 65 years or older, it did not affect this risk in younger women. This result has obvious consequences for physicians' prescription decisions.

Etiological explanations (#1a in Fig. 6.1) abound in public health because they unify explanations that refer to the causes of illness and to the mechanisms that provide the connection between causes and the illness they cause. Thus, *causal* explanations are etiological explanations that clarify the causal origin, while *mechanical* explanations clarify the mechanical origin of disease. Taken together, this is what Wesley C. Salmon called a causal-mechanical or etiological explanation (Salmon, 1984); see also (Dammann, 2020). One simple example of an etiological explanation is the explanation of health disparities by reference to socioeconomic status (cause) and stress (mechanism) (Adler & Rehkopf, 2008).

The causal-mechanical model represents only one of multiple philosophical accounts of *scientific* explanation. The earlier *deductive-nomological* (or "covering law") model proposed by Carl Hempel (Hempel, 1962), the D-N model, as it is now often abbreviated, states that one or more accepted laws, such as those of thermodynamics, in addition to one or more particular contextual facts about a certain event, e.g., a metal lid is stuck on a glass jar and the jar is put in hot water, *jointly explain* the fact that the metal lid comes off the jar easily once the jar is taken out of the water. Another type of explanation, *unificationist* explanation, was introduced by Michael Friedman, who started his 1974 paper with the question of what connects explanation to scientific understanding (Friedman, 1974), a question that Hempel (according to Friedman) shied away from for being psychological and, thus, not to be considered part of logic. Friedman argued that, in essence, providing a scientific explanation is to provide a comprehensive statement that unifies multiple less comprehensive statements. He further argued that since understanding is global, not limited to single instances of phenomena to be explained, we "genuinely increase our understanding of the world" by replacing one statement with a more comprehensive statement, which reduces the total number of accepted statements (Friedman, 1974, p. 19). Friedman's version of unificationist explanation was later modified by Philip Kitcher, who suggested that the number of types of premises accepted as underived can be minimized by reducing the *number* of argument patterns that derive *many* beliefs (Kitcher, 1981).

In the above accounts of explanation, an increased intelligibility and, ultimately, understanding is part of the goal. In our framework of explanation in medicine and public health, a *meta-epistemological* explanation (#4a in Fig. 6.1) is one that increases our knowledge about our knowledge; it increases the number of facts that we know about the number of facts we know. This sounds much more complicated than it is. In our context, a meta-epistemological explanation is nothing more than a clarification of what we have learned from a public health intervention project. This type of explanation would be any explanation that refers to the results of an intervention study that has yielded new knowledge. For example, a community intervention program initiated to reduce smoking among women yielded results that suggest that community involvement improves the success rate of such program (Secker-Walker et al., 2000). Here, the novel piece of information is the community participation bit and any explanation that refers to this bit would count as a meta-epistemological explanation.

Justificatory Explanation

These explanations are given to justify action. Whoever is in a decision-making position for a public health program will require a solid justification for an action to be taken. The response to the request *What justifies this intervention?* is an explanation that is given to justify or warrant the intervention. Ruth Faden and Sirine Shebaya have argued that the broad mission of public health to protect and improve the health of populations is too broad to appropriately justify some public health interventions (Faden & Shebaya, 2019). They identify five justifications that may justify public health interventions: "(1) overall benefit, (2) collective action and efficiency, (3) fairness in the distribution of burdens, (4) prevention of harm (the harm principle), and (5) paternalism".

I will now very briefly refer to three main ways to justify an action in public health: scientific, economic (both are subsumed under the subtype *open;* #1b in Fig. 6.1 and Table 6.1), and moral (#2a).

Scientific justification requires explanations that refer to scientific reasons or desiderata. This type of explanation is not to be confused with scientific explanations (see above). Justificatory explanations of the scientific type simply cite scientific reasons in support of a justificatory statement. In other words, a scientific justificatory explanation refers to a scientific *need* as a justification for action. Perhaps the most frequently employed scientific justificatory explanation is the one given in the background section of scientific grant applications. This usually reads something like: "We want to study the phenomenon P. Previous research has revealed that P is caused by C, but the mechanism M remains to be elucidated. In this application, we propose a series of experiments designed to characterize M".

Economic justification is the purpose of explanations that cite expected economic gains or losses as reasons why some action should or should not be taken in public health. Comparative economic analysis techniques are involved, such as cost-effectiveness, cost-benefit, cost-utility analyses, and so on. A study from the UK revealed that decision-makers apparently prefer to base their decisions on more complex and detailed methods rather than on simpler ones (Phillips et al., 2011). The growing field of public health economics (Edwards et al., 2013) is complex and multifaceted, and represents a formidable target area for further philosophical inquiry.

Moral justification (Fig. 6.1, #2a) can be provided by offering moral reasons why an action is warranted. Ross Upshur has conveniently summarized the principles to be considered in the justification of public health interventions (Upshur, 2002). He discusses the harm, least restrictive means, reciprocity, and transparency principles. These principles can be viewed, individually or together, as reference points for justificatory explanations. The harm principle, as outlined in John Stuart Mill's *On Liberty*, holds that personal freedom cannot be rightfully constrained unless such limitations are imposed in order to prevent others from harm. Upshur suggests that the harm principle is "perhaps the foundational principle for public health ethics in a democratic society" (Upshur, 2002, p. 102). For example, mandatory face masks during the most serious phases of the COVID-19 pandemic can be justified by the argument that the mask-associated reduction of personal comfort is far outweighed by the beneficial population effect on disease incidence and mortality. The least restrictive means principle requires that public health policies should implement and exhaust less invasive interventions before more draconian measures are initiated. To stay with our previous example, mandatory face masks are considered less restrictive than mandatory sheltering in place. Reciprocity refers to the right of the individual to be compensated for losses due to public health interventions. Transparency covers the need to design decision-making processes in a fair manner that includes all stakeholders, free discourse among them, and the absence of political or financial interests, among others.

Methodological Explanation

At first glance, methodological explanations seem to be justifications of why certain methods are used. I think, however, that the primary motivation for this type of explanation is to simply describe methodology, just like etiological explanations describe the causal-mechanical genesis of a phenomenon. In public health, methodological explanations explain the details of intervention procedures and data analysis. To explain why a particular method is used is a *scientific* justificatory explanation that details scientific reasons for such usage.

Any public health intervention will be implemented in a particular way. The creation and provision of an intervention methodology explanation

(#2b in Fig. 6.1) in the form of a detailed intervention implementation plan is necessary for stakeholders to understand what kind of intervention is planned and what its implementation will mean for them and their constituents.

Public health nursing is one of the areas of public health in which a considerable amount of work has been done to specify what kinds of interventions public health entails. Linda Olson Keller and colleagues have developed a framework for public health intervention known as the Intervention Wheel for population-based public health practice (Keller et al., 1998, 2004). The Wheel is a graphical depiction of its three equally important core aspects: interventions are population-based; they are implemented at the level of the individual/family, community, or system; and there are 17 different types of public health interventions that are further specified in the model.

Once a public health program is implemented, its success (or failure) needs to be evaluated. An analysis plan is needed that explains the methods that are to be used in program evaluation (#3b in Fig. 6.1). Bobby Milstein and Scott Wetterhall have proposed a framework for program evaluation that consists of six steps: stakeholder engagement, program description, focusing the evaluation design, evidence gathering, conclusion justification, ensuring usage and lessons learned. Interestingly, the second item (program description) comes rather close to our aforementioned explanation of intervention methodology: "Before stakeholders can talk about evaluating a program, they should agree on what the program is. They must describe the program in enough detail to ensure a solid understanding of its mission, objectives, and strategies" (Milstein & Wetterhall, 2016). Part of the explanation of analysis methods should be whether the data to be analyzed are quantitative, qualitative, or mixed methods.

Anticipatory Explanation

Anticipatory explanations are forward looking by definition. They explain by reference to future events, not to things that have happened in the past (see also Chap. 9 on prospective explanation). In other words, both the explanans and the explanandum of anticipatory explanations have yet to occur. In the context of the healthwork cycle depicted in Fig. 6.1, we can offer *expectational* explanations in public health in the form of statements like, for example, "We expect this program to reduce the number of opioid overdoses by 10% over the next twelve months". *Destinatory* explanations are visionary statements of what the plans are for the future development of affairs.

Expectational explanations (#3a in Fig. 6.1) outline what future state of affairs one expects to be the case under defined circumstances and why. In the public health workflow, they simply explain the results that are expected if a defined intervention is implemented in a certain way. On a superficial level, expectational explanations are merely descriptive, serving the purpose of an outline for the uninformed. On a deeper level, they can also serve as a justificatory explanation, when used to mount an argument in support of the initiation of a program.

The final kind of explanation, *destinatory explanation*, outlines the plan for moving forward after a public health project is completed (#4b in Fig. 6.1). It is exemplified by the questions from the audience to the speaker after a presentation at a scientific conference like "Now that you are done with this project, what are your next steps?" or "What else needs to be done to achieve your long-term research goal?" I would be remiss not to mention that destinatory explanations are not teleological explanations (Stout, 1996; Wright, 1976). The latter explain facts (mainly actions) by reference to the actor's reasons to act. The former are explanations of where things are going or are expected to go in the future. While teleological explanations always have a causal connotation (the reason being the cause of the action), destinatory explanations do not.

EIGHT EXPLANATORY FUNCTIONS

In the previous section I have already touched upon the eight types of explanation used in the healthwork cycle. In this section I outline how they are plugged into the cycle as the work proceeds from beginning to end. It might be helpful if you follow the healthwork process in Fig. 6.1 while reading this section.

Assessment to definition: As a first step in the development of a public health program, public health workers must be able to assess the state of the health of their target population accurately. Usually, those in charge of public health activities work in municipal or regional (in the United States: county or state) departments of public health. They are charged with overseeing public health activities to support the population residing in their catchment area. For their work to be evidence-based, the department has to collect evidence, that is, valid information about the state of health in this population, which is a research activity guided by scientific principles. How is the occurrence of disease explained? An *epistemic/etiological* explanation needs to be provided that tells decision-makers *why* and *how* a certain assessment result occurs (Fig. 6.1, #1a). In the evidence-based public health framework (Brownson et al., 2009), this explanation is based on type 1 scientific evidence, that is, data on the "size and strength of preventable risk—disease relationship (measures of burden, etiologic research)" (Brownson et al., 2009, p. 179).

Before data from surveillance and epidemiological studies can be turned into a definition of public health action, an explanation needs to be given that specifies *why* the collected data justify a certain public health action (#1b). This *justificatory/open* explanation is called "open" because it needs to employ all kinds of justification (scientific, moral, economic, and so on). In the context of dangerous infectious diseases, this seems trivial and is, obviously, done a long time in advance and not just when the need arises. With other health indicators, however, such as a novel clustering of cancer cases in a certain community, the justificatory explanation will be made only after the new data have become available.

Definition to intervention: Public health agencies like the Centers for Disease Control and Prevention (CDC) in the United States are mainly concerned with the definition of health issues for which surveillance measures are to be developed. They have generated a list of criteria that specify the scope of the public health problem, the ability to control it, and the public health system capacity needed to implement proper control measures (CDC, 2012). In the UK, the COVID-19 pandemic triggered the creation of a new agency in 2021, the UK Health Security Agency (UKHSA), which is charged with infectious disease surveillance, prevention, and response. It is government agencies like these that decide how threats to the public's health are to be defined.

To declare a population health measure as an indicator of a health burden that requires amelioration, public health researchers, agencies, and politicians must offer a *justificatory/moral* explanation why an intervention is warranted (#2a). Of course, this also helps justifying the intervention plan and is, therefore, also a justificatory explanation. Next, a *methodological/procedural* explanation is needed to clarify what sort of intervention is likely to ameliorate the situation and how it is supposed to work (#2b).

Intervention to evaluation: The expected results will be explained by means of an *anticipatory/expectational* explanation before the intervention is initiated and such explanation of expected results is sometimes refined while the intervention is implemented (#3a). Concomitantly, it needs to be explained in what ways the outcome of the intervention will be evaluated. This is a *methodological/analytical* explanation that specifies the technical ways of outcome evaluation (#3b).

Evaluation to assessment: When the evaluation is completed, it is time to ask what has been learned. What exactly is the knowledge added by the project? This knowledge gain (if any) is explained in the form of an *epistemic/meta-epistemological* explanation (#4a). Since this is an explanation that increases our knowledge about our knowledge, I count it as a scientific explanation.

One interesting topic in this context is the purported explanatory opacity of some artificial intelligence approaches used in health data analysis (Amann et al., 2020). What can we know about our knowledge gain if it comes from machine learning algorithms whose results are not interpretable? I have argued elsewhere that there might be ways to use computational models of illness occurrence as providers of etio-prognostic explanations (Dammann, 2021a).

The last type of explanation before the workflow cycle arrives back at the beginning is the *anticipatory/destinatory* explanation of what is to come next (#4b). In our current context, this will be an explanation of the next steps (changes to process, especially new forms of assessment, and so on).

Comments & Caveats

What is the role for explanation (broadly construed) in the curbing of medical uncertainty? First and foremost, let me reiterate that explanation cannot reduce A-uncertainty because A-uncertainty cannot be modified but it is what it is. For example, the average response rate to a certain drug will never be exactly the same in different populations simply because it is A-uncertain. It may be that with increasingly large numbers of individuals in said populations the average response rates may approach each other and even converge at some point. However, these are average response rates, not the response to be expected in individual members of the population.

By offering explanations about the etiology, diagnosis, intervention, and prognosis in the medical workflow, it is possible to curb the unwanted consequences of the E-uncertainty about the individual patient's disease history, diagnosis, treatment, and prognosis. While it might not be possible to reduce the component of the E-uncertainty that is due to the A-uncertainty in these contexts, it is certainly possible to curb the component of the E-uncertainty that is due to the lack of knowledge *about* A- and E-uncertainty. I strongly believe that an honest attempt to offer comprehensive explanations in medicine will help patients and medics alike to tackle the uncertainties they face. Again, I do not suggest that offering comprehensive and detailed explanations is capable of removing uncertainty in medicine. I intend to indicate that while it is impossible to remove A-uncertainty, it might be possible to curb E-uncertainty in the sense of keeping it at bay.

The way I have used use the term *explanation* in this chapter is very broad and goes deliberately beyond the definition of scientific explanation, because reference to science is only one component of reasoning in medicine and public health. Thus, the types of explanation I have proposed and discussed include non-scientific explanations that are used for the communication of assumptions, expectations, reasons, as well as knowledge about facts, not for the process of knowledge *generation*, the hallmark of scientific activities. In particular, I have departed appreciably from the traditional philosophical concept of explanation as closely and perhaps *exclusively* related to causal inference. Instead, I have offered a smorgasbord of explanations employed for different purposes in medicine practice.

One important objection to the framework of explanation types offered in this chapter is that one may say that except for scientific explanations, the other types just are not explanations at all, but justifications, descriptions, predictions, outlines of plans, and so on. On my view, the components of these terms (e.g., justification and explanation) are not mutually exclusive, but one specifies what the other does. In this regard, I propose to distinguish between *models* of explanation (e.g., the D-N model, the causal-mechanical model, and unificationist models of explanation) and *kinds* of explanation as those listed in Table 6.1. While models of explanation are defined by how philosophers think explanation works, types of explanation are defined by what explanations do.

Of course, my proposed framework is just one possible view of the medical and population health workflow and the kinds (and types) of explanation used therein. I am certain that many others can be construed and some of these will probably be more helpful than the one presented here. Of note, the framework is not intended for usage in other contexts. Most certainly do I not intend to propose a framework for explanation in general. However, it may very well be that some of the classification of explanations depicted in Table 6.1 can be used in other contexts. However, such usage would need to be justified before the backdrop of that other context. There is just no one-size-fits-all solution.

Maël Lemoine begins his handbook chapter on explanation in medicine with the statement that "the scientific part of medicine seeks explanations" (Lemoine, 2017, p. 296). He continues with a call for inclusion of multiple types of explanation in medicine such as "molecular, epidemiological, psychiatric, pathophysiological, social, ..." explanations. I would like to offer two comments. First, I do not think that there is such a thing as the scientific part of medicine (as outlined in Chap. 3). Medicine has no scientific part. At least, individuals working in medicine *and* science are the exception, not the rule.[10] The vast majority of medics care for patients, organize, and optimize that care, and improve it. While they may use scientific data, they do not generate them; they do not *do* the science. The science is done by medical and health scientists like bioscientists, who generate mechanical explanations, and by epidemiologists, who generate causal explanations (Dammann, 2020). Second, Lemoine's list of "types" of explanation is confused in terms of being based on different classification systems. Molecules are biological entities; psychiatry is part of medicine; and epidemiology, pathophysiology, and sociology are branches of science and thus activities outside clinical medicine. In the remainder of his chapter, Lemoine distinguishes between deductive-nomological, deductive-statistical, and mechanistic models of explanation. While this is clearly in keeping with the traditional accounts of explanation in philosophy of science and certainly a potentially useful approach, I hope that the purpose-driven framework of explanation I propose in this chapter will be helpful in providing a purpose-driven roadmap for explanation in medicine and public health.

We must keep in mind what kinds of stakeholders in medicine offer the explanation and who are the ones supposed to benefit. Who is the explainer and who is the explainee? Assuming that it will most often be the health professionals who do the explaining, while the recipients are patients, health policymakers, and the general public, we may need to consider whether different perceptions of truth and knowledge might affect the explanatory process and success. The attempt to successfully explain a planned public health program—for example, mask wearing in public—to a community whose members subscribe to the notion of "fake news" maybe futile. Public trust is of paramount importance in a healthy public discourse. This has important ramification for medicine and public health, for example, in the context of explaining the benefits of vaccination to individuals and to populations. One important example of philosophical work in this realm is Maya Goldenberg's argument that vaccination hesitancy is not due to science illiteracy but due to lack of trust in science (Goldenberg, 2021).

My discussion in this chapter comes from a western perspective (I trained as a medical doctor in Germany and as an epidemiologist in the United States). Alex Broadbent and Benjamin Smart have made a cogent argument that in public health policy, "ignoring local social and cultural factors is a mistake" (Broadbent & Smart, 2020, p. 405). On this view, it is objectionable if a public health intervention ignores the specific sociocultural background of the population it serves. I suggest that the same is true for medicine. Accordingly, any attempt to curb uncertainty by explanation should include not only scientific and medical facts but also consider "local social and cultural factors".

NOTES

1. See https://www.merriam-webster.com/thesaurus/explanation; accessed 15 September 2021 and https://www.britannica.com/topic/explanation; accessed 16 July 2021.
2. https://en.wikipedia.org/wiki/Explanation; accessed 7/20/2021. The author of the entry cites as the source for this definition Drake, J. *Introduction to Logic*. EP TECH PRESS 2018, pp. 160–161.
3. Explanations of why *and* how are explanations that go beyond causal explanations by providing information about the causes (why) and mechanism (how) some phenomenon occurs. See Chap. 10 in (Salmon, 1984) and (Dammann, 2020).
4. *The American Heritage Dictionary*. Second College edition. Houghton Mifflin, Boston, 1982: 477.
5. See, for example, (Dellsén, 2016; Lange, 2017; Reutlinger & Saatsi, 2018; Ruben, 1990; Skow, 2015).
6. See (Leong, 2019) for a summary of the struggle.

7. In addition to his account of "explanation by constraint", Lange also discusses two other non-causal accounts of explanation, i.e., "really statistical explanations" and "dimensional explanations" (Lange, 2017).
8. I have previously called this kind "scientific explanation" (Dammann, 2022). This was unfortunate because it muddles the terminology with respect to the standard meaning of the term in philosophy of science.
9. I have previously called this "prospective" explanation (Dammann, 2022). This collides with the more general way I now use the term (see Chap. 8).
10. Indeed, the physician-scientist is a vanishing breed (Yeravdekar & Singh, 2022).

References

Adler, N. E., & Rehkopf, D. H. (2008). U.S. disparities in health: Descriptions, causes, and mechanisms. *Annual Review of Public Health, 29*(1), 235–252.

Amann, J., Blasimme, A., Vayena, E., Frey, D., & Madai, V. I. (2020). Explainability for artificial intelligence in healthcare: A multidisciplinary perspective. *BMC Medical Informatics and Decision Making, 20*(1), 310.

Arnauld, A., & Nicole, P. (1964). *The Art of Thinking; Port-Royal Logic.* Indianapolis: Bobbs-Merrill.

Audi, R. (1999). *The Cambridge dictionary of philosophy* (2nd ed.). Cambridge University Press.

Bird, A. (1998). *Philosophy of science.* Routledge.

Broadbent, A., & Smart, B. (2020). Kinds of explanation in public health policy. In J. Sholl & S. Rattan (Eds.), *Explaining health across the sciences* (pp. 405–415). Springer.

Brownson, R. C., Fielding, J. E., & Maylahn, C. M. (2009). Evidence-based public health: A fundamental concept for public health practice. *Annual Review of Public Health, 30*, 175–201.

CDC. (2012). *Public health surveillance: Preparing for the future.*

Dammann, O. (2017). The etiological stance: Explaining illness occurrence. *Perspectives in Biology and Medicine, 60*(2), 151–165.

Dammann, O. (2020). *Etiological explanations: Illness causation theory.* CRC Press.

Dammann, O. (2021a). Agent-based models as etio-prognostic explanations. *Argumenta, 1,* 19–38.

Dammann, O. (2021b). Evidence mapping to justify health interventions. *Perspectives in Biology and Medicine, 64*(2), 155–172.

Dammann, O. (2022). Explanation in Public Health. In S. Venkatapuram & A. Broadbent (Eds.), *Routledge handbook of the philosophy of public health.* Routledge.

Dellsén, F. (2016). There may yet be non-causal explanations. *Journal for General Philosophy of Science, 47*(2), 377–384.

De Regt, H. (2017). *Understanding Scientific Understanding*. Oxford University Press.

Edwards, R. T., Charles, J. M., & Lloyd-Williams, H. (2013). Public health economics: A systematic review of guidance for the economic evaluation of public health interventions and discussion of key methodological issues. *BMC Public Health, 13*, 1001.

Faden, R. R., & Shebaya, S. (2019). Public health programs and policies: Ethical justifications. In A. C. Mastroianni, J. P. Kahn, & N. E. Kass (Eds.), *The Oxford handbook of public health ethics* (pp. 20–32). Oxford University Press.

Friedman, M. (1974). Explanation and scientific understanding. *Journal of Philosophy, 71*(1), 5–19.

Gerwin, M. E. (1985). Bas van Fraassen, the scientific image. *Canadian Journal of Philosophy, 15*(2), 363–378.

Goldenberg, M. (2021). *Vaccine hesitancy*. University of Pittsburg Press.

Hall, H. I., Correa, A., Yoon, P. W., Braden, C. R., & Centers for Disease, C., & Prevention. (2012). Lexicon, definitions, and conceptual framework for public health surveillance. *MMWR Surveillance Summaries, 61*, 10–14.

Hempel, C. G. (1962). Deductive-nomological versus statistical explanation. In H. Feigl & G. Maxwell (Eds.), *Scientific explanation, space, and time* (Vol. III, pp. 98–169). University of Minnesota Press.

Hernán, M. A., & Robins, J. M. (2020). *Causal inference: What if? In*. Chapman & Hall/CRC.

Keller, L. O., Strohschein, S., Lia-Hoagberg, B., & Schaffer, M. (1998). Population-based public health nursing interventions: A model from practice. *Public Health Nursing, 15*(3), 207–215.

Keller, L. O., Strohschein, S., Lia-Hoagberg, B., & Schaffer, M. A. (2004). Population-based public health interventions: Practice-based and evidence-supported. Part I. *Public Health Nursing, 21*(5), 453–468.

Keyes, K. M., & Galea, S. (2016). *Population health science*. Oxford University Press.

Kitcher, P. (1981). Explanatory unification. *Philosophy of Science, 48*(4), 507–531.

Kitcher, P. (1989). Explanatory unification and the causal structure of the world. In P. Kitcher & W. Salmon (Eds.), *Scientific explanation* (Vol. 8, pp. 410–505). University of Minnesota Press.

Kleinbaum, D. G., Kupper, L. L., & Morgenstern, H. (1982). *Epidemiologic research: Principles and quantitative methods*. Lifetime Learning Publications.

Krieger, N. (2001). Theories for social epidemiology in the 21st century: An ecosocial perspective. *International Journal of Epidemiology, 30*(4), 668–677.

Krieger, N. (2011). *Epidemiology and the people's health: Theory and context*. Oxford University Press.

Lange, M. (2017). *Because without cause: Non-causal explanation in science and mathematics*. Oxford University Press.

Lemoine, M. (2017). Explanation in medicine. In M. Solomon, J. R. Simon, & H. Kincaid (Eds.), *The Routledge companion to philosophy of medicine* (pp. 296–309). Routledge.

Leong, A. (2019). The struggle over parcel C: How Boston's Chinatown won a victory in the fight against institutional expansion and environmental racism. *Amerasia Journal, 21*(3), 99–120.

Lewis, D. (1986). Causal explanation. In *Philosophical papers* (Vol. II, pp. 214–240). Oxford University Press.

Lipton, P. (1991). *Inference to the best explanation*. Routledge.

MacMahon, B., & Pugh, T. F. (1970). *Epidemiology; principles and methods* (1st ed.). Little.

Miettinen, O. S. (1985). *Theoretical epidemiology*. John Wiley & Sons.

Milstein, B., & Wetterhall, S. (2016). A framework featuring steps and standards for program evaluation. *Health Promotion Practice, 1*(3), 221–228.

Phillips, C. J., Fordham, R., Marsh, K., Bertranou, E., Davies, S., Hale, J., et al. (2011). Exploring the role of economics in prioritization in public health: What do stakeholders think? *European Journal of Public Health, 21*(5), 578–584.

Reutlinger, A., & Saatsi, J. (2018). *Explanation beyond causation: Philosophical perspectives on non-causal explanations* (1st ed.). Oxford University Press.

Richards, C. L., Iademarco, M. F., & Anderson, T. C. (2014). A new strategy for public health surveillance at CDC: Improving national surveillance activities and outcomes. *Public Health Reports, 129*(6), 472–476.

Ridker, P. M., Cook, N. R., Lee, I. M., Gordon, D., Gaziano, J. M., Manson, J. E., et al. (2005). A randomized trial of low-dose aspirin in the primary prevention of cardiovascular disease in women. *The New England Journal of Medicine, 352*(13), 1293–1304.

Rothman, K. J. (1986). *Modern epidemiology*. Little, Brown & Company.

Rothman, K. J., Lash, T. L., VanderWeele, T. J., & Haneuse, S. (2021). *Modern epidemiology* (4th ed.). Wolters Kluwer.

Ruben, D. H. (1990). *Explaining explanation*. Routledge.

Salmon, W. C. (1984). *Scientific explanation and the causal structure of the world*. Princeton University Press.

Salmon, W. C. (1997). Causality and explanation: A reply to two critiques. *Philosophy of Science, 64*(3), 461–477.

Secker-Walker, R. H., Flynn, B. S., Solomon, L. J., Skelly, J. M., Dorwaldt, A. L., & Ashikaga, T. (2000). Helping women quit smoking: Results of a community intervention program. *American Journal of Public Health, 90*(6), 940–946.

Skow, B. (2015). Scientific explanation. In P. Humphreys (Ed.), *The Oxford handbook of philosophy of science*. OUP.

Skow, B. (2016). *Reasons why*, First edition. ed. Oxford University Press, Oxford, United Kingdom; New York, NY.

Stout, R. (1996). *Things that happen because they should*. Oxford University Press.

Upshur, R. E. (2002). Principles for the justification of public health intervention. *Canadian Journal of Public Health, 93*(2), 101–103.

Van Fraassen Bas, C. (1980). The Scientific Image. Oxford University Press.

VanderWeele, T. J. (2015). *Explanation in causal inference: Methods for mediation and interaction*. Oxford University Press.

Woodward, J. (2017). Scientific explanation. In E. N. Zalta (Ed.), *The Stanford encyclopedia of philosophy* (Fall edn). Metaphysics Research Lab, Stanford University.

Woodward, J., & Ross, L. (2021). Scientific explanation. In E. N. Zalta (Ed.), *The Stanford Encyclopedia of Philosophy* (Summer edn). Metaphysics Research Lab, Stanford University.

Wright, L. (1976). *Teleological explanations: An etiological analysis of goals and functions*. University of California Press.

Yeravdekar, R. C., & Singh, A. (2022). Physician-scientists: Fixing the leaking pipeline — A scoping review. *Medical Science Educator, 32*(6), 1413–1424.

CHAPTER 7

Causometry

Introduction

In the previous chapters, I have analyzed the ways how medics and health scientists tackle the problem of uncertainty by means of inference and explanation. In this chapter, I turn to a third conceptual topic that plays a major role in the set of strategies to curb uncertainty in medicine: "causometry". Running the risk of misusing a neologism created by Aleksandr Kronik for psychological purposes,[1] I suggest its usage for the measurement of causation. Thus conceived, causometry refers to techniques that would allow for the objective qualitative establishment and quantification of causal relationships. Similarly, I use the term "causometrics" as referring to the theoretical analysis of what causometry represents and entails, and what a measurement instrument, i.e., a "causometer", would need to be able to do. Can such an instrument exist? If not, why not? I believe that causometry might be an interesting way to approach the nature and extent of causal relationships in medicine and the health sciences, and perhaps help reduce E-uncertainty.

Causality is one of the central concepts we consider when thinking about how the world works. We refer to causation (the process) and causality (the concept)[2] as an explanatory tool in our everyday lives. Causality is so basic an idea that some have suggested that it is a fundamental, irreducible characteristic of how the universe works:[3] *Ex nihilo nihil*

O. Dammann, *Uncertainty and Explanation in Medicine and the Health Sciences*, https://doi.org/10.1007/978-3-031-82271-1_7

fit—Nothing happens without cause (Parmenides). Everything happens for a reason *because* of something else. Interestingly, causality seems to be a concept that everyone seems to grasp intuitively. However, when pressed, most have difficulty defining it in a way that all can agree with and that does not leave room for scenarios that do not fit the bill. Indeed, one striking and genuinely surprising phenomenon is that authors in the causal data sciences appear to assume that their readers know what causation is even before they start reading. In other words, they seem to assume that a very general, ordinary language, folk notion of causation exists and is shared by readers with no need for explication. They use a particular causal framework that is built on a handful of causal principles that serve as background assumptions and that are essential for causal data science. Some of these have their own set of assumptions that I won't be able to dig into further due to space limitations.

Any event or phenomenon of import in medicine has some kind of origin in the past, a causal story, a natural history (or "etiology"). Be it the occurrence of a sign or symptom, a test result, a sudden change in disease status, a side effect of a drug, or a change in disease trajectory—all such events have a cause that explains *why* they occur as well as a mechanism that explains *how* they occur. I believe it is of utmost importance for medicine to tell etiological stories in the form of etiological explanations, which refer separately to the causal and mechanistic components of the natural history of the phenomenon at hand. Unfortunately, references in medicine to event etiology do not always make a clear-cut distinction between causes and mechanisms. Causal explanation in medicine oftentimes ignores the fact that, technically speaking, causal explanations provide answers to why-questions and mechanical explanations provide answers to how-questions, which are two very different kinds of questions. As already mentioned above, if both causal and mechanical explanations are provided jointly, they constitute a causal-mechanical or etiological explanation (Salmon, 1984).[4] I believe that comprehensive etiologic explanations should be about the entire *etiologic process* that begins with a cause (or set of causes), continues with a mechanism, and leads up to the occurrence of an event or phenomenon. My topic in this chapter, however, will be mainly about causation and the ways medics and scientists could approach causal uncertainty by means of causometry. By zooming in on causation I do not intend to ignore mechanisms. In fact, I think that an analysis of mechanisms and mechanical explanation in medicine is much needed. However, I do not feel competent to provide such an analysis, simply because I am an epidemiologist working on disease causation, not a basic scientist working on disease mechanisms.

The next section will offer some terminological clarification. Thereafter, I offer some brief thoughts on causal metaphysics in medicine and epidemiology. I will put forward the slightly provocative argument that, strictly speaking, modern epidemiology does not define causes by what they do (that would be clarified by causal-mechanical explanations) but by providing a methodological framework that allows risk factors to transition from simple association to causation. This means that, in epidemiology, causes are *defined* by whether they are what epidemiologists require from a risk factor to count as a cause. Epidemiologists do not *find* causes, they *make* them. To find causes, one would need what I call a "causometer" that can objectively identify causation in valid and reliable ways. In the last section of this chapter, I turn to the question whether such causometer can exist and, thus, whether causation can be measured, which would help remove causal uncertainty.

CAUSAL TERMINOLOGY

The scientific and philosophical literature on causation has grown appreciably over the past decades. The topic has gained traction, for example, in biology, epidemiology, statistics, machine learning, and the law.[5] This increasing interest is paralleled by an ongoing and arguably increasing attention to causation in philosophy of science.[6] Although some of these works do attempt to cross the divide between science and philosophy, much of the discourse in these two worlds remains somewhat disjointed. At least in part, I think, this is due to obviously different motivations. Scientists are mainly interested in *causal inference*, the method to find *causes*, because their goal is to extract causal information from data. In essence, they want to devise tools that enable them to move from correlation to causation. Philosophers, on the other hand, appear to focus on grappling with *causation*, the process, and *causality*, the concept. Their main goal is to find ways to characterize and understand causality as a phenomenon.

Indeed, scientists do not appear to be overly interested in the conceptual side of the topic. They apparently assume that we all know what we are talking about when we talk about causal phenomena. They rarely define terms like "cause" and "causation" in their writings. In other words, scientists seem to be more interested in the epistemological aspects of causality, which does not come as a surprise because making knowledge is what scientists do. Philosophers, on the other hand, seem to be more concerned with the metaphysics of causality, trying to get a handle on how to define causes and properly describe causation.

At this point, therefore, a preliminary note about the metaphysics of causation in medicine seems in order. The modern biomedical paradigm is that disease and recovery are predominantly biological processes. A disease is frequently defined by contrast to a typical biological process, e.g., as abnormal tissue growth and repair in contrast to normal tissue growth and repair. For such definition of biomedical phenomena as basically biological in nature, one should keep in mind that any pathological process is piggy backing onto a typical process, the process of typical human development. In other words, much of what happens to patients when they get sick, get diagnosed, get treated, and (ideally) get better is a *developmental biological process*. Human disease is essentially a mix of two processes: the process of regular human development, and a second pathological process that interferes with and disturbs the first. In other words, disease is a kind of *state transition* that is instantiated as an alteration of a regular developmental process, which results in an undesirable version of such process that comes with pain, suffering, sickness, or death.[7]

Before moving on, let me briefly introduce in a bit more detail the terminology regarding the four main concepts I will discuss: causality, causation, cause, and causal inference.

What is *causality*? For starters, I will use the term *causality* as an overarching term for the concept that unifies causes, causing, causation, and causal inference. Causality is, in this book at least, the big box that contains all these related but separable items. We all have a certain idea for what we mean when we use words like cause, causing, causation, and causality. However, an extended search of the philosophical literature reveals a wide and sometimes confusing variety of definitions for these terms. Since most causes (of disease at least) in medicine are identified by epidemiologists, my focus will be on the metaphysics of causality in modern epidemiology. I will explore what epidemiologists refer to when they refer to the *concept* of causality, including what kinds of *things* or *events* causes are, what kind of *activity* causing is, and what kind of *process* causation is. I am not sure we have as of yet achieved a comprehensive metaphysical characterization of causality in epidemiology. Indeed, it comes as a surprise that, except in a few places (e.g., in Susser's and Rothman's work), epidemiologic authors do not provide a definition or even explication of what they consider a cause, causation, and causal inference *to be*. I am, therefore, constrained not so much by existing definitions but by what I can (or cannot) read out of epidemiologic textbooks and scientific publications.

Causes are defined, in this book, as the things or events that do the causing, which is observable as a process of causation. If epidemiology is supposed to identify causes of illness, it should be possible for epidemiologists to define what a cause *is*. Interestingly, most, if not all, epidemiological discussions of causation fail to present such definition. I will take an inclusive view and consider anything to be a cause that contributes to the occurrence of a phenomenon. That contribution may be small or large, endogenous and exogenous, and even what philosophers would *not* call a cause, i.e., a background condition. I have previously argued, with Carmina Erdei, that in order to get a handle on the etiology of autism spectrum disorder among preterm infants, one needs to allow such background conditions to enter the causal framework (Dammann, 2020, pp. 79–93; Erdei & Dammann, 2014). My point is that background conditions contribute to the "causal history" of a phenomenon. In that sense, oxygen is a component cause of cancer per Rothman's model of causation in epidemiology (Rothman, 1976) or a Mackian INUS condition (Mackie, 1974), i.e., an insufficient but non-redundant part of an unnecessary but sufficient conglomerate of causal factors.[8]

When I talk about *causation*, I talk about a process in which causes cause their effects. Illness causation is a complex, multifactorial process. It is an etiological process that consists of many contributors and their interactions: background conditions, initiators, modifiers, mediators, and perhaps other kinds of causally effective factors that, taken together, form such etiological process. One way to identify such factors is to perform epidemiological studies to identify risk factor constellations that allow for the conclusion that the constituent risk factors culminate in illness occurrence. Another way is to perform laboratory experiments to identify biological mechanisms that explain just how the risk factor constellations identified by epidemiologists connect causes with their effects.[9] In what follows, I will argue that while epidemiology does indeed help identify risk factor constellations, it does not help us discover causes of illness. Instead, epidemiology *defines* what counts as a cause by requiring data analysts to follow certain procedural guidelines that lead them to the point where epidemiological theory accepts that a certain risk factor under investigation does indeed qualify as a cause. The discovery work is done prior to the data analysis, during the stage of creating a hypothesis that is testable by epidemiological analysis.

One central recognition in modern epidemiology is that all we do is *observe* health characteristics in populations and *model* the interrelationships between independent and dependent variables using statistical data analytic techniques. Nothing in the data represents causal relationships (correlation is not causation). Nothing in epidemiological data and analysis results is *inherently* causal. As philosopher Nancy Cartwright writes, "The slogan, 'no cause in, no causes out' needs to be taken seriously. Causal inference requires antecedent causal assumptions and cannot otherwise be valid" (Cartwright, 2007, p. 198). The literature on *causal inference* in epidemiology, however, is about methodological approaches that can help us get from observed data to knowledge about causal relationships. The idea appears to be that, somehow, causal information can be extracted from data by means of epidemiological methods. Some causality experts deliberately emphasize that their methods can do just that, à la "data in, causation out". I agree with Cartwright that this is impossible, simply because there is more to causal inference that "association in randomized settings". As mentioned above, epidemiology may contribute to descriptions of illness causation processes but is incapable in and of itself to *identify* such causes (Dammann, 2020). Explaining illness occurrence requires causal-mechanistic (i.e., etiological) explanations, which cannot be provided by the rather simplistic epidemiological (frequentist, observational) approaches *alone*, but requires additional evidence such as experimental, biological, interventional evidence as well (Dammann, 2021).

I want to take the argument one step further and propose that epidemiologists do not *identify* causes of illness from data but *make* them by declaring candidate risk factors to be *causal risk factors* based on certain assumptions and decision rules. To put it even more provocatively, characteristics or exposures are causes only if they pass epidemiological muster, i.e., *because* epidemiologists have granted them that status. On this account, and in keeping with Di Finetti's account of probability, epidemiological descriptions of causation as a certain connection-like relationship between a risk factor and a disease are less like descriptions of objective natural phenomena and more like descriptions of a mental concept that we retreat to in order to enable and simplify the communication about said relationships.

In the next section I shall give an overview of causal metaphysics that is by far not exhaustive and rather superficial from the perspective of philosophy of science, but sufficient for our current context. In the subsequent section I shall turn to causometry, ending on the notion that it is at least partially possible to measure causation using formalizations of causal heuristics such as Hill's. Indeed, I propose that it is possible to conceive of the generation of causal knowledge in medicine as a three-step process, from biological hypothesis, to the generation of causes via the POA and finally to the causometric establishment of causation.

CAUSAL METAPHYSICS

To answer the causometry question we need to have an idea what are we talking about when we talk about causation. The philosophical literature abounds with metaphysical accounts of causation. Unfortunately, philosophical inquiry and discourse have played a minor role in medicine, except in medical and public health ethics. Causality is a topic that has always been at the forefront of philosophy of science and the disinterest in medicine in what current philosophy has to say about it is simply baffling given the importance of causal concepts in medicine. I guess the main reason for this is that philosophy's business is to ask questions, reflect, and debate, while medicine is looking for straightforward, feasible, and effective proposals of what to do. While philosophers are good at identifying problems, medics are interested in finding workable solutions.

A similar desideratum can be stated for epidemiology. As a relatively new area of inquiry, modern epidemiology has grown out of a mix of medical perspective and population statistics methodology to form a comprehensive methodological approach to answer the question, "What causes illness?" (and, of course, other questions that do not feature as prominently in this book). My personal experience is that although epidemiologists rely heavily (if not *entirely*) on methods developed historically out of theory of science, they do not really appreciate the potential benefit philosophy of science still has to offer. The only instance I am aware of where an epidemiologist openly covered philosophical background information in a book on epidemiological causality is chapter 16 in Tyler VanderWeele's formidable book *Explanation in Causal Inference*. Although the philosophy chapter comes at the very end of his book, right before the appendix, one cannot therefore escape the impression that philosophical considerations are something like an afterthought for VanderWeele. A reviewer of a recent paper of mine, probably a genetic epidemiologist, wrote "believe me – scientists don't need philosophers to tell them how to do their work". Granted, philosophy has arguably not much to say about how scientists and medics should do their work, but I think that a case can be made that they have something to say about how to draw inferences, offer explanations, and think about causality in medicine and the health sciences.

The refusal by medical practitioners and health scientists to utilize philosophical insights could be interpreted as a misunderstanding or simply be rooted in ignorance. Or it might be that philosophical considerations really do not matter to them. After all, not all race car pilots are interested in the current discourse in theoretical race car engineering, nor do all priests necessarily follow the latest debates on liberation theology. Nevertheless, I believe that philosophical reflection of how causality is conceptualized in medicine and epidemiology might have an impact on how medics and public health practitioners think about causality if it only mattered to them. Indeed, it might help curb their E-uncertainty about causal relationships, for example, by improving the causal component of etiological explanations. Supporting this notion is rather straight forward. The general assumption is that causes are *responsible* for their effects by means of producing them; they *make* the effect occur. This kind of thinking is deeply engrained in human experience. While learning how their world works, most toddlers discover the magic of the light switch. Flip up, lights on—flip down, lights off. Experiences like this, some simple and some more complex, form our awareness of our capability to *control* the world around us. This idea of control by action underlies much of the conceptions and the idea to control illness occurrence by causal action is one of them. Of course, many will readily acknowledge that illness causation is way more complex than switching lights on and off, but I think it is likely that such simplistic light switch experiences linger in our minds and form the mainstay of statements such as "excessive sunlight exposure is the cause of skin cancer". By now, most scientists acknowledge that all illness causation is multivariable, with causally contributing factors constituting a network of interacting patho-mechanisms that jointly culminate in the development of disease. For example, although some may prefer to think of diseases as exclusively environmental or exclusively genetic in origin, epidemiologist Ken Rothman emphasized in his introductory epidemiology course I took in the 1990s that statements like "40% of cancer is genetic and 60% is environmental" are nonsensical because "100% is genetic and 100% is environmental", stressing the fact that both genetic and environmental causes are part of all patho-mechanisms.

One important upshot of the light switch line of causal thinking is that one needs to determine whether such causal *producers* are deterministic or indeterministic. The question is whether whenever the cause occurs, the effect will *always or almost always* occur as well, or whenever the cause occurs, it is merely *more likely* that the effect will also occur. Falling out of a 15th story window will likely always lead to death (although there are stories about individuals who survived plane crashes and falls from extreme heights[10]) while smoking will *not* always lead to lung cancer. However, the distinction between deterministic and probabilistic causation does not directly translate to the prevention level. It is not correct that whenever we are looking at a deterministic cause, reducing exposure to it will always prevent the effect because there might be other causes that lead to the same effect.

Of course, this focus on causal inference in advanced analytical epidemiology is of utmost importance to my current project. In particular, the joint contributions of Miguel Hernán, James Robins, and Tyler VanderWeele, presented in two excellent books (Hernán & Robins, 2020; VanderWeele, 2015), have prepared the ground for work in causal inference in epidemiology. In terms of etiological reasoning, it needs to be highlighted that some aspects of this work, particularly mediation analysis and interaction (VanderWeele, 2015), are considered relevant to and helpful in causal explanation.

The general paradigm today appears to be that we (a) somehow know what a cause is/does and thus (b) know what it is we are looking for and, therefore, (c) can develop methods to detect causes of illness in the real world. On this view, epidemiologists know what a cause is (or at least what kind of relationship qualifies as a causal one and which doesn't) and thus can devise methods to find causes. Note that all this requires a predefined notion of "cause" that we already have in mind when we start our search. Interestingly, it is not at all clear that epidemiologists have an exact concept of what a cause really is. Indeed, it is difficult to identify a single unified and universal definition of the term and concept in the epidemiological literature, with a few exceptions like (Rothman & Greenland, 2005a; Susser, 1991), inter alia. The most comprehensive and detailed account is Hernán's "Definition of Causal Effect for Epidemiological Research" (Hernán, 2004). However, it is not an account of what epidemiologists mean by "causation" but how Hernán proposes to define "causal effect".

Perhaps, the term "cause" may be so engrained in our everyday thinking that we really don't need to define it because we all intuitively know what it is and we all refer to the same thing when we use the word. As political philosopher Herbert Marcuse noted in his *One Dimensional Man*, some words become cliché and "as cliché, govern the speech or the writing; the communication thus precludes genuine development of meaning" (Marcuse, 1964, p. 87). Marcuse further postulates that "self-validating, analytical propositions appear which function like magic-ritual formulas. Hammered and re-hammered into the recipient's mind, they produce the effect of enclosing it within the circle of the conditions prescribed by the formula. [...] The ritualized concept is made immune against contradiction" (Marcuse, 1964, p. 88). At least to me, it seems as if this has happened with the terms cause, causation, and causal inference in epidemiology. They have become a cliché that not only leaves the terms undefined (or at least ill defined) but also precludes further development of the concepts they are supposed to cover. I hope that this book is at least partially successful in breaking through this barrier erected by our human tendency to *talk cliché*.

Nevertheless, there are a few characteristics of "cause" that seem to be generally accepted. First, a *cause* is thought of something that stands in a relationship to something else, usually called the *effect*. Second, the main temporal characteristic of such relationship is that a cause must precede its effect. Third, the effect cannot cause its cause; thus, the relationship is asymmetrical. Fourth, a causal relationship is thought of being *productive* in that the cause *somehow* produces its effect. A generalized description of this characteristic is that producing an effect is conceived as the cause being responsible for a change in an observed system which is defined as the occurrence of the effect in said system. The main inference in epidemiology and statistics seems to be that although these four characteristics may be features that we have inferred from empirical observation, such observation *alone* cannot establish causation. The main observations supporting the four characteristics would be (1) that the co-occurrence of causes and their effects (Hume's constant connection), (2) that presumed causes occur first, followed by their effect, (3) that the causal process is uni-directional, and (4) that there is a strong indication that without the cause the effect would not have happened (counterfactual reasoning). All this, taken together, supports the conclusion that causes *should be strongly associated* with their effects, but that, alas, such association is not always causation.

Introducing these everyday intuitions raises multiple questions. Do we think that association is one criterion for causation because association is a *natural* characteristic of causal relationships (descriptive empiricist view) or because *we think* that causes *should be* associated with their effects (prescriptive rationalist view). Do we think that time order (causes first, then effects) is another characteristic of causation because there is such a thing we call causation of which time order is a natural characteristic or because we think that causes should precede their effects? Is asymmetry a third characteristic because causation happens to be uni-directional or because we think it should be? And finally, do we think that no effect does occur without the cause being present beforehand or that no effect *should or can* occur without a preceding cause. In short, is epidemiological work descriptive empiricist or prescriptive rationalist?

Causometrics

Some causal theorists have written about "Measuring Causality" (Kathpalia & Nagaraj, 2021). Kathpalia and Nagaraj refer to Granger-causality, transfer entropy, and other methods to infer causal relationships from data. They call such methods "data-driven causality measures" (ibid., p.198), which they contrast with "model-based causality measures", including structural equation modeling and dynamic causal modeling (ibid., p.206). Much of their article, however, suggests that the authors' goal is to discuss methods for causal *inference*. This seems to indicate that the authors consider causal inference to be some kind of causal measurement, just as I do when I distinguish between qualitative from quantitative causal measurement.

Science is based on measurement. We cannot talk intelligently about any phenomenon in science without measuring variables and putting them in relation to each other. Therefore, let us now move to the question whether causation can be measured. I first briefly summarize what can be called causal principles in causal data science, i.e., data observation, quasi-determinism, statistical independence, Bayesian interpretation of probability, manipulation, and randomization based on counterfactualism. I review three causal methods, including causal inference based on randomization, graph-based causal discovery, and coherentist heuristics. Finally, I ask whether it is possible to measure causation and what it would take to do so. Although it is tempting to say that a "causometer" cannot exist in principle because causation is not a physical quantity, it is too heterogeneous a thing to be tackled by a single measurement system, and all quantification of causation would require prior causal inference, which is difficult in and of itself, it is possible, I think, to devise a method that considers multiple aspects of a purported causal relationship à la Hill's coherentist heuristics, thereby establishing causation in a qualitative way (as in causal inference). Moreover, I believe it might be possible to devise a causal scoring system based on said heuristics that comes close to a quantification at least of the strength of the evidence supporting a causal notion, if not of the strength of the causal relationship itself. In conclusion, I consider it likely, or at least possible, that causation can be measured. The upshot of this conclusion is that while it may be impossible to eliminate causal uncertainty in medicine, it is possible to curb it.

To produce novel knowledge, scientists need a reliable methodological framework. With the goal to explain and predict what goes on in the world, this framework involves concepts such as observation, measurement, experiment, inference, and explanation. All of these are things that scientists do and that are designed to discover causal relationships or to make causal inferences based on data. I will use the term *causal data science* to refer to the field of science that employs observed data for causal discovery and inference. While some causal data scientists disagree (Robins & Wasserman, 1999), others insist that causal inference and discovery is, at least to some extent, possible based on observed statistical data without background knowledge (Pearl, 2009; Peters et al., 2017; Spirtes et al., 2000). They have proposed *causal methods*, i.e., algorithms, data operations, inferential principles, etc., that are based on *causal principles* and are supposed to help with causal discovery and inference. Some of these causal methods yield what could be called *causal metrics*, i.e., quantitative estimates of an underlying causal estimand that *measure*, in some way or another, the causal relationship among variables in a causal structure.

My focus in this section is on the question whether causal measurement is possible and my main reference frame is causal data science in medicine and epidemiology. In what follows I first give a brief overview of the causal principles that causal data scientists use as building blocks to generate their causal methods. Next, I briefly outline three causal methods based on randomization, causal graphs, and explanatory coherentism. I then discuss specific items that bear on the question whether causation can be measured and how.

Causal Principles in Causal Data Science

The first thing causal data scientists need are *data*. Most causal methods are about data that come in the form of measurable quantities, be it as the data values of certain measurable quantities in a causal mechanism, e.g., the distance in centimeters between the gas pedal and the car floor and the RPM of the motor, or as data coming from an epidemiological study that includes thousands of participants, for each of whom hundreds of health-related variables have been documented and saved in a large dataset. Of note, this is technically information already, not just data, according to our transitional inference framework outlined in Chap. 5.

What is key about such data is that they come from *empirical observations*, not from experiments.[11] The standard methodology to analyze such data is statistics, but since correlation association is not causation, additional causal principles need to be employed. Most causal methods are rooted in the idea that "deep down" the world has a "quasi-deterministic" causal structure. For example, Pearl states that "human perception of causality has remained quasi-deterministic, and those fallible humans are still the main consumers of causal talk" (Pearl, 2009, p. 257), one of the reasons for his "preference toward Laplace's quasi-deterministic conception of causality" (ibid., 26). On this view, the world seems to function non-deterministically, but the observed causal variability is due to unknown factors in causal functions, not due to an inherently probabilistic (A-uncertain) structure of the world. In other words, at least some causal methods rely on our accepting quasi-determinism as an underlying assumption of causal discovery and inference.

Causal methods rely heavily on the principle that if two variables are statistically independent from each other they cannot be causally related. In other words, the thinking is that if two events are causally related, they must be statistically associated. While association cannot indicate causation, the absence of an association suggests the absence of causation, although exceptions to this rule exist, such as the one arising from limited data on exponential functions. Thus, causal methods rely on statistics as an indicator of independence, often when stepwise algorithms are designed to search for causal relationships in a given causal structure.

Part of causal methods also rely on Bayesian thinking, the core of which is the recognition that our beliefs about, e.g., the chance of rain in the next few hours will change once we know that a huge black storm cloud is coming toward us. In other words, new information updates the evidence available to us in a way that changes our beliefs about the likelihood of events. This and other elements of Bayesian statistics are frequently used in causal data science (Pearl, 2009; Peters et al., 2017; Spirtes et al., 2000).

"Without experimental manipulations, the resolving power of any possible method for inferring causal structure from statistical relationships is limited by statistical indistinguishability" (Spirtes et al., 2000, p. 59). In other words, statistical metrics cannot distinguish among several causal structures that yield the same statistical metric. However, intervention can come to the rescue. Arguably, the whole enterprise of causal inference and discovery is motivated by the desire to predict natural occurrences and the outcomes of interventions: "A joint distribution tells us how probable events are and how probabilities would change with subsequent observations, but a causal model also tells us how these probabilities would change as a result of external interventions" (Pearl, 2009, p. 22). The causal principle here is the assumption that manipulating a cause should change its effect. For example, Peters, Janzing, and Schölkopf argue that if A causes B, intervening on B should *not* change A, while an intervention on A should change B. If, however, both A and B are caused by a third variable (a common cause), intervening on either A or B should *not* change the respective other (Peters et al., 2017, p. 9).

One of the most central assumptions that form the underpinnings of causal reasoning is the idea that causality can be described as a counterfactual contrast. If A causes B, B occurs if A occurs. If A does not occur, B does not occur. (Underlying assumptions here are that the causal relationship is (a) deterministic and (b) sufficient.) In real-life situations, however, each instant of this causal event can occur in only one of two constellations: either A does occur, or it doesn't. In either case, we can observe only one instance of B occurring (or not). If A occurs, we can only observe if B occurs *given that A* occurs. We cannot observe what would have happened had A not occurred. This means that in individual instances we can never decide whether A caused B. However, we can design an experiment in which we let A occur many times (group 1) or not (group 2) in a randomized fashion. Randomization solves the confounder (common cause) problem because all confounders, known *and* unknown, should be distributed equally in the two groups. Members of group 2 are in essence a counterfactual mock version of group 1. Any difference of occurrence of B between the groups can, therefore, be attributed to the presence of A.

Some consider this kind of scenario a litmus test for causal inference based on observational data. Miguel Hernán writes provocatively that "in ideal randomized experiments, association *is* causation" (italics in original)

(Hernán, 2004, p. 267). Philosophers such as Worrall and Cartwright appear to disagree (Cartwright, 2010; Worrall, 2007).

Causal Methods

In medicine and the health sciences, causal discovery is cumulative and based on an explanatory-coherentist model of inference. While single observations do not yet enable causal inference, the convergence of evidence from multiple sources and scientific approaches does. The discovery process usually starts with a clinical observation of a novel phenomenon. A classic example is the observation of Kaposi sarcoma and *Pneumocystis carinii* pneumonia in a case series of homosexual men published in the 1980s (Centers for Disease, 1982). Based on earlier observation of homosexuality and Kaposi sarcoma (Friedman-Kien, 1981) as well as *Pneumocystis carinii* (Gottlieb et al., 1981), the hypothesis was put forward that an infectious agent transmitted via sexual contact among men might be the cause. Jerome Groopman wrote a concise piece for *Nature* in 1984, summarizing the subsequent research with the infection hypothesis based on the finding that an immunosuppressive virus was more frequent than expected in AIDS patients by Essex and colleagues (causal hypothesis), as well as subsequent isolation of such virus (HTLV-III) by Gallo's and Montagnier's research groups (mechanistic hypothesis) (Groopman, 1984). However, this is an example of an infectious disease, where the identification of the infectious agent is key for the establishment of the rather simple cause-effect relationship. The story is much more complicated in non-infectious, chronic disease. Let us consider, for example, the history of the causal link between smoking and lung cancer. In his concise history, Proctor mentions first the published hypothesis by Adler in 1912 that "abuse of tobacco and alcohol" might be responsible for the observed increase in pulmonary cancer in the late nineteenth and early twentieth century (Proctor, 2012). Subsequently, four lines of evidence began supporting the notion. First, evidence in support of a *statistical association* between smoking and lung cancer was provided by population studies conducted by Müller, Schairer, Schöniger in Germany, Wynder and Graham in the United States, and Doll and Hill in the UK. Second, animal research by Roffo in Argentina and Wynder, Graham and Croninger in the United States yielded initial *mechanistic* evidence by showing that juice and tar from tobacco combustion and smoke caused tumors in lab animals. Third, additional *mechanistic* evidence came from cellular pathology studies: Hilding showed that smokers suffered from ciliostasis and the death of cilia in proximity to lung areas where cancer was detected and Auerbach observed precancerous cellular changes in smokers. Fourth, by 1961, chemical analysis of cigarette smoke had revealed a large number of carcinogenic substances. Proctor ends his review on the multivariable notion that

> No causes are themselves uncaused, however, which means that when we think about what causes lung cancer or even smoking, we should think not just in terms of how individuals 'decide' to start smoking, but rather in terms of larger, more weblike threads of causation. We have to look at the cigarette epidemic and therefore lung cancer as facilitated by long causal chains of a sociopolitical, technical, molecular and agricultural nature [...] We need to better understand such webs or networks if we are to be more creative in finding ways to reduce the toll from this, the world's deadliest malignancy. (Proctor, 2012, p. 91)

Let us now focus on three technically different non-experimental kinds of methods for causal reasoning relevant to medicine and the health sciences, i.e., methods based on (1) randomized trials and target trial emulation, (2) graph/probability-based discovery algorithms, and (3) coherentist evaluation of causal heuristics. In each one, the goal is to find out whether we look at a causal system or relationship when we look at data. I interpret causal measurement as the process of establishing a causal relationship or relationships based on these methods, which yield a qualitative or quantitative causal metric that assists in making the leap from association to causation. I will introduce the fundamental ideas for each one in the following four sections as a basis for my discussion in the remainder of this chapter. My description will be concise, and, as always, I will refer to the work written by others whenever it is potentially helpful.

Much of what has been written about causation in causal data science is not about causation but about *causal inference*. Causal inference is the process of establishing a causal relationship between at least two events or characteristics. Causal inference can be understood as establishing the presence of causation in a *single instance* (e.g., between one instance of lightning and the subsequent thunder) or in a *regular relationship* between two (or more) events or characteristics (e.g., exposure to radio frequency radiation and cancer). As such, causal inference is a process with a binary conclusion: either the causal relationship is present, or it is not. Part of my goal in this chapter is to explore whether it is possible to call this qualitative *causal measurement* or *causometrics*.

The parent disciplines of causal data science are statistics and philosophy. Although the goals are rather practical (and mainly about identifying helpful interventions) the technical work is done by theorists which I will call *causal data scientists*. Data science is a catchall term used to refer to data-related scientific or analytic work. Consider it an interdisciplinary field that integrates aspects of mathematics, computer science, as well as data modeling and analysis. The applied sciences in which data science plays an important role are, inter alia, engineering, epidemiology, and statistics. The main motivation for causal data science is rooted in the recognition that gathering data and analyzing them with statistical methods is somehow helpful in establishing causal relationships, but not sufficient ("association is not causation"). Thus, most causal data science is about extracting causal information from observed data. The main task for causal data scientists is to develop methods that "can help with the inference of causal structures" from data (Peters et al., 2017, p. xi).

The need to control for the effect of third variables (confounders) is *in praxi* solved by *randomization*, first implemented by C.S. Peirce at the end of the nineteenth century and then widely promoted since the 1930s by R.A. Fisher (Hall, 2007) as what has now come to be called the "Rothamsted view" of statistics (Cox, 2012). The role of randomization as *the* kernel of the idea of causal inference cannot be underestimated. In fact, it can be said that randomization is considered the gold standard for causal data science.

When a new medical intervention is introduced, it needs to be shown that its application in patients really *causes* the intended health improvement. It does not suffice to give a pill to several individuals and, for example, consider the intervention causal if some of the individuals get better. Over the past hundred years the medical health research community has developed an approach called *randomized-controlled trial* (RCT) which has come to be considered the litmus test for causal inference in the health sciences. The design is to randomize eligible individuals who then, if in the treatment group, receive the intervention or, if in the comparison group, receive standard of care, a placebo, or a different kind or dosage of the same intervention. At the end of the trial, it is inferred that any outcome difference between the study participants in the trial "arms" is caused by the difference in intervention, e.g., is due to the new drug compared to standard of care. The "cause-maker" here is the randomization scheme, which renders the study groups similar on average regarding any possible variable (like age, sex, race, ethnicity, etc.), measured or unmeasured. In other words, it is thought impossible (or at least highly unlikely) that the outcome difference is caused by any factor other than the intervention. The central idea underlying the randomization dogma is the argument structure of counterfactual reasoning (Rubin, 1974, p. 700). In essence, the contrast between the two (or more) arms in an RCT is supposed to emulate what happens had the intervention not occurred (control arm) in contrast to what happens if the intervention does occur (intervention arm). The causal metric in this approach has two components: the above method of data collection and the statistical data analysis, which in turn consists of a measure of association and some sort of statistical test. For example, investigators randomized a total of 847 women with advanced breast cancer to receive a new drug (pembrolizumab; PEM) and standard chemotherapy ($N = 566$) or placebo plus chemotherapy (Cortes et al., 2022). The patients in the PEM group had a median overall survival of 23 months versus 16 months in the placebo arm. The measure of association chosen was the so-called hazard ratio for death, which turned out to be 0.73, indicating that individuals who received PEM had a 27% lower risk of death over a certain time period than individuals in the comparison group (the hazard ratio for no difference would be 1.0; increased risks would yield a hazard ratio >1.0). The risk reduction was statistically significant with a p-value of 0.0185, and the 95% confidence interval ranged from 0.55 to 0.95, indicating with 95% confidence that this interval covers the value of the true (unknown and, indeed, unknowable) risk reduction. In this example, the hazard ratio plays the role of causal metric or effect measure, indicating something like the strength of the risk reduction by PEM exposure. However, it is not just the value of the hazard ratio but also (i) the background information that the hazard ratio comes from a well-conducted RCT and (ii) the additional information from statistical testing, which is to be interpreted as support for a rejection of the notion that the observed risk reduction is due to chance. *Target trial emulation* (Hernán, 2021; Hernán & Robins, 2016) uses observational data to devise a trial protocol similar to one that would have been used to implement a full-fledged, real-life RCT. Eligibility criteria, treatment strategies and assignment, outcomes, follow-up, causal contrast, and data analysis need to be specified and rigorously followed. Hernán has offered a succinct discussion of what target trial emulation can or cannot achieve, e.g., in the absence of information on confounders (Hernán, 2021). Target trial emulation can yield results similar to those of a real RCT, as demonstrated by the PreVent study investigators, who conducted an RCT of positive airway pressure maintenance versus none during intubation (Admon et al., 2019). The effect estimate (risk ratio) for a decrease in severe hypoxia after positive pressure intervention was 0.6 in the emulated trial and 0.48 in the real RCT. Both results achieved formal statistical significance and the inferences drawn for intervention decisions would likely be the same.

Graph-based causal methods employ directed acyclic graphs (DAGs) as their main tool, i.e., graphs in which the purported causal relationship between nodes (variables) is depicted by edges (arrows). A very simple DAG would be A→B, indicating that the originator of the DAG thinks of A as a cause of B. Such DAGs are very useful to outline and communicate the details of a presumably causal structure as the first step of causal search and discovery strategies. Since the 1980s, scientists, engineers, epidemiologists, and philosophers have developed methods for causal discovery and inference using DAGs. Multiple single-volume treatments of the topic are available (Gebharter, 2017; Kleinberg, 2013; Pearl, 2000; Peters et al., 2017; Spirtes et al., 1993; Williamson, 2005). These approaches draw on probability theory, Bayesian reasoning, and computational techniques to run algorithms over the available (observational) data to do the discovery work.

Pearl's approach is heavily influenced by an interventionist view of causation, which holds that only intervention on certain variables in causal structures allows for causal inference (Pearl et al., 2016, p. 54). In a DAG with the two variables X and Y that are both descendants of a common cause variable Z (i.e., being at the receiving end of an arrow coming from Z), holding X constant will demonstrate independence between X and Y, which makes it impossible that X is a cause of Y. A second argument Pearl brings up to support his view is the assumption that "in a properly randomized controlled experiment, all factors that influence the outcome variable are either static, or vary at random, except for one – so any change in the outcome variable *must be* due to that one input variable" (emphasis mine) (Pearl et al., 2016, p. 53). At least in part, this strong (in fact, the strongest possible) causal inference is probably due to Pearl's quasi-deterministic framework. Based on this (and other) assumptions, Pearl has developed his "do-calculus", which denotes the effects of fixing variable values by intervention. While he asserts that "although statistical analysis cannot distinguish genuine causation from spurious covariation in every conceivable case, in many cases it can" (Pearl, 2000, p. 59), Pearl also writes that "causal effects cannot be estimated from the dataset itself without a causal story" (Pearl et al., 2016, p. 56). However, he claims further that his do-calculus represents "an *extra*-statistical method that can be used to [...] mathematically describe causal scenarios of any complexity [...] as swiftly and comfortably as [one] can solve for X in an algebra problem" (cursive in original) (ibid., 5). Pearl's do-calculus is used in a wide range of biomedical research settings, from the search for causal relationships in molecular pathways (Mohammad-Taheri et al., 2022) to causal effects of polysubstance usage on opioid overdose (Mahipal & Alam, 2022). Software has been developed for the implementation of the do-calculus in the health sciences, e.g., CausalTrail (Stockel et al., 2015).

Causal *discovery* is the identification of causal structures from observed data *without a preexisting causal model* (Glymour et al., 2019) by means of algorithms. These are stepwise procedures that analyze the statistical relationships among a given set of variables based on the conditional independence assumption, which assumes that there is no common cause of any two variables in the variable set. Again, causal discovery methods are model-free; they are naïve regarding the nature of the variables, do not pre-assign causal roles (such as x is the purported cause and y the purported effect), and are designed to search for causal structures in the given dataset.

A few underlying assumptions need explication to understand causal search algorithms (Fig. 7.1; adapted from (Glymour et al., 2019)) First, algorithm work starts with the construction of a graphical depiction of all possible relationships between all variables in a variable set as undirected connectors (Fig. 7.1B). The goal is to get from an undirected to a directed graphical causal model (DGCM). Second, to achieve that goal, search algorithms rely on statistical estimates and methods, e.g., probabilities and associations. What distinguishes between association and causation is the way algorithms *exclude* relationships between two variables that turn out to be statistically independent (Fig. 7.1C). Another step involves exclusion of relationships between a variable and a co-variable conditional on their common descendent (Fig. 7.1D). Further steps (details are irrelevant here) lead to a causal model (Fig. 7.1F) that is similar to the "true causal graph" (Fig. 7.1A) unknown to the causal searcher before the algorithm is applied. The algorithm underlying this example is the PC algorithm named after the authors of its original publication (Spirtes & Glymour, 1991). Thus, one main assumption (among others) is that in order to move from

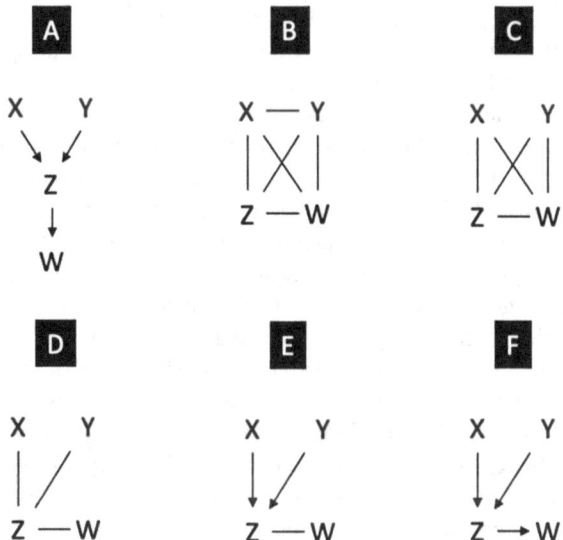

Fig. 7.1   Illustration of PC algorithm (see text for description; modified from Glymour, Zhang 2019)

association to causation (Spirtes et al., 1991) the algorithm works by exclusion of candidate relationships between variables that turn out to be statistically independent.

Second, graph-based discovery algorithms assume that causal relationships depicted in the graphs are deterministic or at least quasi-deterministic. For example, Clark Glymour and colleagues hold that, in the context of structural equation models, "the value of each variable is a deterministic function of its direct causes in the graph and ... unmeasured disturbances" (Glymour et al., 2019, p. 2). This assumption dovetails with the notion that effects *depend* on their causes: "edges between nodes indicate causal dependence" (Kleinberg, 2013, p. 5).

Third, it is important to keep in mind that there is no causality in the graph. Instead, the graph is *interpreted* as depicting a joint probability distribution of events that is causal. Nothing in the graph itself can be used to infer causation without initial clarification of the causal relationships between variables. Koller and Friedman suggest that "a type of reasoning for which a causal interpretation of the (Bayesian) network is critical (are) situations where we *intervene* in the world" (italics in original) (Koller &

Friedman, 2009, p. 1009). The obvious upshot of this motivation is that causal interpretations of DAGs include the assumption that interventions on causes will lead to changes in their effects.

A third approach to causal inference, mainly in epidemiology, is the application of *external standards* to the characteristics and results of individual epidemiological studies. The classic reference in this context is to Austin Bradford Hill's causal viewpoints, a list of nine criteria (in the broader, non-"necessary and sufficient" sense of the term) that are considered helpful in judging the causal nature of an observed association (Hill, 1965), including strength of association, temporality, consistency, dose-response, analogy, specificity, biological plausibility, and experimental evidence. Mervyn Susser (Susser, 1991) and Alfredo Morabia (Morabia, 1991) have pointed out that Hill's work appears to be based on the work of epidemiologists including Yerushalmy and Lilienfeld, as well as similar criteria used by a committee charged by the US Surgeon General with a causal analysis of the data on the health effects of smoking (1964). The approach has been discussed widely in epidemiology (Ioannidis, 2015; Morabia, 2013; Rothman & Greenland, 2005b) and philosophy (Howick et al., 2009; Thygesen et al., 2005; Worrall, 2011), to offer only a few selected references. I have previously suggested that Hill's guidelines can be interpreted as an explanatory-coherentist framework and that it might be possible to implement it computationally (Dammann, 2018). We have subsequently shown that this does indeed work, comparing the results of an in-silico analysis using Paul Thagard's ECHO software to real-life applications of Hill's method in medicine (Dammann et al., 2020).

It would be incorrect to assume that Hill's method is somewhat antiquated and not used in the health sciences. Among the recent examples are studies of the causal relationship between Zika virus and birth defects (Rasmussen et al., 2016), of smoking and multiple sclerosis (Degelman & Herman, 2017), of risk factors for musculoskeletal complaints among female musicians (Borger et al., 2021), and of red meat intake as a causal factor in cardiovascular disease and type-2 diabetes (Hill et al., 2022). However, it should be noted that Hill's method does not provide criteria in the hard-and-fast sense of the term, but rather mere heuristics. Thus, they cannot establish causation but can definitely help making a common-sense argument in support of causal notions (Phillips & Goodman, 2006). Thus, I submit that they can curb, but not eliminate, E-uncertainty about causal relationships relevant to medicine and the health sciences.

Problems with Causometry

Let us now move to the question whether causation can be measured. In what follows I will tackle three issues. First, we need consider what the prerequisites would be for causation to be measurable in principle. I propose that causal measurement is possible in principle if there is at least one property or mark of causation that can be objectively measured. The existence of such aspect (or aspects) could distinguish between instances of causation and no causation. Different forms or kinds of such aspect or mark might even distinguish between different kinds of causation, supporting the notion of causal pluralism.

The second issue of import for our problem is that causation can be considered at two levels, token and type. Most philosophers of science are familiar with the story of Billy and Suzie throwing stones at a glass window. The *cause* is Billie and Suzy throwing their stones, the *mechanism* is the flying stone's rupturing the surface integrity of the glass, and the *effect* is the shattering of the window. This is a token causal event (it happens just once) and the question is what aspect of causation could be *measured* in this token scenario and *how*? From the type causation perspective, we would consider any thrown stone smashing any window in general. What would be measurable about stones smashing windows in general and how?

Third, measurement comes in two forms, qualitative and quantitative. The distinction is important because, as I will show, qualitative measurement amounts to not much more than causal inference, the establishment of causality in a particular event or situation. Quantitative causal measurement, however, would mean to establish a technique to measure *degrees* of causation. Of course, qualitative causal measurement would be a prerequisite for quantitative causal measurement, simply because causation is, trivially, unmeasurable *by definition* if not present.

Before we turn to these issues, however, we first need to briefly introduce the idea of measurement. One basic aspect of measurement is that it is "the objective representation of our empirical knowledge of the world by numbers" (Finkelstein & Leaning, 1984, p. 25). Thus, if causation is part of our empirical knowledge about the world, which it arguably is, the next question would be if causation is also part of the *measurable* component of our empirical world by virtue of being represented objectively by numbers.

A more detailed definition of "measurement" is

the assignment of numbers to properties of objects or events in the real world by means of an objective empirical operation, in such a way as to describe them. The modern form of measurement theory is representational - numbers assigned to objects/events must represent the perceived relations between the properties of those objects/events. (ibid. 26)

By this definition, measurement is conceptualized as an *objective* assignment of numbers to *properties* of objects or events. Two questions arise immediately. First, in keeping with our discussion in previous sections, it seems unlikely that any causal method will make an *objective* assignment of numbers possible. The overall agreement appears to be that, except under extreme deterministic assumptions, no causal inference is entirely watertight. Second, one would need to specify which properties of causation numbers could be assigned to. Thus, measurement of causation in the sense of the above definition might never be entirely reliable, even if measurable properties of causation could be identified.

The question whether causation is measurable *in principle* asks whether causation is something that has at least one measurable property that can be assessed with a measurement instrument that yields objective novel or confirmatory information about causation that was not available before the measurement. Measurement requires a measurable entity. What aspects or properties of causation are measurable, and how? If measurement in its usual sense means to establish a specific physical characteristic, such as length, weight, or velocity, of an object or event in comparison to a standard/norm, what characteristic or property of causation would be measurable and what kind of measurement tool would be needed and compared to what kind of standard? Macro-causal processes (like billiard balls colliding, stones being thrown at windows, remote garage door openings, etiopathogenesis of cancer, etc.) are based on many different kinds of micro-causal mechanisms that are potentially measurable (two hard billiard ball surfaces hitting each other with force; the hard stone surface hitting the glass window forcefully; electromagnetic waves that set the garage door motor in motion as soon as the remote button is pressed; whatever the biological mechanism is that renders body cells cancerous). It seems that one would either need an apparatus that can measure at least one kind of causal micro-event or perhaps even one that targets the one causal feature that underlies all kinds of causation, should one exist.

So, what aspects of causation are potentially measurable? One characteristic of causation that may be of interest for measurement is *causal reliability*. If a cause causes its effect, it should do so reliably. In other words, one should be able to rely on the effect to occur if the cause has occurred. One should be able to trust the remote control to reliably open the garage door. One way to measure reliability is to measure the regularity of the cause-effect sequence. In token causation, this cannot be measured because there is no such thing as regularity in one event. In type causation, however, regularity of the co-occurrence of cause and effect can be assessed by estimating the degree of statistical association between cause and effect. At least some, perhaps even all, causation is probabilistic; thus, not all occurrences of the same cause are always followed by the same effect. Thus, observing multiple potentially causal events and measuring the likelihood of effect occurrence would be a way of measuring the degree of causal success in a frequentist way. In epidemiology, for example, it can be established by measures such as the odds ratio, i.e., the ratio of the odds that the effect occurs in the presence of the cause versus the odds that it occurs in its absence. The more regular the co-occurrence, the higher the odds ratio. While this kind of estimate could be considered a quantitative measure of the strength of the causal relationship, it would still fall prey to the "association is not causation" paradigm. A high value for the odds ratio alone also does not provide qualitative information; nothing in the calculation of the odds ratio ensures that the co-occurrence and its degree is not due to chance. Additional information about the origin of the odds ratio (from RCTs vs. observational studies, adjusted for confounders or not, etc.) is needed for qualitative causal inference. Thus, measuring causal effectiveness is establishing the degree of causal effectiveness across many events of similar nature. But as indicated above, measurement as a concept seems to apply to individual events, not collectives. Counting instances of causal success in a series of events and calculating the percentage of success in that series is just that: counting and calculating the frequency of said event in said series of events. Even if we consider this series of events a token event (which yields the series), counting success and calculating a percentage is not measuring success in that series of token events. It is a derivation of a summary statistic, an estimation of average success in the series based on the individual successes that give rise to the series.

Establishing a statistical association between cause and effect beyond what is expected by chance yields an answer to the question: does the effect reliably occur after the cause has occurred? This is, technically speaking, a qualitative question, yielding a yes or no response. The quantitative measurement of something requires not only the practical availability of an appropriate measuring apparatus/instrument but also the availability, or at least the theoretical possibility, of a quantitative scale that serves as the standard for such measurement. For example, length measurement determines the extent of an object in two dimensions relative to a standard, like the standard meter bar kept in Paris. Weight and time measurement are other basic forms of measurement, while velocity (distance per time) and pressure (force per area) are composite measurements that include multiple measured components. Again, one could suggest that at least some physical measures like Joule, Pascal, or Tesla *are* causal measures. However, there is no physical entity that represents causation. We need to accept that all we can do is follow the procedure: (1) develop a causal hypothesis based on the observation of token events; (2) establish the presence of causation in type settings; (3) estimate the strength/vigor of the purported causal relationship; and (4) apply type data to individual token cases.

A quantitative way to interpret evidence for causal reliability is to look at its *causal strength* or *vigor*. Causal vigor or strength appeals to the intuition that causation is some kind of *force*. Indeed, many of the processes we consider causal (think back to the billiard balls, stones thrown, and garage doors above) are examples of processes in which a physical force produces the causal event we consider to be the defining element of said process. The reference frame would have no causation at one end of the spectrum, quantifiable as 0 (*zero*) causation, i.e., the absence of causation, perhaps best established by the presence of statistical independence. The other end of the spectrum could be represented by constant (perfect, absolute, deterministic) causation, quantifiable as a causal strength of 1 (*one*). Thus conceived, causal vigor would be measured on a scale from 0 to 1, equivalent to the measurement of the strength of a magnet attracting a piece of metal with a certain measurable vigor, with a measurement of 1 being obtained when another magnet of opposite polarization comes close and a measurement of 0 when a piece of paper is brought next to it. In practice, this is done when recording the strength of magnets in units of Gauss or Tesla. Such magnetism-like measurement of causal strength would require that causal strength be not a binary thing, as in "causation is present" or "no causation", but measurable on a continuous scale, like temperature or distance. This would align with the notion of probabilistic causation, where probabilities can vary (between 0 and 1), but not so well with the notion of quasi-determinism that underlies some of the reasoning with causal graphs and causal discovery algorithms. Such measurement of physical causation on a continuous scale might be conceivable for some kinds of causation, like in magnetic attraction and repulsion, or in forces of tension or shear stress. This, however, would be measurement of magnetic strength or degree of tension, i.e., kinds of physical causation, not of causation *simpliciter*. Viewed from this perspective, *some* causal events may be measurable in terms of their physical properties or dispositions, but I would not agree that such measurement would be causal measurement. Opponents may argue that in some sense physical measurements are measures of causal processes and, thus, are measures of causation. My response would be in keeping with Elizabeth Anscombe's view (Anscombe, 1993) and propose that the term "causal measurement" can be added to a language in which are already represented many concepts of physical measurement, such as measurement of attraction, repulsion, friction, and so on. I think it is possible to employ this concept of causal measurement in more complex scenarios, like the causation of accidents, illness, or death, by means of quantification of the association between cause and effect using, e.g., relative risk estimates such as the odds ratio or hazard ratio. Of note, I do not think that such quantitative estimates directly measure causation. Instead, I think that under certain circumstances they can be used to quantify the causal vigor of an association that has already been deemed to be causal. In other words, an odds ratio of 2.5 (given it is adjusted for confounders and the confidence does include 1.0) does not indicate causation, it *measures* the causal vigor of the cause as 2.5 times that of any other cause that contributes to the occurrence to the effect in the absence of the cause, if and only if the association has previously been established as causal.

A second candidate characteristic of causation that might be measurable is *causal responsibility*. Although some philosophical approaches to causality do not center on this aspect, everyday usage of the term causation seems to include the notion that something is a cause if it is responsible for the occurrence of the effect, i.e., for the causal change that characterizes the particular macro-causal event. However, many causal scenarios (some will even say: all causal scenarios) are multicausal. Which one of the multiple causes is responsible for the causal event? Take, for example, a classic car accident scenario. It is after dark in mid-January. The highway in New England is only dimly lit, the rain is freezing over, creating that dangerous thin layer of black ice. The Volvo driver is nervous because he knows he had one shot Tequila too many and—boom—he crashes into the rear end of a disabled Audi standing right behind the curve in the middle of the lane, no warning lights flashing. The Volvo driver suffers severe whiplash, and luckily not much more damage is done because I don't like gruesome examples. Clearly, multiple factors contributed to this accident. The time of day (it was night), the light (it was dim), the weather (it rained), the road condition (black ice), the Volvo driver's inebriation (considerable), the Audi's position (in the lane, behind a curve), and the Audi warning lights (none) all contributed to the Audi driver's whiplash. All the multiple antecedent factors seem to have contributed to the crash, but are all of them causes? To what extent? And are they to be weighed equally in terms of their responsibility for the accident? It seems sensible to ask *to what degree* the putative cause was causally involved. This could be called the *degree of causal responsibility*. Measurement of that degree, however, is probably rather difficult. Still, it is conceivable that such measure would be very helpful in cases of complex causation where multiple causal factors interact in the generation of the effect.

The above discussion suggests that causal measurement might be possible using type level data, while it is less clear that it is possible at the token level. If causal measurement is intended to provide insight into a single causal event, not about the generalizability from a single event or thing to a class of events or things, the measurement would need to yield a single datum, while measurements across classes or populations are summarized as aggregate data (e.g., means or percentages). The length of an individual piece of wood can be measured using a tape measure in inches or centimeters but talk about the average length of hundreds of pieces of wood is not measurement. Such aggregate data are just mathematical derivatives from multiple measurements that can be used for the description of groups of events or things. Either we need to find different ways of measurement for token and type causation or we need to accept the problems that come with the application of type causation evidence to token cases.

One interesting way to measure causation would be to develop a causometer analogue to pain assessment scales as used in medicine. Such scales rely on verbal (interview-based) patient responses or on visual quantification tools such as Likert scales, ranging from "no pain" to "pain as bad as it could be" (Haefeli & Elfering, 2005). However, even though such scales may use numbers to distinguish between degrees of pain, they do not provide an *objective* measurement as defined above simply because they are based on individuals' subjective pain level. Moreover, the numbers used to distinguish between levels of pain reflect just an order of pain levels (3 is higher than 2) but do not allow for the inference that a pain level of, say, 6 is twice as high as a level of 3. How could such semi-quantitative, subjective, human-estimation-based measurement tool be used to measure causation? For the overarching project from causal hypothesis to application of type estimates to individuals one could develop a rating tool based on the Hill's heuristics that allows for the collection of evidence for causation, followed by a data-integration process and scoring the number of criteria that are ticked off as present. The individual criteria could be weighted, and the final score could be interpreted as indicating the degree of belief that the event, process, or result is causal. I am not aware that something like this has been attempted successfully. Of course, such assessment would still be subjective and not objectively watertight. It would also not be about token, only about type causation, and the numerical assignment in this case would simply be assigning the number one for the presence and zero for the absence of causation. Of course, there might be other measurable causal properties that I have neglected here.

My discussion so far suggests that causal measurement might be difficult, but not entirely impossible. In the next section I lay out why I tend to believe the latter is the case. I will argue that causation cannot be measured objectively simply because the necessary "causometer" that would yield causal information is elusive. What measurement system could capture the idea of causation the same way that we have systems to capture time, length, weight, and so forth? One response would be that there just isn't one, in which case causation cannot be measured for just that reason. Another is that there is one, but we just don't know it yet. This would indicate that we may or may not be able to identify it. In the first case, we just need to look harder, for example, come up with a scientific program that has the goal to identify the physical quantity we need to measure to quantify causation. In the second case we are doomed because the entire enterprise is just futile. A third possibility is that causation is measurable only as a mixed quantity, such as speed or pressure. Again, it would take an elaborate research project to find out what the contributing sub-quantities might be.

If measurement is the objective quantification of a physical quantity, such quantity must be a variable, i.e., it must be possible to declare various levels of the measured quantity, either on a continuous scale, e.g., magnetic forces measured as 1, 2, 3 Tesla, or on a categorical scale, e.g., no, low, medium, high temperature measured in centigrade.

Another aspect of the causometer problem is the Anscombian possibility that there are multiple kinds of causality (causal pluralism). This view is reflected in Illari and Russo's mosaicism (Illari & Russo, 2014) and my own defense of etiological pluralism (Dammann, 2020, pp. 53–62). Thus, measurement of one kind of causation, e.g., ligand-receptor binding, might not be possible if applied to another, e.g., measuring the impact of social determinants on health.

The basic underlying requirement for any kind of causal measurement would be the *establishment* of causation before any further measurement can even be considered. Why measure causation if it isn't causation? One would first need to provide evidence that the causal event to be measured actually *is* causation. Only then can causal measurement proceed meaningfully as the quantification of the causal process. However, the problem of causal inference, i.e., the problem how to establish the causal nature of a token event *unequivocally*, is far from being solved. This is the reason why some say "causation cannot be proven" (Weed, 2008). Even the most intricate methods to establish causation are fallible, which makes the question interesting *how* we can ever be sure that some events are indubitably causal.

* * *

In this chapter I have taken the perspective that tackling uncertainty in medicine and the health science requires a serious consideration of questions related to causality. In essence, causality is the concept underlying any explanation of an effect by reference to its causes and, when the explanation also incorporates mechanisms, to the etiological process that explains its occurrence by reference to its causes and mechanisms. To establish causation in a watertight fashion, I hold, one would need to have a way to measure token causation, i.e., to do "causometry". I have summarized what can be called causal principles in causal data science, i.e., data observation, quasi-determinism, statistical independence, Bayesian interpretation of probability, manipulation, and randomization based on counterfactualism. I have reviewed three causal methods, including causal inference based on randomization, graph-based causal discovery, and coherentist heuristics. The chapter ends with the suggestion that a token "causometer" cannot exist but that it is possible to establish the presence of type causation and to quantify the causal vigor of the cause using epidemiological measures.

My discussion in the last three chapters suggests that inference, explanation, and causometry are important conceptual topics to consider when thinking about the puzzle of medical ineffectiveness. Such consideration is needed to curb uncertainty in medicine and the health sciences. Alas, I believe that it might be not possible to remove all uncertainty, simply because life is inherently uncertain and no scientific method can rid us of this A-uncertainty, only reduce E-uncertainty to various degrees.

The next three chapters (Part III of the book) represent three case studies of how the concepts covered in part II can be utilized to tackle various problems in medicine and the health sciences. The first example is from my own work on the etiological explanation of retinopathy of prematurity (ROP). This is an example of how an etiological explanation can benefit from a coherentist approach to causal explanation using the Hill's heuristics as a quasi-causometer. The second is an extension of the conceptual explanatory framework I outlined in Chap. 6. The third offers a vision for an integrated approach to evidence mapping. All three are examples of how the concepts in Part II of this book can be utilized to reduce uncertainty about the etiology of disease (Chap. 8), the explanatory functions of agent-based disease modeling (Chap. 9), and the justification of health interventions (Chap. 10).

NOTES

1. See Kronik (2018).
2. I will distinguish "causation" from "causality" by using the former as the term for the causal process that connects cause and effect, and the latter to denote the overarching concept that juxtaposes cause and effect as the start and finish of causation. Of course, the term "cause" is used in many ways, and I will use it in reference to the generic idea of a cause, whether necessary or sufficient, proximal or distal, single or general.
3. Indeed, it has been proposed that causation is a fundamental property of the world as we know it, like time and space. I will not discuss the issue of causal fundamentality any further. For more on this see (Bombelli et al., 1987; Tamm, 2021). If not fundamental, causation appears to be at least quasi-fundamental as it is very hard to find a definition of causation that is non-circular. By "quasi fundamental" I simply mean not easily reducible to purportedly non-causal entities such as time and space.

4. I have advocated my view on etiological explanations in detail elsewhere (Dammann, 2020).
5. See Berzuini et al. (2012), Hernán and Robins (2020), Imbens and Rubin (2015), Kleinberg (2013), Moore (2009), Pearl (2009), Peters et al. (2017), Shipley (2000), Spirtes et al. (2000), VanderWeele (2015).
6. See Gillies (2019), Hill et al. (2021), Illari and Russo (2014), Mumford and Anjum (2011), Reiss (2015), Williamson (2005), Woodward (2003).
7. Thanks to Ben Smart for alerting me that there are some definitions and accounts of "disease" in the philosophy of medicine that do not include value-related concepts such as "undesirable". Unfortunately, a full account of disease as captured by my working definition offered here will have to wait for another day.
8. A brief explanation of Rothman's accounts is on page 206 and a bit more can be found in (Dammann, 2020, pp. 14–16)
9. In *Etiological Explanations*, I have outlined the constituents of such etiological processes and their functions (Dammann, 2020).
10. See, for example, the list of survival stories provided by American news channel CNN; http://www.cnn.com/2010/WORLD/africa/05/13/libya.planecrash.survivors/index.html
11. I will come back to the idea of experiments and randomized studies further down in the chapter.

References

Admon, A. J., Donnelly, J. P., Casey, J. D., Janz, D. R., Russell, D. W., Joffe, A. M., et al. (2019). Emulating a novel clinical trial using existing observational data. Predicting results of the prevent study. *Annals of the American Thoracic Society, 16*(8), 998–1007.

Anscombe, G. E. M. (1993). Causality and determination. In E. Sosa & M. Tooley (Eds.), *Causation* (pp. 88–104). OUP.

Berzuini, C., Dawid, P., & Bernardinelli, L. (2012). *Causality: Statistical perspectives and applications.* Wiley.

Bombelli, L., Lee, J., Meyer, D., & Sorkin, R. D. (1987). Space-time as a causal set. *Physical Review Letters, 59*(5), 521–524.

Borger, T., Nel, E. J., Kok, L. M., Marinelli, F. E., & Woldendorp, K. H. (2021). Risk factors for musculoskeletal complaints in female musicians: A systematic review and exploration for future studies. *Medical Problems of Performing Artists, 36*(4), 279–296.

Cartwright, N. (2007). *Hunting causes and using them: Approaches in philosophy and economics.* Cambridge University Press.

Cartwright, N. (2010). What are randomised controlled trials good for? *Philosophical Studies: An International Journal for Philosophy in the Analytic Tradition, 147*(1), 59–70.

Centers for Disease, C. (1982). A cluster of Kaposi's sarcoma and Pneumocystis carinii pneumonia among homosexual male residents of Los Angeles and orange counties, California. *MMWR. Morbidity and Mortality Weekly Report, 31*(23), 305–307.

Cortes, J., Rugo, H. S., Cescon, D. W., Im, S.-A., Yusof, M. M., Gallardo, C., et al. (2022). Pembrolizumab plus chemotherapy in advanced triple-negative breast cancer. *New England Journal of Medicine, 387*(3), 217–226.

Cox, D. R. (2012). Statistical causality: Some historical remarks. In C. Berzuini, P. Dawid, & L. Bernardinelli (Eds.), *Causality* (pp. 1–5). John Wiley & Sons.

Dammann, O. (2018). Hill's heuristics and explanatory coherentism in epidemiology. *American Journal of Epidemiology, 187*(1), 1–6.

Dammann, O. (2020). *Etiological explanations: Illness causation theory.* CRC Press.

Dammann, O. (2021). Evidence mapping to justify health interventions. *Perspectives in Biology and Medicine, 64*(2), 155–172.

Dammann, O., Poston, T., & Thagard, P. (2020). How do medical researchers make causal inferences? In K. McCain & K. Kampourakis (Eds.), *What is scientific knowledge? An introduction to contemporary epistemology of science* (pp. 33–51). Routledge.

Degelman, M. L., & Herman, K. M. (2017). Smoking and multiple sclerosis: A systematic review and meta-analysis using the Bradford Hill criteria for causation. *Multiple Sclerosis and Related Disorders, 17*, 207–216.

Erdei, C., & Dammann, O. (2014). The perfect storm: Preterm birth, neurodevelopmental mechanisms, and autism causation. *Perspectives in Biology and Medicine, 57*(4), 470–481.

Finkelstein, L., & Leaning, M. S. (1984). A review of the fundamental concepts of measurement. *Measurement, 2*(1), 25–34.

Friedman-Kien, A. E. (1981). Disseminated Kaposi's sarcoma syndrome in young homosexual men. *Journal of the American Academy of Dermatology, 5*(4), 468–471.

Gebharter, A. (2017). *Causal nets, interventionism, and mechanisms: Philosophical foundations and applications, synthese library, studies in epistemology, logic, methodology, and philosophy of science* (1st edn, p. 1). Springer International Publishing (VII, 184 pages 155 illustrations). https://doi.org/10.1007/978-3-319-49908-6

Gillies, D. (2019). *Causality, probability, and medicine (1st edn).* Routledge.

Glymour, C., Zhang, K., & Spirtes, P. (2019). Review of causal discovery methods based on graphical models. *Frontiers in Genetics, 10*, 524.

Gottlieb, M. S., Schroff, R., Schanker, H. M., Weisman, J. D., Fan, P. T., Wolf, R. A., et al. (1981). Pneumocystis carinii pneumonia and mucosal candidiasis in previously healthy homosexual men: Evidence of a new acquired cellular immunodeficiency. *The New England Journal of Medicine, 305*(24), 1425–1431.

Groopman, J. E. (1984). Causation of AIDS revealed. *Nature, 308*(5962), 769.

Haefeli, M., & Elfering, A. (2005). Pain assessment. *European Spine Journal, 15*(S1), S17–S24.

Hall, N. S. (2007). R. A. Fisher and his advocacy of randomization. *Journal of the History of Biology, 40*(2), 295–325.

Hernán, M. A. (2004). A definition of causal effect for epidemiological research. *Journal of Epidemiology and Community Health, 58*(4), 265–271.

Hernán, M. A. (2021). Methods of public health research — Strengthening causal inference from observational data. *New England Journal of Medicine, 385*(15), 1345–1348.

Hernán, M. A., & Robins, J. M. (2016). Using big data to emulate a target trial when a randomized trial is not available. *American Journal of Epidemiology, 183*(8), 758–764.

Hernán, M. A., & Robins, J. M. (2020). *Causal inference: What if? In.* Chapman & Hall/CRC.

Hill, A. B. (1965). The environment and disease: Association or causation? *Proceedings of the Royal Society of Medicine, 58*, 295–300.

Hill, B., Lagerlund, H., & Psillos, S. (2021). *Reconsidering causal powers: Historical and conceptual perspectives.* Oxford University Press.

Hill, E. R., O'Connor, L. E., Wang, Y., Clark, C. M., McGowan, B. S., Forman, M. R., et al. (2022). Red and processed meat intakes and cardiovascular disease and type 2 diabetes mellitus: An umbrella systematic review and assessment of causal relations using Bradford Hill's criteria. *Critical Reviews in Food Science and Nutrition, 64*, 1–18.

Howick, J., Glasziou, P., & Aronson, J. K. (2009). The evolution of evidence hierarchies: What can Bradford Hill's 'guidelines for causation' contribute? *Journal of the Royal Society of Medicine, 102*(5), 186–194.

Illari, P. M., & Russo, F. (2014). *Causality: Philosophical theory meets scientific practice* (1st ed.). Oxford University Press.

Imbens, G., & Rubin, D. B. (2015). *Causal inference for statistics, social, and biomedical sciences - an introduction.* CUP.

Ioannidis, J. P. (2015). Exposure-wide epidemiology: Revisiting Bradford Hill. *Statistics in Medicine, 35*(11), 1749–1762.

Kathpalia, A., & Nagaraj, N. (2021). Measuring causality. *Resonance, 26*(2), 191–210.

Kleinberg, S. (2013). *Causality, probability, and time.* Cambridge University Press.

Koller, D., & Friedman, N. (2009). *Probabilistic graphical models: Principles and techniques.* MIT Press.

Kronik, A. (2018). *How young are you? Understanding psychological age, time, causometry, to create meaningful, harmonious, productive lives.* New Academia Pub.

Mackie, J. L. (1974). *The cement of the universe; a study of causation.* Clarendon Press.

Mahipal, V., & Alam, M. A. U. (2022). Estimating heterogeneous causal effect of polysubstance usage on drug overdose from large-scale electronic health record. In *2022 44th Annual International Conference of the IEEE Engineering in Medicine & Biology Society (EMBC).*

Marcuse, H. (1964). *One-dimensional man; studies in the ideology of advanced industrial society.* Beacon Press.

Mohammad-Taheri, S., Zucker, J., Hoyt, C. T., Sachs, K., Tewari, V., Ness, R., et al. (2022). Do-calculus enables estimation of causal effects in partially observed biomolecular pathways. *Bioinformatics, 38*(Supplement_1), i350–i358.

Moore, M. S. (2009). *Causation and responsibility: An essay in law, morals, and metaphysics.* Oxford University Press.

Morabia, A. (1991). On the origin of Hill's causal criteria. *Epidemiology, 2*(5), 367–369.

Morabia, A. (2013). Hume, Mill, Hill, and the sui generis epidemiologic approach to causal inference. *American Journal of Epidemiology, 178*(10), 1526–1532.

Mumford, S., & Anjum, R. L. (2011). *Getting causes from powers.* Oxford University Press.

Pearl, J. (2000). *Causality - models, reasoning and inference.* Cambridge University Press.

Pearl, J. (2009). *Causality: Models, reasoning, and inference.* Cambridge University Press.

Pearl, J., Glymour, M., & Jewell, N. P. (2016). *Causal inference in statistics: A primer.* Wiley.

Peters, J., Janzing, D., & Schölkopf, B. (2017). *Elements of causal inference: Foundations and learning algorithms.* The MIT Press.

Phillips, C. V., & Goodman, K. J. (2006). Causal criteria and counterfactuals; nothing more (or less) than scientific common sense. *Emerging Themes in Epidemiology, 3,* 5.

Proctor, R. N. (2012). The history of the discovery of the cigarette-lung cancer link: Evidentiary traditions, corporate denial, global toll. *Tobacco Control, 21*(2), 87–91.

Rasmussen, S. A., Jamieson, D. J., Honein, M. A., & Petersen, L. R. (2016). Zika virus and birth defects--reviewing the evidence for causality. *The New England Journal of Medicine, 374*(20), 1981–1987.

Reiss, J. (2015). *Causation, evidence, and inference.* Routledge.

Robins, J., & Wasserman, L. (1999). On the impossibility of inferring causation from association without background knowledge. In C. Glymour & G. F. Cooper (Eds.), *Computation, causation, discovery* (pp. 305–321). AAAI/MIT Press.

Rothman, K. J. (1976). Causes. *American Journal of Epidemiology, 104,* 87–92.

Rothman, K. J., & Greenland, S. (2005a). Causation and causal inference in epidemiology. *American Journal of Public Health, 95*(Suppl 1), S144–S150.

Rothman, K. J., & Greenland, S. (2005b). *Hill's criteria for causality* (0470011815). (Encyclopedia of biostatistics), Online, Issue.

Rubin, D. B. (1974). Estimating causal effects of treatments in randomized and nonrandomized studies. *Journal of Educational Psychology, 66*(5), 688–701.

Salmon, W. C. (1984). *Scientific explanation and the causal structure of the world.* Princeton University Press.

Shipley, B. (2000). *Cause and correlation in biology.* Cambridge University Press.

Spirtes, P., & Glymour, C. (1991). An algorithm for fast recovery of sparse causal graphs. *Social Science Computer Review, 9*(1), 62–72.

Spirtes, P., Glymour, C., & Scheines, R. (1991). From probability to causality. *Philosophical Studies: An International Journal for Philosophy in the Analytic Tradition, 64*, 1–36.

Spirtes, P., Glymour, C., & Scheines, R. (2000). *Causation, prediction, and search* (2nd ed.). MIT Press.

Spirtes, P., Glymour, C. N., & Scheines, R. (1993). *Causation, prediction, and search.* Springer-Verlag.

Stockel, D., Schmidt, F., Trampert, P., & Lenhof, H. P. (2015). CausalTrail: Testing hypothesis using causal Bayesian networks. *F1000Res, 4.*

Susser, M. (1991). What is a cause and how do we know one? A grammar for pragmatic epidemiology. *American Journal of Epidemiology, 133*, 635–648.

Tamm, M. (2021). Is causality a necessary tool for understanding our universe, or is it a part of the problem? *Entropy, 23*(7), 886.

Thygesen, L. C., Andersen, G. S., & Andersen, H. (2005). A philosophical analysis of the Hill criteria. *Journal of Epidemiology and Community Health, 59*(6), 512–516.

VanderWeele, T. J. (2015). *Explanation in causal inference: Methods for mediation and interaction.* Oxford University Press.

Weed, D. L. (2008). Truth, epidemiology, and general causation. *Brooklyn Law Review, 73*(3), 943–957.

Williamson, J. (2005). *Bayesian nets and causality: Philosophical and computational foundations.* Oxford University Press.

Woodward, J. (2003). *Making things happen - A theory of causal explanation.* Oxford University Press.

Worrall, J. (2007). Why there's no cause to randomize. *British Journal for the Philosophy of Science, 58*(3), 451–488.

Worrall, J. (2011). Causality in medicine: Getting back to the Hill top. *Preventive Medicine, 53*(4–5), 235–238.

PART III

Application

CHAPTER 8

Etiological Explanation

INTRODUCTION

In the preceding chapters I have outlined my views about inference, explanation, and causometry as elements of an approach to tackle uncertainty in medicine and the health sciences. I have stressed that I do not think that it is possible to eliminate uncertainty, but that these techniques play important roles in curbing its negative effects. In this chapter, I will provide an example of how uncertainty about the origin of a neonatal disorder, retinopathy of prematurity (ROP), can be reduced.

Over the past two decades I have worked on the clinical epidemiology of ROP (Chen et al., 2010, 2011; Dammann, 2010; Dammann et al., 2009, 2021; Dammann & Leviton, 2006; Holm et al., 2017; Ingvaldsen et al., 2021; Lee & Dammann, 2012; Lee et al., 2013; Morken et al., 2019; Rivera et al., 2017). Since my main interest is in ROP causation and explanation, I have also published in the philosophy of science literature (Dammann, 2017, 2020, 2021; Dammann et al., 2020; Dammann & Smart, 2019). In this chapter, I bring these two lines of research together.

This chapter is a modification of an early (single author) version of a paper previously published in *Progress in Retina and Eye Research*. The final version was co-authored with Brian Stansfield.

O. Dammann, *Uncertainty and Explanation in Medicine and the Health Sciences*, https://doi.org/10.1007/978-3-031-82271-1_8

Retinopathy of prematurity (ROP) is a neonatal neurovascular disorder of the retina and associated visual structures (Dammann et al., 2022; Hartnett, 2015; Hellstrom et al., 2013). The disorder is characterized by a two-phase course. Early after premature birth, retinal blood vessel growth is slowed down due to relative overexposure to exogenous oxygen in the delivery suite and neonatal intensive care unit (NICU). In preterm newborns, the immature lung tissue lacks a surface-active agent (surfactant) that is supposed to keep the lung open during exspiration. Although it is possible to administer surfactant exogenously after birth, some preterm infants still have relatively low oxygen levels in their blood so that exogenous oxygen is administered as well, with the unwanted side effect of retinal blood vessel growth inhibition. According to tissue requirements, developing blood vessels growth slows down when oxygen is abundant. In the second phase, exogenous oxygen supplementation is reduced when the newborn's lung begins to work better. This relative hypoxia (relative to elevated levels earlier) induces an overshoot in retinal blood vessel growth, which can have detrimental effects of partial or complete blindness. Since ROP can reach such sight-threatening stages and even lead to blindness, effective screening and early intervention is needed. Once the disease is diagnosed, treatment options (secondary prevention) include laser ablation and intravitreal injection of anti-vascular endothelial growth factor (VEGF) agents (VanderVeen & Cataltepe, 2019). However, both these interventions are rather invasive. Thus, primary prevention of ROP (reducing its incidence) remains an important goal. This, in turn, means that finding ways to identify and intervene on causes of the disease is paramount.

According to the above causal explanation, exposure to excessive and/or uncontrolled administration of exogenous oxygen is considered the main causal culprit. Part of my goal in this chapter is to demonstrate that evidence can be mounted in support of the hypothesis that oxygen is not the only cause of ROP. More specifically, my main claim is that, above and beyond being one of many clinical risk factors for ROP, neonatal sepsis, an overwhelming systemic infection, is also an independent cause, i.e., apart from oxygen. The upshot of this notion is that not only interventions targeting oxygen exposure but also interventions on neonatal sepsis and the associated systemic inflammatory response might help reduce the disease burden associated with ROP.

In the next section I will first briefly introduce ROP, neonatal sepsis, the idea of a "risk factor", and the central hypothesis of this chapter. I will then turn to the theoretical concepts of etiological explanation and combined contribution. Readers interested mainly in the biological component of my argument can skip this section and move on to a more detailed exposition of the main argument, which I support by contrasting the current "standard model of ROP" centered on oxygen with an alternative causal "infection → inflammation → ROP" model. Finally, I will apply Hill's heuristics as a quasi-causometer rooted in explanatory-coherentist reasoning.

RETINOPATHY OF PREMATURITY

Retinopathy of prematurity is a complex neonatal disorder with multiple factors contributing to the development of the disease. In this chapter I intend to mount the evidence in support of the proposal that neonatal sepsis meets all requirements for being a cause of ROP (not a just a precondition, mechanism, or innocent bystander) by means of initiating the early stages of the patho-mechanism of ROP occurrence, i.e., systemic inflammation.

I will use the model of etiological explanation as previously discussed, distinguishing between two overlapping processes in ROP causation: the causation process which includes cause and mechanism, and the disease process which includes the mechanism and the resulting features of the disorder itself (Fig. 8.1).

It can be shown that sepsis can initiate the early stages of the patho-mechanism via systemic inflammation (causation process) and that systemic inflammation can contribute to growth factor aberrations and the retinal characteristics of ROP (disease process). The combination of these factors with immaturity at birth (as intrinsic risk modifier) and prenatal

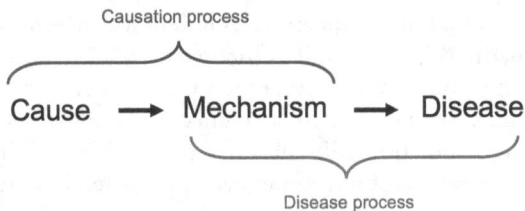

Fig. 8.1 Etiological explanation based on reference to the cause of a disease and the mechanism that connects cause and disease. Note that the disease mechanism is part of both the causation process and the disease process

inflammation (as extrinsic facilitator) seems to provide a cogent functional framework of ROP occurrence. Taken together, the above evidence supports the notion that neonatal sepsis is a causal initiator of ROP.

Among preterm infants, *sepsis* is a frequent and potentially life-threatening disease. Overall, sepsis is characterized as a "systemic infection that prompts a cascade of often fatal inflammatory immune responses" (Coggins & Glaser, 2022). Neonatal sepsis is defined as sepsis occurring within the first 28 days of postnatal life and is further divided into early onset (EOS) when occurring at day 2 or 3 after birth and late onset sepsis (LOS) when occurring later than 72 hours after birth (Hayes et al., 2021). In 2017, the annual worldwide number of new cases of neonatal sepsis was estimated at 1.327 million (James et al., 2018). In a comprehensive literature analysis of 26 articles accounting for almost 3 million live births, investigators calculated 2824 sepsis cases per 100,000 live births (Fleischmann et al., 2021). Among preterm newborns, the risk for EOS (~13%) is considerably higher than for LOS (~0.3%). Not all cases of sepsis are confirmed by a positive blood culture ("culture-proven sepsis"). If not "culture-proven", sepsis is considered to be "culture-negative" and sometimes called "clinical sepsis" (Coggins & Glaser, 2022). Among extremely low gestational age newborns, one of three infants with LOS does not survive. Both EOS and LOS have been identified as risk factors for ROP (Huang et al., 2019), and it is not yet clear if one is a stronger risk factor than the other.

For the purported causal relationship between LOS and ROP, the neonatal systemic inflammatory response to the bacterial initiator of a septic episode is crucially important (Dammann & Leviton, 2014). For the time being, it suffices to say that the systemic mediators of inflammation generated in neonatal sepsis, such as pro-inflammatory cytokines and chemokines, are likely mediators between infection and ROP by interfering with retinal growth factors that regulate vasculogenesis, thereby affecting retinal vessel growth. With the limit of neonatal viability now down to 22 weeks gestation at birth due to improved perinatal care in high resource settings, and the known increasing incidence of ROP with decreasing gestational age, the population at highest risk for ROP is growing.

The search for causes of illness begins with epidemiological risk factor studies. A whole host of risk factors for ROP has been identified *beyond* oxygen, including intrauterine growth restriction (Chu et al., 2020), low birthweight (Lundgren et al., 2014), being small for gestational age (Fortes Filho et al., 2009), surfactant administration (Termote et al., 1994), poor postnatal weight gain (Wallace et al., 2000), ethnicity (Aralikatti et al., 2010), hyperglycemia (Mohamed et al., 2013), sepsis (Tolsma et al., 2011), blood transfusions (Chalmers et al., 2020), and maternal conditions like usage of reproductive technologies (Trifonova et al., 2018), chorioamnionitis (Mitra et al., 2014), preeclampsia (Shulman et al., 2017), iron deficiency (Dai et al., 2015), diabetes (Opara et al., 2020), and smoking (Hudalla et al., 2021), among others.[1] However, most of these publications refrain from calling these risk factors *causes*. For example, in what is perhaps the most comprehensive review of risk factors for ROP to date, the term "cause" is used to refer to the relationship between ROP and blindness, between ROP examination and morbidity, between missing ROP at screening and its consequences, between the causes of preterm birth and ROP, and between surfactant deficiency and respiratory distress, but not for the relationship between risk factors and ROP (Kim et al., 2018). One reason might be that authors believe there can be only one cause of ROP and that this place is reserved for oxygen. Another reason might be that authors think that none of the risk factors they write about comes with a plausible mechanism that would connect cause and effect. And yet another might be that authors subscribe to the tenet "association is not causation" and think of non-randomized, observational risk factor studies of ROP as providing evidence only for the former but not for the latter.

A *risk factor* is, according to the National Cancer Institute,[2] "something that increases the chance of developing a disease". This definition requires the demonstration that the chance of developing disease is higher among individuals with the risk factor than among individuals without, which can only be ascertained using statistical approaches because "chance" and "risk" are quantitative concepts. This is a scenario of population risk, not personal risk. Granted, to have an increased chance of disease in a population, an association between risk factor and disease can only arise if more individuals with the risk factor develop the disease than those without. This would indicate that an increased *individual* risk for the disease gives rise to an increased *population* risk merely by accumulation. While the inference from one person (individual) to multiple (population) by means of accumulation seems straight forward, the inference backward from population to individual is more difficult (see Chap. 5). Another difficulty arises from the fact that in both individuals and populations the disease has already occurred in some without and more with the risk factor. Thus, risk estimation works backward in population studies if one does not look at prospective cohort studies where true incidence (new occurrence) of disease is compared between those with versus without the risk factor.

In general, risk analyses require large studies that involve many individuals with and without the purported risk factor, which deserves this appellation only if it is statistically associated with the disease in models that adjust for confounders. Thus, technically speaking, a risk factor is something that is associated with an increased disease *presence* (which we can observe in various kinds of studies), not really something that increases the chance of disease *occurrence* (which is an inference about future events based on prospective, adjusted data.) While the NCI definition appears to require a risk factor to increase the likelihood of disease *prospectively* (the disease has not yet occurred), my definition simply refers to available data from the past (disease has occurred and we can compare its prevalence or incidence among individuals with and without the risk factor).

One additional point is crucial: risk factors are not causes simply because they are first and foremost statistical associations and "association is not causation" without further ado. Theoretical (Hill, 1965) and mathematical (Hernán & Robins, 2006) tools have been developed to help decide when it is time to move from talk about a statistical risk factor to talk about a causal one. One of the few definitions of "cause" offered by health scientists is Mervyn Susser's of a cause as what makes a difference (Susser, 1991). I take Susser's difference-making to really mean the *making* (creation, production) of a difference, not just *being associated* with a difference. Of course, the question arises how to distinguish between risk factors that are just associated with ROP and factors that are causally involved in its occurrence? Among the methods that are supposed to help distinguish between the two kinds of risk factors, i.e., to move a risk factor from association to causation is confounder adjustment in multivariable risk analyses, propensity score adjustment or matching, target trial emulation, and Mendelian randomization. Of note, all of these are statistical methods that still rely on associations. The causal ingredient that is considered to reveal that an association is causal does not come directly from the data, but from study design (e.g., randomization) and analysis (e.g., rearrangement of observational data as a "target trial"). However, some of us are not entirely convinced that causal information can be extracted from statistical data at all (see Chap. 7). As philosopher of science Nancy Cartwright recognized many years ago, "No causes in, no causes out" (Cartwright, 1994).

The other method very familiar to epidemiologists and in fact often used is what may be called "explanatory coherence analysis" (ECA). In the most frequently cited paper about this method, the author describes how to evaluate causal hypotheses from data generated by observational studies (Hill, 1965). In essence, the method suggests taking nine viewpoints that would make causation a better explanation for the observed effect than a mere association. These viewpoints are temporality, strength of association, consistency, specificity, biological gradient, consistency, plausibility, coherence, and analogy. I will use this method to look at the evidence in support of a causal role for oxygen in ROP occurrence later in this chapter.

Still, a cause is usually taken to be a factor that *induces* an effect by means of a mechanism. To explain the occurrence of a disease using both causal and mechanical evidence is what I have called an "etiological explanation" (Dammann, 2020) (see Chap. 6). Indeed, it is important to not only ask *why* ROP occurs (this is a causal question) but also *how* a candidate risk factors contribute to ROP occurrence (this is a mechanical question). It is also important to recognize that the causal-mechanical *function* of risk factors may be very different in ROP causation. While all the risk factors for ROP listed above may make a difference to the risk for ROP in multivariable analyses, they are unlikely to have the same kind of initiating and productive function in ROP etiopathogenesis as oxygen does. In keeping with the causal-mechanical model for etiological explanations, it needs to be clarified for each risk factor whether it is a cause (initiator) of ROP occurrence (this is sometimes being called the "root cause"), part of the mechanism leading from cause to ROP, or simply an innocent bystander that happens to be associated with both the risk factor and ROP. One way of doing this is to use the concept I have come to call *combined contribution* (Dammann, 2017), in which risk factors of a disease are classified by the way *how* they contribute causally to illness occurrence.

The central hypothesis defended in this chapter has been a long way coming. The idea that neonatal sepsis might be a cause of ROP was induced by our work on systemic inflammation as a potential mechanism that connects prenatal intrauterine infection with neonatal brain white matter abnormalities (Dammann & Leviton, 1997, 1998). As a conceptual analogy, we first reviewed the information available in 2006 (Dammann & Leviton, 2006) and 2010 (Dammann, 2010) that supported the contention that a similar relationship might exist between perinatal infection, systemic inflammation, and ROP. Based on this rationale, we also suggested that there might in fact be a prenatal "pre-phase" of ROP that influences the occurrence and/or severity of the two postnatal phases of ROP (Dammann et al., 2021; Hellstrom et al., 2013; Lee & Dammann, 2012). Using this overarching theoretical framework, we then undertook clinical epidemiologic analyses using the data from the ELGAN (Extremely Low Gestational Age Newborn) study (Dammann et al., 2021) and found associations between placental infection/inflammation and ROP (Chen et al., 2011) and between neonatal systemic inflammation and ROP (Holm et al., 2017). At that time, we also joined forces with colleagues in Canada and reviewed the literature on inflammation in the progression of ROP. As part of that work, we suggested that ROP should not just be considered a disease of the central retina but also includes choroidal degeneration (Rivera et al., 2017). Finally, we expanded our framework to include long-term abnormal visual outcomes (AVO) (Ingvaldsen et al., 2021). Our suggestion is that both prenatal intrauterine infection and inflammation (IUI) as well as neonatal intermittent or sustained systemic inflammation (ISSI) may contribute to the etiology of both ROP and AVO, such as structural changes visible on magnetic resonance images, dorsal stream dysfunction, and retinal architecture changes (Morken et al., 2019). In order to redirect perinatal researchers' gaze from "just ROP" to "beyond ROP", we proposed that this entire scenario with pre- and postnatal exposures, ROP, and AVOs could be called "visuopathy of prematurity" (Ingvaldsen et al., 2021). A large, multi-center ROP-focused cohort study is needed (and in planning) that will allow us to test this hypothesis in a large dataset of preterm newborns. Let me now shift gears and move to the philosophical component of this chapter, and briefly introduce causation and causal inference with a focus on etiological explanation and combined contribution.

ETIOLOGICAL EXPLANATION AND COMBINED CONTRIBUTION

Two main aspects of my previous work are relevant for this chapter: first, the *etiological stance* I proposed (Dammann, 2017) as the basis for a more overarching account of the structure of *etiological explanations* (Dammann, 2020), the topic of the remainder of this section. Second, I proposed to view the classic qualitative causal method in epidemiology, the "Hill viewpoints" (Hill, 1965) as a heuristic for causal inference (Dammann, 2018) based on the framework of explanatory coherence as championed by Ted

Poston (Poston, 2014). This method for causal inference will be applied to the hypothesis that neonatal sepsis causes ROP in the last section of this chapter.

Etiological Explanation

Prevention of a disease such as ROP requires the ability to explain its etiology (causal origin) and pathogenesis (disease mechanism). In medicine, these terms are not very well defined. One way is to look at etiology as restricted to the cause in question and at the mechanism as what connects cause and effect. Simply put, flipping the light switch is usually viewed as the cause of the bulb beginning to emit light and the electricity flowing through the wiring from its energy source all the way to the bulb is viewed as the mechanism. This comes close to what Wesley Salmon called a "causal-mechanical explanation", in which the occurrence of an event is explained by reference to both causes and mechanisms (Salmon, 1984). However, the processes that lead to the occurrence of human disease are almost always more complex than flipping a light switch. To accommodate such complexity, I have previously developed a process framework of etiological explanations (Dammann, 2017, 2020) (see Chap. 6). In brief, the concept of "etiological explanation" holds that the term "etiology" (causal history) includes the entire process of disease occurrence, i.e., the etiological process. The *etiological process* consists of two overlapping sub-processes, i.e., the causation process and the disease process (Fig. 8.1). While the causation process includes initiating causes and the mediating patho-mechanism that connects causes with disease, the disease process includes the (subclinical) patho-mechanism and the (clinical) disease from start (very first signs or symptoms) to finish (recovery or death). The idea is that interfering with the causal process will eliminate or at least reduce the incidence of its effect, thereby promoting *primary prevention*, i.e., prevention before the disease process has begun. Interfering with the disease process leads to *secondary prevention*, i.e., prevention by interruption of the disease mechanism. Intervention that targets the adverse consequences of the disease is *tertiary prevention*. Thus, robust knowledge about the etiologic and disease processes of ROP would maximize intervention options.

In keeping with John Stuart Mill's multivariable model of causation (Mill, 1856), and with the view that each sufficient cause of any disease consists of a number of non-sufficient component causes (Rothman,

1976), I have proposed that taking a comprehensive and inclusive etiological stance when explaining illness occurrence by reference to the combination of contributors might be more informative than simply talking about "the cause" of a disease (Dammann, 2017). Rothman's sufficient-component cause model purports that diseases can have one or more constellations of *component causes* (think pieces of pizza) that jointly form *sufficient causes* of disease (think whole pizzas). The model is widely used to visualize how causation is conceptualized in epidemiology. One core message of the model is its multivariable view of causation. Another is that none of the sufficient causes is necessary to cause the disease because we can have multiple sufficient causes (multiple complete but different pizzas can lead to disease). The third is that only those component causes that are part of each possible kind of sufficient cause are a *necessary* component cause, simply because it is necessary to complete every one of the sufficient causes (pizzas). Without a necessary component cause disease will not occur because none of the sufficient causal constellations is complete. One of the downsides of the model is its terminology because it uses the word "cause" for both sufficient causes (constellations) and component causes, although both represent different causal concepts. While sufficient causes are constellations of multiple individual component causes, these component causes are individual causal contributors that are, in and of themselves, insufficient to cause the effect.

Combined Contribution

What the sufficient-component cause model does not specify is *how* individual component causes *contribute* to the etiological process. I therefore proposed to consider the *combined contribution* of several factors with different etiologic and pathogenetic functions. According to that model, component causes can be initiators, mediators, modifiers, and facilitators (Dammann, 2017). Attributing one or more of these roles to individual risk factors can provide a context-aware view of the combined contribution of said factors to the occurrence of illness, in our present case, ROP.[3]

Causal *initiators* are causes that start the etiological process. Consider the etiology of skin cancer due to excessive sun exposure (Fig. 8.2). In this example, the sun is what is usually considered a *root cause* of an event, the factor that started the first part of the etiological process, i.e., the causation process. In ROP research, exposure to excessive exogenous oxygen currently plays this role in the standard etiological explanation of ROP

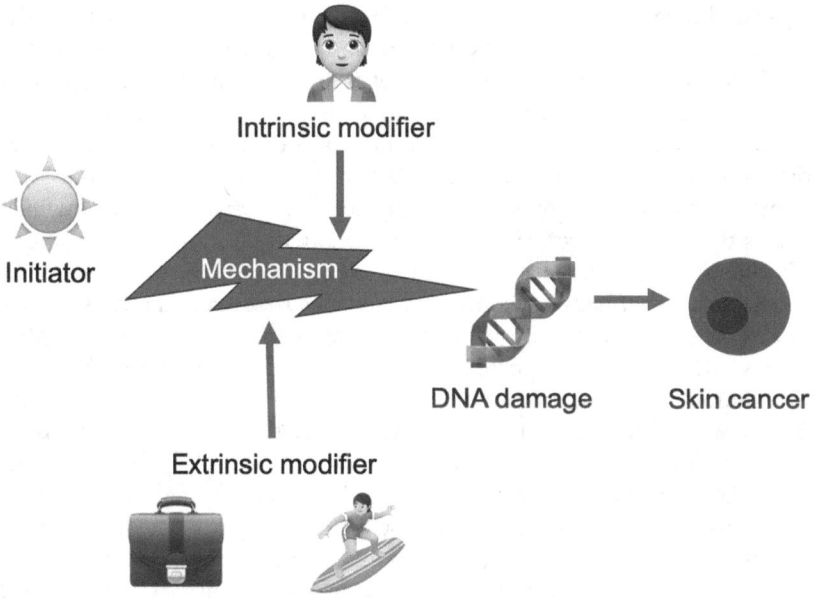

Fig. 8.2 Combined contribution initiator (sun), mechanism (UV-radiation), and intrinsic (skin color) and extrinsic (environment) to the development of skin cancer

occurrence. I submit that it is plausible that neonatal sepsis can play this role as well.

Causal *mediators* are the *mechanisms* that connect the initiators with the subsequent components of the etiological process, i.e., the way *how* an initiator exerts its effect on the illness of interest. We know that sun exposure comes with ultraviolet radiation that can damage skin cell DNA. In medical terminology mechanisms are often called patho-mechanism or pathogenesis. Work on the patho-mechanism of ROP focuses on the oxygen-dependent fluctuations of growth factors, mainly insulin-like growth factor (IGF) and vascular endothelial growth factor (VEGF), which connect oxygen exposure and blood vessel abnormalities in the preterm retina (Chen & Smith, 2007; Hartnett, 2015). It is possible that not just oxygen fluctuations but also sepsis-induced inflammatory signals (cytokines) can lead to dysregulation of growth factors that in turn affect retinal vessel growth.

Causal *modifiers* come in two varieties. *Intrinsic* modifiers are preexisting conditions that are characteristics of an individual, such as their genes. Intrinsic modifiers change the impact of an initiator and/or mechanism at the level of the individual. For example, having pale skin increases the negative impact of sunlight and UV radiation on someone's skin cancer risk compared to individuals with darker skin tones. In ROP etiology, immaturity at birth is almost certainly such an intrinsic modifier which makes the immature retina more vulnerable than the retinas of gestationally older infants (Dammann, 2023).

Extrinsic modifiers are events or conditions that make the causal story more (or less) likely to unfold. For example, working in a profession that comes with prolonged exposure to sunlight. In ROP etiology, such extrinsic condition could be intrauterine exposure to infection (Dammann et al., 2021), which may alter the risk for ROP associated with oxygen exposure and/or sepsis.

In the next two sections I will first apply this conceptual framework to the standard etiological explanation of ROP first with oxygen, then with infection inflammation as the causal initiator. Both sections offer detailed scientific evidence; readers not interested in such detail may skip forward to the section on Hill's heuristics.

THE CURRENT CAUSAL MODEL: OXYGEN

Among infants born preterm excessive exposure to high or volatile oxygen level is being viewed as *the* (and often the only) causal initiator of the etiological process that culminates in ROP occurrence (Rodriguez et al., 2023; Saugstad, 2006). Some authors assert this causal role for oxygen verbatim. For example, Weinberger and colleagues write that "oxygen also induces aberrant physiologic responses that can be damaging in premature infants. For example, vasoconstriction in the retina is an early response to oxygen that can lead to vasoobliteration, neovascularization, and retinal traction (retinopathy of prematurity)" (Weinberger et al., 2002). Claxton and Fruttiger write that "exposure to hyperoxia causes vaso-obliteration of capillaries in the retinal center" (Claxton & Fruttiger, 2003). My point here is not that the notion is wrong, merely that oxygen is viewed as the initiator of the causation process, not as a secondary contributor to ROP risk. The search for plausible causes of ROP began with the advent of modern neonatology when the disease was first observed in the 1940s. T.L. Terry is frequently quoted as the first author describing what he called "retrolental fibroplasia" (RLF) in the first half of the 1940s (Terry,

1942a, 1942b, 1944). A decade later some authors still wrote that "we know nothing about the etiology of the disease and, at present, we have no clue whatsoever to the factor that may cause retrolental fibroplasia" (Blodi & Parke, 1953).

The recognition that the exposure to excessive levels of oxygen plays a causal role in the development of ROP emerged in the early 1950s (Ashton, 1954; Campbell, 1951). Experimental oxygen-induced retinopathy (OIR) models were developed in the kitten (Ashton et al., 1954). In this model, a decrease in oxygen was associated with vessel budding in the retina and into adjacent tissue (Ashton et al., 1954) and intermittent hyperoxia in mice led to pathological signs of RLF, such as retinal folding and detachment (Gyllensten & Hellström, 1952).[4] Ever since V.E. Kinsey and A. Patz received the Albert Lasker Clinical Medical Research Award in 1956[5] "for discovering that excessive oxygen administration is the cause of retinopathy of prematurity in premature babies", the main etiologic focus of research, both in the laboratory and in clinical epidemiology, has been on oxygen as *the* cause of ROP (Rodriguez et al., 2023).

Dissenting voices surfaced in the early 1980s. Always a fierce critic of simplistic thinking, Bill Silverman referred to the fallacy of assuming that oxygen is the sole cause of ROP already in 1982, when he wrote that "[t]he watertight case in support of 'hyperoxia is the cause of ROP' has been leaking for years, the leaks are now so large they can no longer be dismissed" (Silverman, 1982). He doubled down in 1986 with the statement that "[n]othing is so dangerous as an idea – when it's the only one you have [such as the one that] supplemental oxygen is the sole necessary and sufficient cause of all instances of cicatricial retinopathy of prematurity" (Silverman, 1986). In important ways, the situation has not much changed until today and it is my explicit goal to open the discussion up for sepsis to be included as playing a causal role in the etiological explanation of ROP occurrence.

The successful development of OIR models in the rat (Ricci, 1990), mouse (Smith et al., 1994), and beagle (McLeod et al., 1996) has cemented exposure to excessive oxygen as the leading causal paradigm for ROP occurrence (Hartnett and Lane, 2013; Higgins, 2019; Saugstad, 2006). In keeping with this reasoning, many past and current preventive efforts have been directed at limiting exposure to exogenous oxygen.

Unfortunately, focusing experimental research on just one single cause may yield undesired consequences. Consider the introduction of the first rat model for neonatal brain damage using hypoxia-ischemia as the causal damage initiator (Rice et al., 1981). This animal model was introduced based on the assumption that perinatal brain damage is due to lack of oxygen and disrupted blood flow. This assumption was, in turn, based on the publication of a paper, among others, that described neuropathological changes in newborns that "had trouble breathing at birth" (Banker & Larroche, 1962)—no direct evidence of hypoxia or ischemia whatsoever. It is plausible to assume that at least some of the rationale for an animal model of hypoxia-ischemia came from adult neurology with its focus on ischemia and hemorrhage as major causes of stroke. While the "Vannucci-Model", as it is now called (Vannucci & Back, 2022), has remained very successful, its exclusive focus on oxygen and blood flow may have diverted both clinicians' and investigators' attention away from other possible causal scenarios. For more than three decades, for instance, the idea that perinatal (and even prenatal) infection might induce neonatal brain damage as well (Gilles et al., 1976; Leviton & Gilles, 1973) remained unexplored in the shadows of "hypoxic-ischemic encephalopathy". Only the recognition of pro-inflammatory cytokines as plausible mechanistic mediators (Dammann & Leviton, 1997; Leviton, 1993) led to the development of experimental models in the rabbit (Debillon et al., 2000) and rat (Cai et al., 2000) that demonstrated the causal potential of infection and inflammation in neonatal brain damage. I believe there is strong reason to speculate that something similar has happened in ROP research. The exclusive attention paid to the causal OIR model may have delayed investigators from using other causal paradigms, which have now been developed using lipopolysaccharide (LPS) in sheep (Loeliger et al., 2011), rats (Hong et al., 2014), and mice (Tremblay et al., 2013) after initial clinical findings had suggested that perinatal infection and systemic inflammation might play a role in the etiology of ROP as well (Dammann, 2010; Lee & Dammann, 2012).

The standard etiological explanation of ROP occurrence refers to a multifactorial sequence of events that begins with preterm birth, which often makes artificial ventilation and oxygen supplementation necessary (Schulzke et al., 2021). Oxygen saturation has effects on a functional network of growth factors including insulin-like growth factor-1 (IGF-1), hypoxia-inducible factor 1-alpha (HIF1-alpha), vascular endothelial growth factor (VEGF), placental growth factor-1 (PlGF-1). Prolonged administration of oxygen can lead to excessively high oxygen levels, and/ or oxygen fluctuations lead to changes in angiogenic growth factor patterns IGF and VEGF (Hartnett & Lane, 2013; Saugstad, 2006) that lead to early cessation of retinal vessel growth in phase 1 and a subsequent overshoot of vessel growth in phase 2 (Chen & Smith, 2007; Hartnett & Penn, 2012). This network, in turn, regulates retinal blood vessel growth and cessation thereof (Hartnett & Lane, 2013; Saugstad, 2006). Oxygen-induced growth factor imbalance has thus been identified as the main pathogenetic mechanism of ROP occurrence (Chen & Smith, 2007; Hartnett, 2015). In this etiological explanation, exogenous oxygen is the causal initiator of ROP occurrence, changes in retinal vascular growth factor patterns represent the mediating patho-mechanism, and preterm birth is a modifier.

Despite its long history as an etiologic factor in ROP, the clinical association between oxygen and ROP is far from trivial. Oxygen exposure defined by saturation targets (Liu et al., 2022), oxygen fluctuations (McColm et al., 2004), and number of days on oxygen (Estrada et al., 2022), among others, have been identified as being associated with an increased risk for treatment-requiring ROP. On the other hand, some investigators did not identify a contribution of multiple variables of oxygen burden to ROP risk beyond that contributed by low gestational age (Chen et al., 2021).

The currently predominant view that low gestational age plays an important role in the etiopathogenesis of ROP is based on the cumulative evidence over many decades pointing to low gestational age as the strongest predictor of ROP (Yu et al., 2022). Indeed, the disease occurs predominantly among infants born at extremely low gestational age (Hong et al., 2021; Quinn et al., 2018), although it can also occur in newborns >34 wks gestation at birth (Azad et al., 2020; Padhi et al., 2014; Quinn, 2016; Ratra et al., 2017; Shah et al., 2012).

Sometimes, low gestational age is considered a risk factor for ROP, simply because the incidence of ROP increases with decreasing gestational age and preterm infants are at greater risk of ROP than term infants. However, low gestational age *in and of itself* is just an indicator of immaturity at birth, and immaturity at birth *alone* is unlikely to be sufficient for ROP to occur. Therefore, I have argued elsewhere that prematurity "per se" does not cause ROP in preterm infants, while prenatal and postnatal factors associated with preterm birth are more likely the causal initiator (Dammann, 2023). Neonatal sepsis may be just such a postnatal cause.

Still, low gestational age at birth (preterm birth) is an interesting causal contributor because it is a marker for multiple other causal contributors. Thus, low gestational age is probably better viewed as a background condition for ROP rather than a causal risk factor of ROP, just as we think of advanced age as a condition for Alzheimer's disease, not as a cause of it. Instead, it is an antecedent of postnatal interventions and events that might be considered causes of ROP (e.g., oxygen exposure and neonatal sepsis; see next sections). In turn, preterm birth is caused by prenatal conditions that might be associated with different levels of ROP risk (Lee et al., 2013). In other words, low gestational age is not only an indicator for biological immaturity at birth but also a marker for causes of preterm birth and for neonatal consequences of preterm birth. Whether it is an intrinsic or extrinsic modifier remains to be clarified. I tend toward thinking it is both. From the perspective of prevention, it still makes sense to suggest that reducing the incidence of preterm birth would lead to less ROP (Kim et al., 2018). However, the preventive mechanism would not be an intervention on risk factors for ROP but an intervention that reduces the population at risk.

ALTERNATIVE MODEL: SEPSIS

As outlined above, there is little doubt that exposure to excessive and/or fluctuating oxygen levels play a role as causal initiator in the natural history of ROP. However, there is no reason to believe that oxygen is *the only* causal initiator. Let me echo the questions that Silverman asked in 1982 (Silverman, 1982): Why does ROP occur in infants who never received supplemental oxygen? Why are there so many infants with prolonged and volatile oxygen exposure who never develop ROP? And why are there still so many infants with ROP after so many changes have been made to neonatal clinical oxygen policies based on decades of clinical studies on optimal oxygen saturation targets?

According to Manschot, infection was considered an etiological factor in the natural history of RLF as early as 1951 by Houlton and Crosse, and by Szewczyk (Manschot, 1954). However, these were inferences based on limited observations in case series, not yet supported by systematic analyses of larger datasets like those available a few decades later. By the mid-1980s, neonatal sepsis had become known as a risk factor for ROP for more than five years (Gunn et al., 1980). Of note, investigators had found that among infants who needed resuscitation with oxygen, sepsis was still significantly associated with ROP, indicating an impact of sepsis above and beyond oxygen. In one of the earlier trials designed to assess the effect of Vitamin E on the occurrence of RLF, sepsis was among the significant risk factors for RLF (Hittner et al., 1981). In the National Collaborative Study on Patent Ductus Arteriosus in Premature Infants, infants with a birth-weight <1750g admitted to 1 of 13 participating hospitals were recruited (Purohit et al., 1985). Among those discharged alive, sufficient data were available for 3025 infants. The overall percentage of RLF (the authors used the previous term for the disorder now called ROP) was 11%. Sepsis was one of the significant risk factors in a multivariable analysis.

Cats and Tan remarked in 1985 that the finding of a difference in sepsis incidence between infants with ROP and without "has evoked little comment" (Cats & Tan, 1985). To some degree, this remains true today. Apart from the scattered studies in which the association between sepsis and ROP was one among many findings and two meta-analyses (Huang et al., 2019; Wang et al., 2019), we do not yet have a comprehensive concept about whether and how sepsis might qualify as a causal initiator of ROP occurrence, and whether and how sepsis and oxygen may play inter-related roles in ROP etiology. In the remainder of this section, I begin mounting the evidence in support of the notion that sepsis is a cause of ROP.

When we previously proposed a role for infection and inflammation in ROP and abnormal visual outcomes (AVO) in preterm infants (Dammann, 2010; Dammann & Leviton, 2006; Rivera et al., 2017), our focus was on the hypothesis that *prenatal* infection and inflammation might modify the risk for ROP (Hellstrom et al., 2013; Lee & Dammann, 2012) and AVO (Ingvaldsen et al., 2021). However, multiple lines of evidence support the hypothesis that *postnatal* neonatal sepsis might also be a risk factor for ROP in addition to oxygen and perhaps even qualify as a causal initiator apart from oxygen.

The association between neonatal sepsis and ROP is documented in many studies (Huang et al., 2019; Wang et al., 2019). Both bacterial or fungal sepsis remain relevant in multivariable risk analyses adjusting for gestational age and oxygen exposure (Bonafiglia et al., 2022; Huncikova et al., 2023; Manzoni et al., 2006; Tolsma et al., 2011; Wang et al., 2019). This suggests that sepsis might be a "second hit" in addition to oxygen (Chen et al., 2011) or perhaps even trigger the postnatal phases of ROP without oxygen being involved at all. The notion that sepsis is a second, independent cause of ROP might be particularly important in light of our finding that oxygen is a stronger risk factor for ROP in infants born at 23–25 weeks gestation than in older infants, while sepsis is a stronger risk factor among infants born at 28–29 weeks gestation (Chen et al., 2011). This raises the possibility that while both oxygen and sepsis play a role in both stages, oxygen might have a stronger influence on stage 1 ROP than sepsis, while sepsis might have more influence on stage 2 than oxygen.

Fungal sepsis emerged as a risk factor for ROP in the 1990s (Kremer et al., 1992; Mittal et al., 1998). However, subsequent studies differ considerably regarding cohort definition and data analytic strategy (Giannantonio et al., 2012; Haroon Parupia & Dhanireddy, 2001; Karlowicz et al., 2000; Manzoni et al., 2006; Noyola et al., 2002; Tadesse et al., 2002). A meta-analysis published in 2008 resulted in a pooled relative risk estimate (odds ratio) of 3.4 (95% CI 2.3–5) for any ROP and 4.1 (3.1–5.4) for severe ROP (Bharwani & Dhanireddy, 2008). The odds ratios in all six studies with any ROP as the outcome ranged from 2 to 10, and in the seven studies on severe ROP from 3 to 5.3. These data indicate that the more than two-fold risk increase for ROP and severe ROP with exposure to candida sepsis is very unlikely to be due to chance alone.

In some studies, late onset sepsis (LOS) appears to be a stronger risk factor than early onset sepsis (EOS). In one of our own analyses, the risk for retinal indicators of severe ROP (e.g., in zone 1 at the center of the retina, prethreshold/threshold, and plus disease) was considerably higher in infants with definitive late bacteremia (11%, 21%, and 16%, resp.) than in infants without (5%, 11%, 8%). We did not observe such differential for early onset bacteremia (7%, 17%, 14%) compared to no early bacteremia (8%, 14%, 9%) (Tolsma et al., 2011). In a study that also identified LOS as a risk factor for ROP above and beyond oxygen and low gestational age, none of the 60 infants with ROP had EOS while 3% of those without did (Manzoni et al., 2006). In a very large study comparing 1597 infants with severe ROP to 10,657 infants with no or mild ROP, the exposure to EOS was not associated with a risk increase (OR 1.0, 95% CI 0.76–1.32) while the exposure to LOS was (1.39, 1.26–1.52) adjusting for confounders including gestational age, but not supplemental oxygen (Goldstein et al., 2019). Although the timing of ROP development may vary among infants, it is likely that late sepsis preferentially affects the second, vasoproliferative phase of ROP.

According to the model of combined contribution in etiological explanations, several factors contribute to ROP in a combined fashion. In what follows I think of sepsis as the inducing cause, inflammation as the first-level mediator (part 1 of the mechanism), and growth factor dysregulation as the second-level mediator (part 2 of the mechanism).

If sepsis can initiate the pathophysiologic process of ROP independent of oxygen, one should expect that (1) preterm infants not exposed to oxygen can develop ROP and (2) exposure to substances mimicking systemic infection such as lipopolysaccharide (LPS) should lead to an ROP-like phenotype without oxygen supplementation being involved. The first contention is supported by early case reports of term infants without oxygen exposure who had "fundus changes consistent with retrolental fibroplasia" (Schulman et al., 1980) and by Bill Silverman's above-quoted statement in 1982 (Silverman, 1982). More recently, oxygen has become so prominent a risk factor that published studies rarely include tables that provide pertinent supportive information.

The second conjecture finds support from animal experiments that suggest the possibility that intraperitoneal injection of LPS during the first five postnatal days leads to systemic inflammation, retinal ROP-like abnormalities (Hong et al., 2014; Tremblay et al., 2013), and subsequently to reduced retinal function (Tremblay et al., 2013). In a neonatal OIR mouse model, pro-inflammatory cytokines are upregulated in the retina and reduced by magnolol treatment, which also leads to reduced retinal HIF-1α and VEGF expression and a significant reduction of neovascular tufts (Yang et al., 2016). Exposure to systemic LPS is associated with elevated levels of inflammatory cytokines in the retinas of neonatal rats (Hong et al., 2014) and with retinal microglia activation and increased levels of inflammatory cytokines in neonatal mice (Tremblay et al., 2013). The hypothesis that retinal microglia might be the link between infection and retinal inflammation is further supported by the finding that after exposure to LPS, pig retinal primary microglial cell cultures respond with an increased production of IL-1β and other pro-inflammatory cytokines (Lim et al., 2019). A study in chronically instrumented fetal sheep suggests that prenatal i.v. LPS administration over three days does not lead to changes in retinal vascularized area, blood vessel width, or neovascularization (Loeliger et al., 2011). However, total thickness of both central and peripheral retina was reduced, and ganglion cell number as well as cell somal areas in the inner nuclear layer were smaller compared to controls (Loeliger et al., 2011).

The above-referenced experimental findings (Hong et al., 2014; Tremblay et al., 2013) raise the possibility that inflammation plays a mechanistic role in infection-associated retinal abnormalities. In keeping with this hypothesis, Wang and colleagues have offered three possibilities how sepsis can lead to ROP, all involving sepsis-induced inflammatory responses (Wang et al., 2019). First, they refer to pathogenetic work done in diabetic retinopathy (Joussen et al., 2004) that points toward *inflammation*-induced endothelial damage, vessel obstruction and leakage, and subsequent non-perfusion of retinal areas. Second, they raise the possibility that systemic inflammation induces an *oxidative stress* response, which in turn activates VEGF pathways (Ushio-Fukai, 2007) and retinal vaso-proliferation. Third, they refer to *inflammation*-induced upregulation of HIF1-alpha (Malkov et al., 2021), which in turn contributes to ROP (Sun et al., 2020). Thus, it seems plausible that oxidative stress and systemic inflammation might contribute to ROP either separately or jointly.

When Cats and Tan found sepsis and exchange transfusions to be significantly associated with ROP in the mid-1980s (Cats & Tan, 1985), they did not think of sepsis as a pointer to oxygen as the main risk factor for ROP. Instead, they thought of sepsis-induced hemolysis as a common cause of ROP (via oxidative stress) and the need for transfusion, another prominent risk factor for ROP (Chalmers et al., 2020). When comparing 31 infants with ROP and 95 controls, the variable indicating total antioxidant status (TAS) was lower in cases than controls, while total oxidant status (TOS) was higher in cases compared to controls (Erdal et al., 2023). The hypothesis that oxidative stress might be a contributor to ROP occurrence was tested by Chemtob and coworkers in a neonatal piglet model (Hardy et al., 1994). They found that activation of the cyclooxygenase pathway causes the occurrence of free radicals in the retinal and choroidal vasculature. Subsequent studies confirmed that reactive oxygen species stimulate the release of thromboxane, a mediator of retinal vasoconstriction implicated in the neovascularization process that is part of ROP (Chemtob et al., 1995).

While it seems plausible that oxidative stress is the mediator between oxygen exposure and ROP (Saugstad, 2006), it might not be the mediator between sepsis and ROP. Indeed, an oxidative stress response does not necessarily seem to be associated with sepsis. For example, Seema et al. found that levels of TNF but not of free radical scavengers differed between 30 infants with neonatal sepsis and 20 controls (Seeema et al., 1999). The view that oxidative stress plays a role in phase 1 ROP (Fevereiro-Martins et al., 2023) while the impact of inflammation might be stronger in phase 2 dovetails with the above proposal that the impact of hyperoxia might be stronger in gestationally younger infants, while sepsis is a more prominent risk factor in gestationally slightly older infants (Chen et al., 2011).

Just like oxygen elicits an oxidative stress response, neonatal sepsis elicits an intermittent or sustained systemic inflammation (ISSI), the worst form sometimes being called a "cytokine storm" (Dammann & Leviton, 2014). If ISSI connects sepsis and ROP, systemically elevated markers of inflammation should be associated with an increased risk for ROP. Multiple studies suggest that exactly that is the case. Silveira et al. found median plasma levels of interleukin (IL) -6, -8, and -10 (but not of IL-1β and tumor necrosis factor (TNF)-α) elevated on postnatal day (d)1 in 8 infants with severe ROP compared to 49 infants who did not develop ROP (Silveira et al., 2011). Sood and colleagues compared inflammatory cytokine levels in whole blood from 877 infants with a birthweight below 1000g (Sood et al., 2010). They found that IL-6 levels were elevated on d1 in infants with mild versus no ROP and the same when comparing infants with severe versus mild ROP. After d3, C-reactive protein (CRP) levels distinguished between no and mild ROP on d3 and d21, while IL-18 was elevated in infants with severe ROP (compared to no ROP) on d7, 14, and 21. In a small case-control study, Yu and coauthors matched 30 infants with a gestational age <32wks with 62 infants without ROP on gestational age and birthweight. In serum obtained by umbilical cord venipuncture they found levels of IL-7, monocyte chemotactic protein (MCP)-1, as well as macrophage inflammatory protein (MIP)-1α and -1β elevated in cases compared to controls (Yu et al., 2014). Since these measurements were made at birth, the biomarker elevations are unlikely to be due to oxygen exposure, unless the inverse is true and infants with elevated markers of inflammation in their umbilical cord blood are at increased need for postnatal supplemental oxygen administration. In our own ELGAN-study cohort (Dammann et al., 2021), we measured 27 cytokines, chemokines, and growth factors on postnatal d1, d7, d14 (early epoch), and d21 and d28 (late epoch) in 1205 infants <28wks gestational age who had at least one eye exam (Holm et al., 2017). In the early epoch, top quartile levels of myeloperoxidase (MPO) and IL-8 on ≥2 days were associated with an increased risk for ROP. In the late epoch (on both d21 and d28) elevated levels of MPO, IL-8, IL-6, serum amyloid A (SAA), and TNF-receptor (TNF-R)1 and 2 were associated with an increased risk for ROP. Again, this finding supports the hypothesis that systemic inflammation plays a more prominent role in stage 2 of ROP etiology than in stage 1. A recent comprehensive analysis of the literature on systemic cytokines and ROP still focuses on oxygen exposure as the root cause and sees cytokine production only as a characteristic of neonatal sepsis, which in turn is listed as one of multiple neonatal "related disorders" that happen to be associated with systemic inflammation (Wu et al., 2023). The hypothesis that neonatal sepsis is a causal risk factor for ROP is further supported by the observation that inflammatory systemic cytokines generated in the context of sepsis may regulate or interfere with the vasculogenic growth factor network that can be viewed as the final molecular pathway to ROP (Pierce et al., 1995; Ramshekar & Hartnett, 2021; Tsai et al., 2022), whether that pathway started with oxygen or sepsis.

Perhaps the most important regulator of retinal neovascularization in oxygen-induced retinopathy (OIR) models is vascular endothelial growth factor (VEGF) (Ramshekar & Hartnett, 2021), which has led to the development of injectable intra-ocular anti-VEGF molecules as the most recent innovation in ROP treatment (Hartnett, 2020). The main regulator of VEGF is hypoxia-inducible factor (HIF) (Penn et al., 2008). Inhibition of the HIF/VEGF pathway by celastrol, a vine plant extract with anti-inflammatory properties, inhibits retinal microglia activation and inflammation and reduces retinal neovascularization and the avascular areas in a mouse OIR model (Zhao et al., 2022). Recombinant thrombomodulin domain 1 (Huang et al., 2021) and melatonin (Xu et al., 2018) appear to exert similar protective effects.

In one of the two papers on LPS-induced retinopathy reference above, VEGF was upregulated in whole retina extracts (Tremblay et al., 2013) but remained unaltered on postnatal day 7 in the other (Hong et al., 2014). Instead, the expression of endogenous inhibitor of angiogenesis thrombospondin (TSP)-1 was increased (Hong et al., 2014). In a murine uveitis model of intravitreous peptidoglycan (PGN, mimicking gram-positive infection) or LPS injection (mimicking gram-negative infection), both exposures led to VEGF upregulation (Lafreniere et al., 2019). Although the authors do not report on the differential of inflammatory cytokine expression after PGN/LPS administration, they show a reduced expression after bevacizumab administration in PGN- but not in LPS-induced uveitis. I am not aware that such differential effect has been studied in the immature retina.

In sum, there is ample evidence in support of an etiological explanation of the occurrence of ROP that includes neonatal sepsis as the causal initiator, inflammation and subsequent growth factor perturbation as mechanism, and preterm birth as a modifier. In the next section I will check the available evidence on sepsis as a candidate cause of ROP against one of the epidemiological quasi-causometers, i.e., Bradford Hill's nine heuristics for causal inference (Hill, 1965) that Alfredo Morabia has called the "sui generis" approach to causal inference in epidemiology (Morabia, 2013).

Hill's Heuristics Applied to Sepsis and ROP

In the 1950s and 1960s it was still a matter of debate whether smoking might cause lung cancer. In 1964, the US Surgeon General's office published a committee report that listed a handful of "criteria for causation" that, taken together, supported the notion that cigarette smoke might indeed be a cause of pulmonary malignancies (United States. Surgeon General's Advisory Committee on Smoking and Health, 1964). One year later, medical statistician and epidemiologist Sir Austin Bradford Hill published a lecture on similar causal heuristics (he called them "viewpoints") that, as Hill suggested, cannot prove causation but offer support for a causal hypothesis based on characteristics of epidemiological data in comparison to other evidence (Hill, 1965).

Hill's paper can be counted among the most influential in all of epidemiology and still remains in use today. For example, it has been used by multiple teams of investigators to assess the evidence in support of the hypothesis that Zika virus causes microcephaly (Awadh et al., 2017; Frank et al., 2016; Rasmussen et al., 2016). Hill's notion that his heuristics can support a causal claim but not offer causal proof makes them, I believe, a "quasi-causometer".

Hill's heuristics draw on the concept of explanatory coherence, meaning "good explanatory fit". One piece of information coheres with others if it fits well with the overarching picture or story. Coherence is strongly context-dependent. For example, a French word in a text that is otherwise written in English may seem incoherent if considered from the language perspective but might be coherent from the content perspective (as in "Bon weekend!"). Although coherence is also one of Hill's nine individual viewpoints, I have previously pointed out that, taken together, all nine represent a set of heuristics that can be seen as an explanatory-coherentist evidence network when brought together with models of explanatory coherence (Poston, 2014; Thagard, 2006), mutually supporting each other in their joint support of a causal hypothesis (Dammann, 2018).[6]

In the present context, Hill's heuristics can offer support for the hypothesis that neonatal sepsis causes ROP based on the degree to which they can be "checked off" against the available evidence connecting neonatal sepsis and ROP. In what follows, I show how evidence from ROP research supports most of Hill's nine viewpoints, thereby indicating that causation is a better explanation for the sepsis-ROP relationship than mere statistical association. For each viewpoint I will give only a summary of the evidence; much of the supporting detail can be found in the previous sections of this chapter.

Temporality is the viewpoint that to establish a cause-effect relationship the purported cause must precede the effect to avoid a wrong causal conclusion in cases where the causal relationship is inverse. Most studies of sepsis as a risk factor of ROP do not speak to the issue whether sepsis or ROP occurred or was diagnosed first. However, it would not make sense to assume that reverse causation is a viable explanation of the association because ROP (retinal dys-vascularization) cannot cause sepsis (an overwhelming systemic infection and inflammatory response), other than in the indirect and unlikely scenario where the eye exam performed by the ophthalmologist for the purpose of ROP screening contributes to a systemic infection.

Strength of association: Hill proposed that it is more likely that we are looking at causation if the association is strong rather than weak. This is what I have previously called "causal vigor". The pooled odds ratio for any ROP and severe ROP in one meta-analysis (Wang et al., 2019) were 1.6 and 2.3, respectively, representing a 60% and 130% risk increase. In another meta-analysis these estimates were 2.2 and 1.9, respectively (Huang et al., 2019). These data, together with those summarized above, can be seen as indicating a strong association.

Consistency of association: The two available meta-analyses on sepsis as a risk factor for any/severe ROP refer to 11/6 (Wang et al., 2019) and 20/22 (Huang et al., 2019) studies. Most of these studies show a risk increase of ROP with neonatal sepsis. I conclude that the association between sepsis and ROP is consistent across many if not most studies.

Specificity of association: This viewpoint refers to the idea promoted by Robert Koch and Jacob Henle: "one bug, one disease" and "one disease, one bug". In our present scenario this would mean that sepsis and nothing else but sepsis causes ROP and that sepsis causes ROP but nothing else. Of course, this kind of specificity does not hold in the case of sepsis and ROP, and it probably does not hold for *any* other cause of complex disease. Thygesen and coworkers have pointed out that multiple authors have criticized this viewpoint and even suggested that it is useless (Thygesen et al., 2005), while Fedak and coauthors hold that it "may have new and interesting implications in the broader context of data integration" (Fedak et al., 2015). I believe it is, therefore, prudent not to put too much weight on this viewpoint.[7]

Biological gradient: This is about dose-response relationships. In an analysis based on a national dataset from Germany, currently published only in abstract form in German. We found in 12,563 preterm infants (22–28 completed weeks of gestation) that the relative risk for the association between sepsis increases from 1.4 (1.2–1.6) if children had one sepsis episode to 1.8 (1.2–2.3) if children had two episodes and further to 4.7 (2.3–9.7) (Glaser et al., 2024). I consider these data strong evidence in support of the notion that a "dose-response" relationship exists between the number of sepsis episodes and the risk for ROP.

Experiment: We have results from animal experiments that model the sepsis exposure and ROP outcome using lipopolysaccharide (LPS) as the exposure in rats (Hong et al., 2014) and sheep (Loeliger et al., 2011). In both studies, the exposure led to ROP-like abnormalities in the retina of the exposed animals.

Plausibility: Much of the plausibility must come by reference to the mechanism that connects sepsis and ROP. Multiple previous papers by us (Dammann, 2010; Lee & Dammann, 2012; Rivera et al., 2017) and others (Fevereiro-Martins et al., 2022) have reviewed the accumulating evidence in support of the argument that systemic inflammation is a plausible mediator between neonatal sepsis and ROP. In tandem with systemic inflammation, oxidative stress also appears to play a mechanistic role; the differential or joint role of the two mechanisms in ROP production remains to be clarified.

Coherence: A causal role for sepsis in ROP is coherent with other pieces of information about ROP, because sepsis does result in ROP-like retina abnormalities in animal experiments (Hong et al., 2014), is associated with ROP in many observational studies (Huang et al., 2019; Wang et al., 2019), and generates inflammatory responses that are likely involved in the pathogenesis of ROP and adverse visual outcomes in preterm infants (Ingvaldsen et al., 2021). The conjecture that ROP is a causal initiator of ROP "fits" with other kinds of evidence that support the same notion.

Analogy: Neonatal sepsis is associated with adverse neurodevelopmental outcomes such as cerebral palsy (Alshaikh et al., 2013) and cognitive abnormalities (Cai et al., 2019) among preterm newborns. The analogy with ROP becomes eminently clear when considering the role of inflammation in the pathogenesis of adverse visual outcomes beyond ROP among preterm infants, which led us to postulate a "visuopathy of prematurity" that shares causes (oxygen, sepsis) and mechanisms (oxidative stress, inflammation) with ROP (Ingvaldsen et al., 2021). Another analogy would be that not only bacterial but also fungal sepsis is associated with an increased risk for ROP.

In sum, all of Hill's viewpoints (except specificity which may have achieved the status of irrelevance in a post-Koch-Henle world of causal inference) support the notion that neonatal sepsis is a cause of ROP, not just an innocent bystander. If Hill's quasi-causometer works, the available evidence suggests that the observed statistical association between sepsis and ROP reflects biological causation.

*   *   *

Retinopathy of prematurity is a complex neonatal disorder with multiple contributing factors. In this chapter I have used the model of etiological explanation and combined contribution to mount the evidence in support of the proposal that neonatal sepsis meets all requirements for being a cause of ROP (not a condition, mechanism, or innocent bystander) by means of initiating the early stages of the patho-mechanism of ROP occurrence, systemic inflammation (causation process), which can contribute to growth factor aberrations and the retinal characteristics of ROP (disease process). The combined contribution of these factors with immaturity at birth (as intrinsic risk modifier) and prenatal inflammation (as extrinsic modifier) seems to provide a cogent functional framework of ROP occurrence. Finally, I have applied the Bradford Hill's heuristics to the available evidence as a quasi-causometer. Taken together, the above suggests that neonatal sepsis is a causal initiator of ROP.

For the sheer complexity of the etiological explanation of ROP, future research will need to be performed using the approach of a prospective cohort study. Important questions to clarify are, for example, whether prenatal infection/inflammation modifies the oxygen- and sepsis-associated risk for ROP in similar or different ways and how oxidative stress and systemic inflammation interact as patho-mechanisms. Moreover, the differential effect of oxygen and sepsis at different post-conceptional ages on the two phases of ROP should be clarified using novel measures of oxygen exposure and retinal diagnosis based on advanced imaging. Regarding the timing of neonatal sepsis, the relative contribution of early and late onset sepsis deserves further study. It is my hope that such work will motivate investigators to develop novel interventions that target neonatal sepsis and will be helpful in designing strategies to reduce the burden associated with ROP.

Finally, this chapter was an example for how the concepts of etiological explanation and causometry can be applied in a complex biomedical context, thereby reducing etiological uncertainty. Indeed, the process might even be considered generating knowledge, but note that all we have done is mount an argument and run published data by Hill's heuristics. In this sense, the chapter has not accomplished a scientific goal, but merely an explanatory one.

NOTES

1. I have offered only one reference for each of these risk factors while multiple or even many are available for most of them.
2. https://www.cancer.gov/publications/dictionaries/cancer-terms/def/risk-factor
3. Note that on this view, the causal contribution of background conditions is considered a causal factor, albeit some philosophers distinguish between causes and conditions (Broadbent, 2008).
4. Neonatologist Bill Silverman has told the fascinating story of this early research on RLF in the Scientific American in 1977 (Silverman, 1977).
5. https://laskerfoundation.org/winners/excessive-oxygen-as-cause-of-blindness-in-premature-infants/
6. Together with philosophers Ted Poston and Paul Thagard, I have shown that Hill's heuristics can be mapped onto other systems of causal explanation (Dammann et al., 2020).
7. In philosophy of medicine this viewpoint has come to be called "the doctrine of specific etiology"; see (Ross, 2018).

REFERENCES

Alshaikh, B., Yusuf, K., & Sauve, R. (2013). Neurodevelopmental outcomes of very low birth weight infants with neonatal sepsis: Systematic review and meta-analysis. *Journal of Perinatology, 33*(7), 558–564.

Aralikatti, A. K., Mitra, A., Denniston, A. K., Haque, M. S., Ewer, A. K., & Butler, L. (2010). Is ethnicity a risk factor for severe retinopathy of prematurity? *Archives of Disease in Childhood. Fetal and Neonatal Edition, 95*(3), F174–F176.

Ashton, N. (1954). Pathological basis of retrolental fibroplasia. *The British Journal of Ophthalmology, 38*(7), 385–396.

Ashton, N., Ward, B., & Serpell, G. (1954). Effect of oxygen on developing retinal vessels with particular reference to the problem of retrolental fibroplasia. *The British Journal of Ophthalmology, 38*(7), 397–432.

Awadh, A., Chughtai, A. A., Dyda, A., Sheikh, M., Heslop, D. J., & MacIntyre, C. R. (2017). Does Zika virus cause microcephaly - Applying the Bradford Hill viewpoints. *PLoS Currents, 9*.

Azad, R., Gilbert, C., Gangwe, A. B., Zhao, P., Wu, W.-C., Sarbajna, P., et al. (2020). Retinopathy of prematurity: How to prevent the third epidemics in developing countries. *Asia-Pacific Journal of Ophthalmology, 9*(5), 440–448.

Banker, B. Q., & Larroche, J. C. (1962). Periventricular leukomalacia of infancy. *Archives of Neurology, 7*, 386–410.

Bharwani, S. K., & Dhanireddy, R. (2008). Systemic fungal infection is associated with the development of retinopathy of prematurity in very low birth weight infants: A meta-review. *Journal of Perinatology: Official Journal of the California Perinatal Association, 28*, 61–66.

Blodi, F. C., & Parke, P. C. (1953). Retrolental fibroplasia. *The American Journal of Nursing, 53*(6), 718–720.

Bonafiglia, E., Gusson, E., Longo, R., Ficial, B., Tisato, M. G., Rossignoli, S., et al. (2022). Early and late onset sepsis and retinopathy of prematurity in a cohort of preterm infants. *Scientific Reports, 12*(1), 11675.

Broadbent, A. (2008). The difference between cause and condition. *Proceedings of the Aristotelian Society, 108*(1pt3), 355–364.

Cai, S., Thompson, D. K., Anderson, P. J., & Yang, J. Y.-M. (2019). Short- and long-term neurodevelopmental outcomes of very preterm infants with neonatal sepsis: A systematic review and meta-analysis. *Children, 6*(12), 131.

Cai, Z., Pan, Z. L., Pang, Y., Evans, O. B., & Rhodes, P. G. (2000). Cytokine induction in fetal rat brains and brain injury in neonatal rats after maternal lipopolysaccharide administration. *Pediatric Research, 47*(1), 64–72.

Campbell, K. (1951). Intensive oxygen therapy as a possible cause of retrolental fibroplasias: A clinical approach. *The Medical Journal of Australia, 2*, 48–50.

Cartwright, N. (1994). No causes in, no causes out. In *Nature's capacities and their measurement* (pp. 39–90). Oxford University Press.

Cats, B. P., & Tan, K. E. (1985). Retinopathy of prematurity: Review of a four-year period. *British Journal of Ophthalmology, 69*(7), 500–503.

Chalmers, J., Zhu, Z., Hua, X., Yu, Y., Zhu, P., Hong, K., et al. (2020). Effect of red blood cell transfusion on the development of retinopathy of prematurity: A systematic review and meta-analysis. *PLoS One, 15*(6), e0234266.

Chemtob, S., Hardy, P., Abran, D., Li, D. Y., Peri, K., Cuzzani, O., et al. (1995). Peroxide-cyclooxygenase interactions in postasphyxial changes in retinal and choroidal hemodynamics. *Journal of Applied Physiology, 78*(6), 2039–2046.

Chen, J., & Smith, L. E. (2007). Retinopathy of prematurity. *Angiogenesis, 10*(2), 133–140.

Chen, J. S., Anderson, J. E., Coyner, A. S., Ostmo, S., Sonmez, K., Erdogmus, D., et al. (2021). Quantification of early neonatal oxygen exposure as a risk factor for retinopathy of prematurity requiring treatment. *Ophthalmology Science, 1*(4), 100070.

Chen, M. L., Allred, E. N., Hecht, J. L., Onderdonk, A., Vanderveen, D. K., Wallace, D. K., et al. (2011). Placenta microbiology and histology and the risk for severe retinopathy of prematurity. *Investigative Ophthalmology & Visual Science, 52*, 7052–7058.

Chen, M. L., Citil, A., McCabe, F., Leicht, K. M., Fiascone, J., Dammann, C. E. L., et al. (2011). Infection, oxygen, and immaturity: Interacting risk factors for retinopathy of prematurity. *Neonatology, 99*, 125–132.

Chen, M. L., Guo, L., Smith, L. E., Dammann, C. E., & Dammann, O. (2010). High or low oxygen saturation and severe retinopathy of prematurity: A meta-analysis. *Pediatrics, 125*(6), e1483–e1492.

Chu, A., Dhindsa, Y., Sim, M. S., Altendahl, M., & Tsui, I. (2020). Prenatal intra-uterine growth restriction and risk of retinopathy of prematurity. *Scientific Reports, 10*(1), 17591.

Claxton, S., & Fruttiger, M. (2003). Role of arteries in oxygen induced vaso-obliteration. *Experimental Eye Research, 77*(3), 305–311.

Coggins, S. A., & Glaser, K. (2022). Updates in Late-Onset Sepsis: Risk Assessment, Therapy, and Outcomes. *NeoReviews, 23*(11), 738–755.

Dai, A. I., Demiryurek, S., Aksoy, S. N., Perk, P., Saygili, O., & Gungor, K. (2015). Maternal iron deficiency anemia as a risk factor for the development of retinopathy of prematurity. *Pediatric Neurology, 53*(2), 146–150.

Dammann, O. (2010). Inflammation and retinopathy of prematurity. *Acta Paediatrica, 99*(7), 975–977.

Dammann, O. (2017). The etiological stance: Explaining illness occurrence. *Perspectives in Biology and Medicine, 60*(2), 151–165.

Dammann, O. (2018). Hill's heuristics and explanatory coherentism in epidemiology. *American Journal of Epidemiology, 187*(1), 1–6.

Dammann, O. (2020). *Etiological explanations: Illness causation theory.* CRC Press.

Dammann, O. (2021). Agent-based models as etio-prognostic explanations. *Argumenta, 1*, 19–38.

Dammann, O. (2023). Does prematurity "per se" cause visual deficits in preterm infants without retinopathy of prematurity? *Eye (London, England), 37*, 2587–2589.

Dammann, O., Brinkhaus, M. J., Bartels, D. B., Dordelmann, M., Dressler, F., Kerk, J., et al. (2009). Immaturity, perinatal inflammation, and retinopathy of prematurity: A multi-hit hypothesis. *Early Human Development, 85*, 325–329.

Dammann, O., & Leviton, A. (1997). Maternal intrauterine infection, cytokines, and brain damage in the preterm newborn. *Pediatric Research, 42*(1), 1–8.

Dammann, O., & Leviton, A. (1998). Infection remote from the brain, neonatal white matter damage, and cerebral palsy in the preterm infant. *Seminars in Pediatric Neurology, 5*(3), 190–201.

Dammann, O., & Leviton, A. (2006). Inflammation, brain damage and visual dysfunction in preterm infants. *Seminars in Fetal & Neonatal Medicine,* *11*(5), 363–368.

Dammann, O., & Leviton, A. (2014). Intermittent or sustained systemic inflammation and the preterm brain. *Pediatric Research, 75*(3), 376–380.

Dammann, O., Leviton, A., O'Shea, T. M., & Paneth, N. (Eds.). (2021). *Extremely preterm birth and its consequences.* Mac Keith Press.

Dammann, O., Mezinska, S., & Gefenas, E. (2022). Health humanities in medicina: The auxiliary stance. *Medicina (Kaunas, Lithuania), 58*(3), 411.

Dammann, O., Poston, T., & Thagard, P. (2020). How do medical researchers make causal inferences? In K. McCain & K. Kampourakis (Eds.), *What is scientific knowledge? An introduction to contemporary epistemology of science* (pp. 33–51). Routledge.

Dammann, O., Rivera, J. C., & Chemtob, S. (2021). The prenatal phase of retinopathy of prematurity. *Acta Paediatrica, 110*(9), 2521–2528.

Dammann, O., & Smart, B. (2019). *Causation in population health informatics and data science.* Springer.

Debillon, T., Gras-Leguen, C., Verielle, V., Winer, N., Caillon, J., Roze, J. C., et al. (2000). Intrauterine infection induces programmed cell death in rabbit periventricular white matter. *Pediatric Research, 47,* 736–742.

Erdal, H., Demirtas, M. S., Kılıcbay, F., & Tunc, G. (2023). Evaluation of oxidative stress levels and dynamic thiol-disulfide balance in patients with retinopathy of prematurity. *Current Eye Research 48*(11), 1026–1033.

Estrada, M. M., Tomlinson, L. A., Yu, Y., Ying, G.-S., & Binenbaum, G. (2022). Daily oxygen supplementation and risk of retinopathy of prematurity. *Ophthalmic Epidemiology, 30,* 1–9.

Fedak, K. M., Bernal, A., Capshaw, Z. A., & Gross, S. (2015). Applying the Bradford Hill criteria in the 21st century: How data integration has changed causal inference in molecular epidemiology. *Emerging Themes in Epidemiology, 12*(1), 14.

Fevereiro-Martins, M., Guimarães, H., Marques-Neves, C., & Bicho, M. (2022). Retinopathy of prematurity: Contribution of inflammatory and genetic factors. *Molecular and Cellular Biochemistry, 477*(6), 1739–1763.

Fevereiro-Martins, M., Marques-Neves, C., Guimarães, H., & Bicho, M. (2023). Retinopathy of prematurity: A review of pathophysiology and signaling pathways. *Survey of Ophthalmology, 68*(2), 175–210.

Fleischmann, C., Reichert, F., Cassini, A., Horner, R., Harder, T., Markwart, R., et al. (2021). Global incidence and mortality of neonatal sepsis: A systematic review and meta-analysis. *Archives of Disease in Childhood, 106*(8), 745–752.

Fortes Filho, J. B., Valiatti, F. B., Eckert, G. U., Costa, M. C., Silveira, R. C., & Procianoy, R. S. (2009). Is being small for gestational age risk factor for retinopathy of prematurity? A study with 345 very low birth weight preterm infants. *Jornal de Pediatria, 85*(1), 48–54.

Frank, C., Faber, M., & Stark, K. (2016). Causal or not: Applying the Bradford Hill aspects of evidence to the association between Zika virus and microcephaly. *EMBO Molecular Medicine, 8*(4), 305–307.

Fuller, J. (2022). Epidemiological Evidence: Use at Your 'Own Risk'? *Philosophy of Science, 87*(5), 1119–1129.

Giannantonio, C., Papacci, P., Cota, F., Vento, G., Tesfagabir, M. G., Purcaro, V., et al. (2012). Analysis of risk factors for progression to treatment-requiring ROP in a single neonatal intensive care unit: Is the exposure time relevant? *The Journal of Maternal-Fetal & Neonatal Medicine, 25*(5), 471–477.

Gilles, F. H., Leviton, A., & Kerr, C. S. (1976). Endotoxin leucoencephalopathy in the telencephalon of the newborn kitten. *Journal of the Neurological Sciences, 27*(2), 183–191.

Glaser, K., Hartel, C., Klingenberg, C., Herting, E., Fortmann, M. I., Speer, C. P., Stensvold, H. J., Huncikova, Z., Ronnestad, A. E., Nentwich, M. M., Stahl, A., Dammann, O., Gopel, W., German Neonatal Network, t.N.N.N.I., the Infection, I.I., Immunisation section of the European Society for Paediatric, R. (2024). Neonatal Sepsis Episodes and Retinopathy of Prematurity in Very Preterm Infants. JAMA Netw Open 7, e2423933.

Goldstein, G. P., Leonard, S. A., Kan, P., Koo, E. B., Lee, H. C., & Carmichael, S. L. (2019). Prenatal and postnatal inflammation-related risk factors for retinopathy of prematurity. *Journal of Perinatology, 39*(7), 964–973.

Gunn, T. R., Easdown, J., Outerbridge, E. W., & Aranda, J. V. (1980). Risk factors in retrolental fibroplasia. *Pediatrics, 65*(6), 1096–1100.

Gyllensten, L. J., & Hellström, B. E. (1952). Retrolental fibroplasia - animal experiments - the effect of the eyes of fullterm mice. a preliminary report. *Acta Paediatrica, 41*(6), 577–582.

Hardy, P., Abran, D., Li, D. Y., Fernandez, H., Varma, D. R., & Chemtob, S. (1994). Free radicals in retinal and choroidal blood flow autoregulation in the piglet: Interaction with prostaglandins. *Investigative Ophthalmology & Visual Science, 35*(2), 580–591.

Haroon Parupia, M. F., & Dhanireddy, R. (2001). Association of postnatal dexamethasone use and fungal sepsis in the development of severe retinopathy of prematurity and progression to laser therapy in extremely low-birth-weight infants. *Journal of Perinatology, 21*(4), 242–247.

Hartnett, M. E. (2015). Pathophysiology and mechanisms of severe retinopathy of prematurity. *Ophthalmology, 122*(1), 200–210.

Hartnett, M. E. (2020). Retinopathy of prematurity: Evolving treatment with anti–vascular endothelial growth factor. *American Journal of Ophthalmology, 218*, 208–213.

Hartnett, M. E., & Lane, R. H. (2013). Effects of oxygen on the development and severity of retinopathy of prematurity. *Journal of AAPOS, 17*(3), 229–234.

Hartnett, M. E., & Penn, J. S. (2012). Mechanisms and management of retinopathy of prematurity. *The New England Journal of Medicine, 367*(26), 2515–2526.

Hayes, R., Hartnett, J., Semova, G., Murray, C., Murphy, K., Carroll, L., et al. (2021). Neonatal sepsis definitions from randomised clinical trials. *Pediatric Research, 93*(5), 1141–1148.

Hellstrom, A., Smith, L. E., & Dammann, O. (2013). Retinopathy of prematurity. *Lancet, 382*(9902), 1445–1457.

Hernán, M. A., & Robins, J. M. (2006). Estimating causal effects from epidemiologic data. *Journal of Epidemiology and Community Health, 60*, 578–586.

Higgins, R. D. (2019). Oxygen saturation and retinopathy of prematurity. *Clinics in Perinatology, 46*(3), 593–599.

Hill, A. B. (1965). The environment and disease: Association or causation? *Proceedings of the Royal Society of Medicine, 58*, 295–300.

Hittner, H. M., Godio, L. B., Rudolph, A. J., Adams, J. M., Garcia-Prats, J. A., Friedman, Z., et al. (1981). Retrolental fibroplasia: Efficacy of vitamin E in a double-blind clinical study of preterm infants. *New England Journal of Medicine, 305*(23), 1365–1371.

Holm, M., Morken, T. S., Fichorova, R., VanderVeen, D., Allred, E. N., Dammann, O., et al. (2017). Systemic inflammation-associated proteins and retinopathy of prematurity in infants born before the 28th week of gestation. *Investigative Ophthalmology & Visual Science, 58*, 6419–6428.

Hong, E. H., Shin, Y. U., Bae, G. H., Choi, Y. J., Ahn, S. J., Sobrin, L., et al. (2021). Nationwide incidence and treatment pattern of retinopathy of prematurity in South Korea using the 2007–2018 national health insurance claims data. *Scientific Reports, 11*(1), 1451.

Hong, H. K., Lee, H. J., Ko, J. H., Park, J. H., Park, J. Y., Choi, C. W., et al. (2014). Neonatal systemic inflammation in rats alters retinal vessel development and simulates pathologic features of retinopathy of prematurity. *Journal of Neuroinflammation, 11*, 87.

Huang, J., Tang, Y., Zhu, T., Li, Y., Chun, H., Qu, Y., et al. (2019). Cumulative evidence for association of sepsis and retinopathy of prematurity. *Medicine (Baltimore), 98*(42), e17512.

Huang, Y.-H., Kuo, C.-H., Peng, I. C., Chang, Y.-S., Tseng, S.-H., Conway, E. M., et al. (2021). Recombinant thrombomodulin domain 1 rescues pathological angiogenesis by inhibition of HIF-1α-VEGF pathway. *Cellular and Molecular Life Sciences, 78*(23), 7681–7692.

Hudalla, H., Bruckner, T., Poschl, J., Strowitzki, T., & Kuon, R. J. (2021). Maternal smoking as an independent risk factor for the development of severe retinopathy of prematurity in very preterm infants. *Eye (London, England), 35*(3), 799–804.

Huncikova, Z., Vatne, A., Stensvold, H. J., Lang, A. M., Stoen, R., Brigtsen, A. K., et al. (2023). Late-onset sepsis in very preterm infants in Norway in

2009–2018: A population-based study. *Archives of Disease in Childhood. Fetal and Neonatal Edition, 108*(5), 478–484.

Ingvaldsen, S. H., Morken, T. S., Austeng, D., & Dammann, O. (2021). Visuopathy of prematurity: Is retinopathy just the tip of the iceberg? *Pediatric Research, 91*(5), 1043–1048.

James, S. L., Abate, D., Abate, K. H., Abay, S. M., Abbafati, C., Abbasi, N., et al. (2018). Global, regional, and national incidence, prevalence, and years lived with disability for 354 diseases and injuries for 195 countries and territories, 1990–2017: A systematic analysis for the Global Burden of Disease Study 2017. *The Lancet, 392*(10159), 1789–1858.

Joussen, A. M., Poulaki, V., Le, M. L., Koizumi, K., Esser, C., Janicki, H., et al. (2004). A central role for inflammation in the pathogenesis of diabetic retinopathy. *The FASEB Journal, 18*(12), 1450–1452.

Karlowicz, M. G., Giannone, P. J., Pestian, J., Morrow, A. L., & Shults, J. (2000). Does candidemia predict threshold retinopathy of prematurity in extremely low birth weight (</=1000 g) neonates? *Pediatrics, 105*(5), 1036–1040.

Kim, S. J., Port, A. D., Swan, R., Campbell, J. P., Chan, R. V. P., & Chiang, M. F. (2018). Retinopathy of prematurity: A review of risk factors and their clinical significance. *Survey of Ophthalmology, 63*(5), 618–637.

Kremer, I., Naor, N., Davidson, S., Arbizo, M., & Nissenkorn, I. (1992). Systemic candidiasis in babies with retinopathy of prematurity. *Graefe's Archive for Clinical and Experimental Ophthalmology, 230*(6), 592–594.

Lafreniere, J. D., Toguri, J. T., Gupta, R. R., Samad, A., O'Brien, D. M., Dickinson, J., et al. (2019). Effects of intravitreal bevacizumab in Gram-positive and Gram-negative models of ocular inflammation. *Clinical & Experimental Ophthalmology, 47*(5), 638–645.

Lee, J., & Dammann, O. (2012). Perinatal infection, inflammation, and retinopathy of prematurity. *Seminars in Fetal & Neonatal Medicine, 17*(1), 26–29.

Lee, J. W., McElrath, T., Chen, M., Wallace, D. K., Allred, E. N., Leviton, A., et al. (2013). Pregnancy disorders appear to modify the risk for retinopathy of prematurity associated with neonatal hyperoxemia and bacteremia. *The Journal of Maternal-Fetal & Neonatal Medicine, 26*(8), 811–818.

Leviton, A. (1993). Preterm birth and cerebral palsy: Is tumor necrosis factor the missing link? *Developmental Medicine and Child Neurology, 35*(6), 553–558.

Leviton, A., & Gilles, F. H. (1973). An epidemiologic study of perinatal telencephalic leucoencephalopathy in an autopsy population. *Journal of the Neurological Sciences, 18*(1), 53–66.

Lim, R. R., Hainsworth, D. P., Mohan, R. R., & Chaurasia, S. S. (2019). Characterization of a functionally active primary microglial cell culture from the pig retina. *Experimental Eye Research, 185*, 107670.

Liu, T., Tomlinson, L. A., Yu, Y., Ying, G. S., Quinn, G. E., Binenbaum, G., et al. (2022). Changes in institutional oxygen saturation targets are associated with an increased rate of severe retinopathy of prematurity. *Journal of AAPOS, 26*(1), 18.

Loeliger, M. M., Mackintosh, A., De Matteo, R., Harding, R., & Rees, S. M. (2011). Erythropoietin protects the developing retina in an ovine model of endotoxin-induced retinal injury. *Investigative Opthalmology & Visual Science, 52*(5), 2656–2661.

Lundgren, P., Kistner, A., Andersson, E. M., Hansen Pupp, I., Holmstrom, G., Ley, D., et al. (2014). Low birth weight is a risk factor for severe retinopathy of prematurity depending on gestational age. *PLoS One, 9*(10), e109460.

Malkov, M. I., Lee, C. T., & Taylor, C. T. (2021). Regulation of the Hypoxia-Inducible Factor (HIF) by pro-inflammatory cytokines. *Cells, 10*(9), 2340.

Manschot, W. A. (1954). Etiology of retrolental fibroplasia. *Archives of Ophthalmology, 52*(6), 833–845.

Manzoni, P., Maestri, A., Leonessa, M., Mostert, M., Farina, D., & Gomirato, G. (2006). Fungal and bacterial sepsis and threshold ROP in preterm very low birth weight neonates. *Journal of Perinatology, 26*(1), 23–30.

McColm, J. R., Cunningham, S., Wade, J., Sedowofia, K., Gellen, B., Sharma, T., et al. (2004). Hypoxic oxygen fluctuations produce less severe retinopathy than hyperoxic fluctuations in a rat model of retinopathy of prematurity. *Pediatric Research, 55*(1), 107–113.

McLeod, D. S., Brownstein, R., & Lutty, G. A. (1996). Vaso-obliteration in the canine model of oxygen-induced retinopathy. *Investigative Ophthalmology & Visual Science, 37*(2), 300–311.

Mill, J. S. (1856). *A system of logic* (4th ed.). John W. Parker & Son.

Mitra, S., Aune, D., Speer, C. P., & Saugstad, O. D. (2014). Chorioamnionitis as a risk factor for retinopathy of prematurity: A systematic review and meta-analysis. *Neonatology, 105*(3), 189–199.

Mittal, M., Dhanireddy, R., & Higgins, R. D. (1998). Candida sepsis and association with retinopathy of prematurity. *Pediatrics, 101*(4 Pt 1), 654–657.

Mohamed, S., Murray, J. C., Dagle, J. M., & Colaizy, T. (2013). Hyperglycemia as a risk factor for the development of retinopathy of prematurity. *BMC Pediatrics, 13*, 78.

Morabia, A. (2013). Hume, Mill, Hill, and the sui generis epidemiologic approach to causal inference. *American Journal of Epidemiology, 178*(10), 1526–1532.

Morken, T. S., Dammann, O., Skranes, J., & Austeng, D. (2019). Retinopathy of prematurity, visual and neurodevelopmental outcome, and imaging of the central nervous system. *Seminars in Perinatology, 43*(6), 381–389.

Noyola, D. E., Bohra, L., Paysse, E. A., Fernandez, M., & Coats, D. K. (2002). Association of candidemia and retinopathy of prematurity in very low birth-weight infants. *Ophthalmology, 109*(1), 80–84.

Opara, C. N., Akintorin, M., Byrd, A., Cirignani, N., Akintorin, S., & Soyemi, K. (2020). Maternal diabetes mellitus as an independent risk factor for clinically significant retinopathy of prematurity severity in neonates less than 1500g. *PLoS One, 15*(8), e0236639.

Padhi, T. R., Rath, S., Jalali, S., Pradhan, L., Kesarwani, S., Nayak, M., et al. (2014). Larger and near-term baby retinopathy: A rare case series. *Eye, 29*(2), 286–289.

Penn, J. S., Madan, A., Caldwell, R. B., Bartoli, M., Caldwell, R. W., & Hartnett, M. E. (2008). Vascular endothelial growth factor in eye disease. *Progress in Retinal and Eye Research, 27*(4), 331–371.

Pierce, E. A., Avery, R. L., Foley, E. D., Aiello, L. P., & Smith, L. E. (1995). Vascular endothelial growth factor/vascular permeability factor expression in a mouse model of retinal neovascularization. *Proceedings of the National Academy of Sciences of the United States of America, 92*(3), 905–909.

Poston, T. (2014). *Reason and explanation: A defense of explanatory coherentism* [text]. Palgrave Macmillan.

Purohit, D. M., Ellison, R. C., Zierler, S., Miettinen, O. S., & Nadas, A. S. (1985). Risk factors for retrolental fibroplasia: Experience with 3,025 premature infants. *Pediatrics, 76*(3), 339–344.

Quinn, G. (2016). Retinopathy of prematurity blindness worldwide: Phenotypes in the third epidemic. *Eye and Brain, 8,* 31–36.

Quinn, G. E., Ying, G.-s., Bell, E. F., Donohue, P. K., Morrison, D., Tomlinson, L. A., et al. (2018). Incidence and early course of retinopathy of prematurity. *JAMA Ophthalmol, 136*(12), 1383–1389.

Ramshekar, A., & Hartnett, M. E. (2021). Vascular endothelial growth factor signaling in models of oxygen-induced retinopathy: Insights into mechanisms of pathology in retinopathy of prematurity. *Frontiers in Pediatrics, 9,* 796143.

Rasmussen, S. A., Jamieson, D. J., Honein, M. A., & Petersen, L. R. (2016). Zika virus and birth defects--reviewing the evidence for causality. *The New England Journal of Medicine, 374*(20), 1981–1987.

Ratra, D., Akhundova, L., & Das, M. (2017). Retinopathy of prematurity like retinopathy in full-term infants. *Oman Journal of Ophthalmology, 10*(3), 167–172.

Ricci, B. (1990). Oxygen-induced retinopathy in the rat model. *Documenta Ophthalmologica, 74*(3), 171–177.

Rice, J. E. d., Vannucci, R. C., & Brierley, J. B. (1981). The influence of immaturity on hypoxic-ischemic brain damage in the rat. *Annals of Neurology, 9*(2), 131–141.

Rivera, J. C., Holm, M., Austeng, D., Morken, T. S., Zhou, T. E., Beaudry-Richard, A., et al. (2017). Retinopathy of prematurity: Inflammation, choroidal degeneration, and novel promising therapeutic strategies. *Journal of Neuroinflammation, 14*(1), 165.

Rodriguez, S. H., Ells, A. L., Blair, M. P., Shah, P. K., Harper, C. A., Martinez-Castellanos, M. A., et al. (2023). Retinopathy of prematurity in the 21st century and the complex impact of supplemental oxygen. *Journal of Clinical Medicine, 12*(3), 1228.

Ross, L. N. (2018). The doctrine of specific etiology. *Biology and Philosophy, 33,* 37.

Rothman, K. J. (1976). Causes. *American Journal of Epidemiology, 104*, 87–92.

Salmon, W. C. (1984). *Scientific explanation and the causal structure of the world.* Princeton University Press.

Saugstad, O. D. (2006). Oxygen and retinopathy of prematurity. *Journal of Perinatology, 26* (Suppl 1), S46–50; discussion S63–44.

Schulman, J., Jampol, L. M., & Schwartz, H. (1980). Peripheral proliferative retinopathy without oxygen therapy in a full-term infant. *American Journal of Ophthalmology, 90*(4), 509–514.

Schulzke, S. M., Stoecklin, B., & von Ungern-Sternberg, B. (2021). Update on ventilatory management of extremely preterm infants—A Neonatal Intensive Care Unit perspective. *Pediatric Anesthesia, 32*(2), 363–371.

Seema, R. K., Mandal, R. N., Tandon, A., Randhawa, V. S., Mehta, G., et al. (1999). Serum TNF-alpha and free radical scavengers in neonatal septicemia. *The Indian Journal of Pediatrics, 66*(4), 511–516.

Shah, P. K., Narendran, V., & Kalpana, N. (2012). Aggressive posterior retinopathy of prematurity in large preterm babies in South India. *Archives of Disease in Childhood - Fetal and Neonatal Edition, 97*(5), F371–F375.

Shulman, J. P., Weng, C., Wilkes, J., Greene, T., & Hartnett, M. E. (2017). Association of maternal preeclampsia with infant risk of premature birth and retinopathy of prematurity. *JAMA Ophthalmol, 135*(9), 947–953.

Silveira, R. C., Fortes Filho, J. B., & Procianoy, R. S. (2011). Assessment of the contribution of cytokine plasma levels to detect retinopathy of prematurity in very low birth weight infants. *Investigative Ophthalmology & Visual Science, 52*, 1297–1301.

Silverman, W. A. (1977). The lesson of retrolental fibroplasia. *Scientific American, 236*(6), 100–107.

Silverman, W. A. (1982). Retinopathy of prematurity: Oxygen dogma challenged. *Archives of Disease in Childhood, 57*(10), 731–733.

Silverman, W. A. (1986). Epoche in retinopathy of prematurity. *Archives of Disease in Childhood, 61*(5), 522–525.

Sjoberg, E.A., 2017. Logical fallacies in animal model research. *Behavioral and Brain Functions, 13*(1), Article No. 3.

Smith, L. F., Wesolowski, E., McLellan, A., Kostyk, S. K., D'Amato, R., Sullivan, R., et al. (1994). Oxygen-induced retinopathy in the mouse. *Investigative Ophthalmology & Visual Science, 35*(1), 101–111.

Sood, B. G., Madan, A., Saha, S., Schendel, D., Thorsen, P., Skogstrand, K., et al. (2010). Perinatal systemic inflammatory response syndrome and retinopathy of prematurity. *Pediatric Research, 67*(4), 394–400.

Stockel, D., Schmidt, F., Trampert, P., Lenhof, H.P., 2015. *CausalTrail: Testing hypothesis using causal Bayesian networks.* F1000Res 4.

Sun, M., Wadehra, M., Casero, D., Lin, M.-C., Aguirre, B., Parikh, S., et al. (2020). Epithelial Membrane Protein 2 (EMP2) Promotes VEGF-induced pathological neovascularization in murine oxygen-induced retinopathy. *Investigative Opthalmology & Visual Science, 61*(2), 3.

Susser, M. (1991). What is a cause and how do we know one? A grammar for pragmatic epidemiology. *American Journal of Epidemiology, 133*, 635–648.

Tadesse, M., Dhanireddy, R., Mittal, M., & Higgins, R. D. (2002). Race, Candida sepsis, and retinopathy of prematurity. *Biology of the Neonate, 81*(2), 86–90.

Termote, J. U., Schalij-Delfos, N. E., Wittebol-Post, D., Brouwers, H. A., Hoogervorst, B. R., & Cats, B. P. (1994). Surfactant replacement therapy: A new risk factor in developing retinopathy of prematurity? *European Journal of Pediatrics, 153*(2), 113–116.

Terry, T. L. (1942a). Extreme prematurity and fibroblastic overgrowth of persistent vascular sheath behind each crystalline lens. *American Journal of Ophthalmology, 25*, 203–204.

Terry, T. L. (1942b). Fibroblastic overgrowth of persistent tunica vasculosa lentis in infants born prematurely: II. Report of cases-clinical aspects. *Transactions of the American Ophthalmological Society, 40*, 262–284.

Terry, T. L. (1944). Retrolental fibroplasia in the premature infant: V. further studies on fibroplastic overgrowth of the persistent tunica vasculosa lentis. *Transactions of the American Ophthalmological Society, 42*, 383–396.

Thagard, P. (2006). Evaluating explanations in law, science, and everyday life. *Current Directions in Psychological Science, 15*(3), 141–145.

Thygesen, L. C., Andersen, G. S., & Andersen, H. (2005). A philosophical analysis of the Hill criteria. *Journal of Epidemiology and Community Health, 59*(6), 512–516.

Tolsma, K. W., Allred, E. N., Chen, M. L., Duker, J., Leviton, A., & Dammann, O. (2011). Neonatal bacteremia and retinopathy of prematurity: The ELGAN study. *Archives of Ophthalmology, 129*(12), 1555–1563.

Tremblay, S., Miloudi, K., Chaychi, S., Favret, S., Binet, F., Polosa, A., et al. (2013). Systemic inflammation perturbs developmental retinal angiogenesis and neuroretinal function. *Investigative Ophthalmology & Visual Science, 54*(13), 8125–8139.

Trifonova, K., Slaveykov, K., Mumdzhiev, H., & Dzhelebov, D. (2018). Artificial reproductive technology - a risk factor for retinopathy of prematurity. *Open Access Macedonian Journal of Medical Sciences, 6*(11), 2245–2249.

Tsai, A. S., Chou, H. D., Ling, X. C., Al-Khaled, T., Valikodath, N., Cole, E., et al. (2022). Assessment and management of retinopathy of prematurity in the era of anti-vascular endothelial growth factor (VEGF). *Progress in Retinal and Eye Research, 88*, 101018.

United States. Surgeon General's Advisory Committee on Smoking and Health. (1964). *Smoking and health; report of the advisory committee to the Surgeon General of the Public Health Service.* U., S. Dept. of Health, Education, and Welfare, Public Health Service; for sale by the Superintendent of Documents, U.S. Govt. Print. Off.

Ushio-Fukai, M. (2007). VEGF signaling through NADPH oxidase-derived ROS. *Antioxidants & Redox Signaling, 9*(6), 731–739.

VanderVeen, D. K., & Cataltepe, S. U. (2019). Anti-vascular endothelial growth factor intravitreal therapy for retinopathy of prematurity. *Seminars in Perinatology, 43*(6), 375–380.

Vannucci, S. J., & Back, S. A. (2022). The Vannucci model of hypoxic-ischemic injury in the neonatal rodent: 40 years later. *Developmental Neuroscience, 44*(4–5), 186–193.

Wallace, D. K., Kylstra, J. A., Phillips, S. J., & Hall, J. G. (2000). Poor postnatal weight gain: A risk factor for severe retinopathy of prematurity. *Journal of AAPOS, 4*(6), 343–347.

Wang, X., Tang, K., Chen, L., Cheng, S., & Xu, H. (2019). Association between sepsis and retinopathy of prematurity: A systematic review and meta-analysis. *BMJ Open, 9*(5), e025440.

Weinberger, B., Laskin, D. L., Heck, D. E., & Laskin, J. D. (2002). Oxygen toxicity in premature infants. *Toxicology and Applied Pharmacology, 181*(1), 60–67.

Wu, P. Y., Fu, Y. K., Lien, R. I., Chiang, M. C., Lee, C. C., Chen, H. C., et al. (2023). Systemic cytokines in retinopathy of prematurity. *Journal of Personalized Medicine, 13*(2), 291.

Xu, Y., Lu, X., Hu, Y., Yang, B., Tsui, C.-K., Yu, S., et al. (2018). Melatonin attenuated retinal neovascularization and neuroglial dysfunction by inhibition of HIF-1α-VEGF pathway in oxygen-induced retinopathy mice. *Journal of Pineal Research, 64*(4), e12473.

Yang, B., Xu, Y., Yu, S., Huang, Y., Lu, L., & Liang, X. (2016). Anti-angiogenic and anti-inflammatory effect of Magnolol in the oxygen-induced retinopathy model. *Inflammation Research, 65*(1), 81–93.

Yu, C. W., Popovic, M. M., Dhoot, A. S., Arjmand, P., Muni, R. H., Tehrani, N. N., et al. (2022). Demographic risk factors of retinopathy of prematurity: A systematic review of population-based studies. *Neonatology, 119*, 1–13.

Yu, H., Yuan, L., Zou, Y., Peng, L., Wang, Y., Li, T., et al. (2014). Serum concentrations of cytokines in infants with retinopathy of prematurity. *APMIS, 122*(9), 818–823.

Zhao, K., Jiang, Y., Zhang, J., Shi, J., Zheng, P., Yang, C., et al. (2022). Celastrol inhibits pathologic neovascularization in oxygen-induced retinopathy by targeting the miR-17-5p/HIF-1α/VEGF pathway. *Cell Cycle, 21*(19), 2091–2108.

CHAPTER 9

Etio-Prognostic Explanation

Introduction

In medicine, explanation by reference to the past helps clarify why events have occurred. If the associated uncertainty is reduced to a comfortable level, the content of such backward-looking explanations can be used to create forward-looking, prognostic explanations. Prognostic explanations are of the anticipatory-expectational type (see Chap. 6, Table 6.1); they explain by referring to what can be expected given knowledge about the past. Briefly, prognostic explanations predict future events based on knowledge about (a) causes of effects and (b) effects of causes. For example, if we know that past exposure X has caused instances of disease Y, we can prognosticate that future instances of exposure to X should result in future instances of Y. And if we know that past instances of pancreatic cancer frequently came with a very short survival time, we can prognosticate that future instances of pancreatic cancer should also come with a short survival time. It is important to note that prognostic explanations do have an explanatory value even if the prognosticated event has not yet occurred, simply by reference to the sum of past experiences that has led to the prognostic explanation at hand. If the prognosis turns out to be correct it will gain additional explanatory oomph. In other words, the prognosis does not need to be confirmed before it can be considered explanatory; confirmation just makes it stronger.

O. Dammann, *Uncertainty and Explanation in Medicine and the Health Sciences*, https://doi.org/10.1007/978-3-031-82271-1_9

In the first part of this chapter, I will propose that prognostic explanations explain by reference to correct prediction. My argument is that just having evidence of replication (confirmation) and having evidence of correct prediction are two very different things, just like "it just so happened" and "I predicted it and I was right" are two very different things. In the second part I discuss, as an example of etio-prognostic explanations, a research approach that delivers data to medicine and public health about events to be expected in infectious disease scenarios such as epidemics: agent-based models (ABMs). Medical and public health professionals need such data to design interventions that help prevent the spread of infection. Mathematical models of epidemics help with this process and agent-based models are one kind of mathematical model that can be used for this purpose. My goal for this chapter is to show that agent-based models can be viewed as devices that offer etio-prognostic explanations about infectious disease scenarios.

PROGNOSTIC EXPLANATION

Let me begin by introducing and defending the concept of *prognostic explanation*, i.e., explanation by reference to evidence from correct prediction. This idea appears to fly in the face of current concepts of explanation, scientific explanation in particular. However, it is compatible with the explanatory pluralism I have advocated for in Chap. 6. Explanation from correct prediction is an explanation based on evidence that comes from successful forecasting of occurrence. For example, if one epidemiological study finds a strong association between a healthy diet and prolonged lifespan, it can be predicted that a similar association will be found in a different population. If this happens, two different kinds of evidence become available. First, the fact that a similar result was obtained in a different population provides confirmatory evidence. Second, the fact that the prediction was successful provides evidence of correct prediction. This evidence is supported by a predictive hypothesis, which supports the causal-mechanical hypothesis that explains why and how the association between healthy diet and longevity arose in the first place. In this sense, prognostic explanation is different from but supported by causal-mechanical (etiological) explanations of disease occurrence. It takes an etiological explanation and makes a prediction based on it, and if confirmed, the prognostic explanation explains by having correctly predicted future events. In essence, etiological explanations explain backward in time, while prognostic explanation explain forward in time. While an etiological explanation explains the occurrence of disease, i.e., why the disease occurs, with reference to its cause and mechanism, a prognostic explanation refers to the same etiological explanation by saying "if that etiological explanation is true we are to expect future instances of disease occurrence in situations where cause and mechanism are in place". In essence, a prognostic explanation *uses* an etiological explanation to make a prediction. If that prediction comes true, the knowledge gained by both etiological and prognostic explanations being valid goes beyond the knowledge gained by etiological explanation alone, thereby increasing the explanatory value.

Heather Douglas has suggested that ignoring prediction has led to impoverished conceptions of scientific explanation (Douglas, 2009). She holds that because explanation is widely considered the main goal of science, prediction has been unjustifiably ignored from recent discourse about explanation. She shows that what unifies the current models of scientific explanation is that they are "useful for producing that other important goal of science: testable predictions" (457). She proposes that the capacity of explanations to generate new predictions is a unifying characteristic of useful scientific explanations. In keeping with and moving beyond Douglas' proposal, I argue that evidence from correct prediction provides predictive explanations, that they are qualitatively different from etiological (causal and mechanical) explanations, and that they add to the justificatory thrust of overarching etiological claims in epidemiology and medicine.

What kind of evidence does prognostic explanation deliver? Among the different kinds of evidence that are needed to justify health interventions (see also the next chapter for more about this issue), one needs not only causal and mechanical evidence but also *confirmatory evidence* from separate epidemiological studies that replicate the causal evidence in populations other than, and different from, the initial epidemiological observation. As discussed above, confirmation is the first benefit that prognostic explanations deliver. In this context, I take confirmation to be just the fact that a similar result emerges from a similar study or research project. This is just confirmation by replication. Predicting such result correctly adds another explanatory level to this scenario. While confirmatory evidence provides an answer to the question "Does a similar study produce a similar result?", prognostic evidence emerges when the hypothesis "A similar study will produce similar results" is answered in the affirmative.

Howick et al. (2009) have called confirmatory evidence *parallel evidence*, referring to concepts like consistency and coherence among studies, as well as replication and their well-known epistemological benefits. Others hold that one needs *interventional evidence* that, in keeping with recent discussions offered by Gillies (2019) and Campaner and Cerri (2020), provides further support for the overarching justification of intervention by reference to demonstrated efficacy and effectiveness. This leaves us with four kinds of evidence that can help support the justification of health interventions: causal, mechanistic, confirmatory (parallel), and interventional. I would argue that adding prognostic evidence would make the rationale for health interventions even stronger. Of course, these kinds of evidence are not mutually exclusive and perhaps also not jointly exhaustive. For example, parallel evidence from separate epidemiological studies that confirm original observations is also causal evidence, just like the initial causal evidence from the initial study.

In the last chapter of this book I will propose a framework for the mapping of evidence that supports the notion that a health intervention is scientifically justified (Dammann, 2021b). The framework employs as a first *explanatory* step the collection of *evidence of association* between candidate cause and effect produced by observational epidemiological research (evidence type A) as well as *biological* evidence produced by laboratory experiments (type B). Evidence of association is explained by a causal hypothesis such that a statistical association between X and Y is explained by the hypothesis that X causes Y. Biological evidence is explained by a mechanistic hypothesis such that the biological observations are explained by the hypothesis that X causes Y via a mechanism M that involves the experimentally generated phenomena. In a second step the model utilizes (type C) confirmatory evidence of subsequent observational epidemiological studies. This is essentially again evidence of association between X and Y, but this time it comes from subsequent research in independent populations, which is Howick's *parallel evidence* (Howick et al., 2009). Just like the initial type A evidence, it is explained by a causal hypothesis. Finally, evidence of difference-making (type D) from clinical or population trials. After X has occurred, evidence that an intervention on M reduces or prevents the occurrence of Y is explained by a mechanistic hypothesis. Let me propose that the second step also cashes in on the added benefit provided by type C and D evidence if it demonstrates that its correct prediction is possible. For example, if type A evidence from a single epidemiological study suggests that X is associated with Y, type C evidence would be evidence of a similar association from a subsequent similar study. Before this parallel type C evidence becomes available, however, a prediction can be made based on the initial type A evidence that type C evidence will become available if additional similar studies are conducted. Once this prediction turns out to be correct, one would not only have confirmed type A evidence but one would also have *evidence from correct prediction.* This parallel type C evidence is explained by the same causal hypothesis that explains the initial type A evidence. A similar scenario plays out if type B (experimental biological) evidence suggests that a certain mechanism is the connection between healthy diet and longevity. Intervening on that mechanism in clinical or population trials would generate type D evidence which is evidence from intervention. Before this type D evidence becomes available, however, a prediction based on the initial type B evidence would be that such type D evidence of difference-making will become available if such trials are conducted. Once this prediction turns out to be correct, one would not only have evidence from intervention but also evidence from correct prediction.

Accepting Douglas' invitation to bring prediction back into explanation, I think that evidence from correct prediction provides *prognostic explanations.* In other words, I offer the proposal that correct prediction *is* explanation. The occurrence of type C and D evidence may be considered evidence that is explained by the same causal and mechanical hypotheses that explain the occurrence of type A and B evidence, respectively. However, the successful correct prediction that type B and C evidence will become available from proper studies is supported by a *predictive* hypothesis, which states that it is possible to make a correct prediction based on type A and B evidence.

In other words, confirmatory (parallel) evidence and interventional evidence provide an opportunity to test predictions. A *correct* causal prediction provides parallel causal evidence if epidemiological studies yield a strong statistical association between an exposure (cause) and a health outcome (effect) that confirm the results of previous similar studies. The data themselves may serve as confirmatory evidence, but the fact that the prediction turned out to be correct provides additional evidence from correct prediction. Similarly, a *correct* mechanistic prediction, based on initial mechanistic evidence from experimental laboratory science, that a clinical or population trial will establish the efficacy of an intervention that blocks or interrupts the patho-mechanism (interventional evidence) yields not only confirmatory evidence as well as interventional evidence but also evidence from correct prediction.

If evidence from correct prediction provides prognostic explanations, what is their explanatory value above and beyond that coming from causal and mechanical evidence? Is prognostic explanation *fundamentally different* from these other kinds of explanation? I think that correct prediction can be viewed as a kind of explanation that is distinct from causal and mechanistic explanation. It does not explain by reference to elements of the etiological process of illness occurrence but by reference to the prognostic success (correctness) of predictions, which would not be possible, or at least much less likely, if the overarching etiological claim were not true. Therefore, it qualifies as an explanation of the predictive evidence (of the fact that a prediction turns out to be correct) by the predictive hypothesis that a correct prediction is possible based on previous type A and B evidence.

Etiological (causal-mechanical) explanations explain why and how diseases occur, thereby providing a cognitive tool that allows us to formulate predictions. However, my proposal is not about the capability of making predictions but about the capability of making *correct* predictions, which then serve as evidence that is explained by a predictive hypothesis, "we are capable of correctly predicting the occurrence of Y". While it is true that etiological explanations assist us in formulating the prediction by clarifying the purported relationship between cause X and effect Y, we could have posited the predictive hypothesis completely independently of type A and B evidence, i.e., without any preceding etiological explanation. Therefore, the generation of a predictive hypothesis does not *depend* on causal or mechanistic evidence but can stand all by itself.

However, it can also be added as a predictive explanation to an existing causal-mechanical explanation, which states that disease Y is caused by cause X by means of mechanism M. Once added, the causal-mechanical explanation (CME) becomes a causal-mechanical-prognostic explanation (CMPE), a constellation of causal, mechanical, and prognostic hypotheses that jointly explain the evidence that (1) X and Y are associated because X causes Y (type A evidence), (2) X and Y are causally connected by mechanism M (type B evidence), and (3) it is possible to correctly predict the re-occurrence of an association in a separate setting (type C evidence) and/or the outcome of an intervention study (type D evidence). Stated more formally, a causal explanation (CE), a mechanistic explanation (ME), and a prognostic explanation (PE) are three components of a CMPE such that

CE   X causes Y

Causal explanations say that the observed epidemiological (type A) evidence is explained by a causal hypothesis. They state that the reason why we can observe the evidence in the first place is *because* the exposure causes the outcome. In other words, they say that because the exposure X_A is a cause of the outcome Y_A, we can observe their association in the first place.

ME   M is the mechanism that connects X and Y

Mechanical explanations say that the observed bio-experimental laboratory (type B) evidence is explained by a mechanistic hypothesis. This means that the observed evidence becomes available *because* there is a mechanism between the experimental intervention (X_B, representing X) and the outcome of the experiment (Y_B, representing Y), which supports the overarching etiological notion that X causes Y. In other words, because the intervention X_B is mechanistically connected with the outcome of the experiment Y_B, we understand *how* X causes Y.

PE   We can correctly predict the re-occurrence of the X-Y association as well as the outcome of interventions on M.

Prognostic explanations say that if the prediction turns out to be correct, the occurrence of such evidence is explained by a *prognostic hypothesis* which states that a correct prediction is possible. The argument here is that we can make such correct prediction, because we understand the *etiology* of why and how Y comes about, namely, because it is caused by X via mechanism M. Thus, the fact that the prediction turns out to be correct supports the causal component of the CMPE (X causes Y) if the evidence from correct prediction is of type C, or its mechanistic component (M being the link between X and Y) if the evidence from correct prediction is of type D. Taking this one step further, it seems reasonable to assume that a prediction out of thin air, without prior causal or mechanistic evidence, will be less likely to be correct than a prediction based only on causal or mechanistic evidence only. We can also presume that the best predictions (most likely correct) will be made based on both causal and mechanistic evidence.

Let me outline the proposed distinction between causal, mechanical, and prognostic explanation a bit more formally:

Causal Explanation

1. Causal hypothesis (CH): X causes Y.
2. Evidence of causation (EC): X and Y pass quasi-causometry requirements.
3. Causal explanation (CE): CH is valid because EC is true.
4. Conclusion: CE strengthens belief in truth of CH.
5. New Predictions

   (a) EC will re-occur.
   (b) Intervening on X will change Y.

Mechanical Explanation

1. Mechanistic hypothesis (MH): M is a mechanism that leads from X to Y.
2. Evidence of mechanism (EM): Lab experiments show how mechanism M connects X and Y.
3. Mechanistic explanation (ME): MH is valid because EM is true.
4. Conclusion: ME strengthens belief in truth of MH.
5. New predictions:

   (a) EM will re-occur.
   (b) Intervening on M will change Y.

Prognostic Explanation

1. Prognostic hypothesis (PH): We can, based on EC and EM, correctly predict the occurrence of future instances of EC and EM.
2. Evidence from correct prediction (ECP): Prediction of epidemiological or experimental study results turns out to be correct.
3. Prognostic Explanation (PE): PH is valid because ECP is true.
4. Conclusion: PE strengthens belief in truth of PH.
5. New Predictions:

   (a) ECP will re-occur.
   (b) Improving CH and MH will lead to better (more precise) PH.

Let's now consider some possible objections.

The symmetry thesis established by Hempel and Oppenheim (1948) says that explanation and prediction are symmetric. In other words, every proper explanation offers a prediction and every prediction generates an explanation. This view has been rejected by, e.g., Scheffler, Rescher, Hanson, and Scriven (see discussion in Douglas, 2009). The idea that explanation and prediction have the same logical form has been abandoned since the 1960s. According to this view, explanation and prediction may be related but are separate concepts. For example, Heather Douglas has reviewed the history of this separation of explanatory versus predictive power and suggests that "[e]xplanation should be understood as a cognitive tool that assists us in generating new predictions" (Douglas, 2009, p. 444). On this view, explanatory evidence supports the process of prediction generation but is still considered a different kind of animal. In other words, explanation helps making predictions, but prediction is not explanation.

Another objection to my proposal could be that confirmatory (type C) evidence is just that: a second (third, fourth, etc.) occurrence of the initially observed association between an exposure and an outcome, albeit in a separate study. Therefore, the objection would continue, it is just a second (third, fourth, etc.) set of data that are explained by a causal hypothesis—the same causal hypothesis that explains type A evidence. Therefore, type C evidence is just that: confirmation, but not explanation of the occurrence of an association between X and Y. A correct prediction of type C evidence would thus qualify as helping with the confirmation, but not the explanation of such occurrence. Indeed, I agree that we need to distinguish between *confirmation* and *prediction success* by reference to (a) the data they are based upon and (b) the different and separate roles they play in strengthening etiological beliefs.

Let's assume we are working on a causal-mechanical explanation of the occurrence of abnormalities in the retina of preterm newborns called ROP as outlined in detail in the previous chapter. We have a *causal* explanation that is supported by data that show a strong statistical association between neonatal sepsis (systemic infection) and ROP. Another research team has offered a mechanistic explanation, supported by data from a laboratory study on animals that show that neonatal inflammation could be the mechanism that connects the infection with ROP. Moreover, a third team has observed a statistical association between circulating markers of inflammation in the bloodstream of preterm babies and ROP. At this point, we have a causal explanation supported by statistical associations in human infants and successful quasi-causometry (sepsis → ROP) and a mechanistic hypothesis (inflammation → ROP), supporting the overarching hypothesis that sepsis might cause ROP by initiating an inflammatory response. We also have a mechanistic explanation from animal studies in the lab (inflammation → ROP), supporting the hypothesis that inflammation can produce ROP. Based on the causal-mechanistic evidence, we predicted that circulating markers of inflammation should be associated with ROP *in our own* data from human newborns. An analysis of our existing data reveals that this is indeed the case. This finding *confirms* that the predicted association is indeed demonstrable in our own data, thereby strengthening previous evidence of the same sort by showing that the finding is *consistent* with previous evidence. Such replication of findings is valued strongly among epidemiologists charged with the identification of causes of disease (Hill, 1965). Here, the body of evidence is comprised of the *data themselves*, the statistical association between inflammation and ROP, which confirms by repetition that *there is something*.

However, such finding has additional explanatory value by virtue of being a *correct prediction*. We had predicted, based on the findings of others, that there should be an association between inflammation and ROP in our own data. The data that support this claim is the observation of prediction success, as defined by the fact that our prediction was correct, not the raw data themselves. It is also not the same as the original hypothesis that an association exists, because that hypothesis was just that: an initial hypothesis of an association not yet observed. Our replication study was based on that initial hypothesis *and* the previous data. However, the main point here is that the explanatory value of predictive evidence arises from two explanatory virtues, i.e., confirmation and successful prediction, not just one. By way of *succeeding* in predicting the event *correctly*, the prediction adds to the existing evidence in a qualitatively distinct way.

What if a prediction is correct by chance? It is eminently reasonable to suggest that any correct prediction of the occurrence of type C or D evidence might be correct solely based on chance. My simple response to this objection is that although this might be true, it is true of all explanations. A correct prediction may occur by chance, simply because the world is wobbly, but that doesn't necessarily make the predictive explanation wrong. It may be wrong by chance, but it may also be by chance correct.

AGENT-BASED MODELS[1]

Computational modeling and simulation of real-life scenarios have become a mainstay in health research and the biosciences. My goal in this section is to provide an analysis of the explanatory scope of agent-based models (ABMs). In contrast to equation-based models (EBMs), ABMs are algorithms that simulate individual agents and attribute changing characteristics to each one, multiple times during multiple iterations over time. Agent-based models were frequently employed in the context of the COVID-19 pandemic (Cuevas, 2020; Hoertel et al., 2020; Kerr et al., 2021; Shamil et al., 2021; Silva et al., 2020; Staffini et al., 2021; Truszkowska et al., 2021). It is not my intent to review these papers in detail; suffice it to say that they are all part of the general endeavor to tackle important population health problems posed by the COVID-19 pandemic and have made considerable contributions to our understanding of epidemiological dynamics of this global health crisis. Instead, I will focus on three philosophical aspects of ABMs as models of causal mechanisms, as generators of emergent phenomena, and as providers of explanations. Based on my discussion, I conclude that while ABMs cannot help much with causal inference, they can be viewed as etio-prognostic explanations of illness occurrence and outcome.

I will begin by introducing ABMs and why they are generally considered helpful. Part of their epistemological value is that they are thought to provide explanations of biological and social mechanisms. One account of ABMs, featured prominently on the Columbia School of Public Health website, has ABMs as models of causal mechanisms of interactions of characteristics that may include impossible or unethical connections and that generate emergent phenomena. The section ends with the proposal to consider ABMs as helpful in generating etio-prognostic explanations.

ABMs: A Primer

As any other computational model, an ABM is an algorithm with inputs, computations, and outputs. In public health, ABMs are generally conceptualized as "a computational approach in which agents with a specified set of characteristics interact with each other and with their environment according to predefined rules" (Tracy et al., 2018, p. 77). What exactly does that mean and why should this be helpful?

An ABM (sometimes also called individual-based model or IBM) is a computer program that simulates changes in populations over time based on the "behavior" of "agents" who have a set of characteristics and who "interact" in predefined and stochastically modeled ways. This kind of simulation is often called *microsimulation* because phenomena are modeled at the level of the individual agent or *micro-level*, and results are observed at the *macro-level*, i.e., the level of the simulated population. Starting values and conditions for transition of agents from one state to another (e.g., from non-infected to infected or from alive to dead) are defined by the programmer. Running the program will result in iterations of changes in these conditions over time. Ending conditions at the macro-level are the outcome of the model. Since the attribution of particular values to individual agents is done by randomly allocating values selected from a probability distribution with set constraints, each run of the algorithm will result in a different outcome. Multiple, oftentimes many runs need to be performed to arrive at a range of outcomes that define an outcome distribution. The results of ABMs are indeterministic (stochastic) as opposed to those of most equation-based models (EBMs).[2]

Agent-based modeling is frequently used in theoretical infectious disease epidemiology (Venkatramanan et al., 2018). As outlined by Hunter and colleagues, ABMs are considered superior to EBMs (such as those that generate the now very familiar COVID-19 incidence and mortality curves) because they allow for the modelling of the behavior of individuals based on social interaction rules and a probabilistic attribution of such behaviors to the agents in a model (Hunter et al., 2017). Agent-based models have to consider four major related aspects: disease, society, movement, and environment. They have to model disease-specific conditions of occurrence and duration, characteristics of the society (population) and how its members move through virtual space and interact with one another in the environment that population is situated in. The result is a highly complex representation of how population parameters change over time with regard to, e.g., disease incidence or mortality rates. Let me note right here that ABMs involve equations as well. However, the underlying equations let a set of variables undergo iterative stochastic changes over a predefined timeframe so that such changes over time *in each agent* contribute to an overall change at the population level.

Let us go through the published description of one ABM-based microsimulation and parse out its individual observational and inferential components. For example, Hoertel and coworkers published *a stochastic agent-based microsimulation model of the COVID-19 epidemic in France. [They] examined the potential impact of post-lockdown measures, including physical distancing, mask-wearing and shielding individuals who are the most vulnerable to severe COVID-19 infection, on cumulative disease incidence and mortality, and on intensive care unit (ICU)-bed occupancy. While lockdown is effective in containing the viral spread, once lifted, regardless of duration, it would be unlikely to prevent a rebound. Both physical distancing and mask-wearing, although effective in slowing the epidemic and in reducing mortality, would also be ineffective in ultimately preventing ICUs from becoming overwhelmed and a subsequent second lockdown. However, these measures coupled with the shielding of vulnerable people would be associated with better outcomes, including lower mortality and maintaining an adequate ICU capacity to prevent a second lockdown.* (Hoertel et al., 2020, p. 1417)

The goal of the model was to simulate the effect of changing measures after the first lockdown in France such as social distancing, mask-wearing, and shielding the most vulnerable. Outcomes measured (variables) at the population level (macro-level) were a rebound, second lockdown, epidemic slow down, intensive care unit admission rates, mortality, as well as combinations of the above. In order to arrive at their results, investigators needed to model events at the individual level (micro-level), including

194 parameters related to French population characteristics (n = 140), social contacts (n = 33) and SARS-CoV-2 characteristics (n = 21) [...]. Parameter values on population characteristics were based on data from the French National Statistical Institute (INSEE) and Santé Publique France. Parameters related to social contacts were based on prior studies (n = 11) or assumptions when no data were available (n = 22). Finally, parameters on disease characteristics were based on data from Institut Pasteur and London Imperial College, except for two unknown key parameters of the epidemic: contamination risk and proportion of undiagnosed COVID-19 cases, which were simultaneously estimated through model calibration. (Hoertel et al., 2020)[3]

In essence, almost two hundred individual and population characteristics were modeled over time and the resulting changes at the population level were observed. Circling back to my tripartite goal in this section to explore ABMs as (a) models of mechanisms, (b) generators of emergent phenomena, and (c) providers of explanation, the (a) mechanisms would be the joint changes over time among the agents of the ABM that (b) lead to certain population-based emergent phenomena, and (c) observing the model values change and results emerge would provide an explanation. The central question I ask in this chapter is an explanation of *what* exactly this might be.

Why are ABMs considered helpful? Obviously, ABMs are created for a purpose. In the general context of our current discussion, any modeler of an epidemic (pandemics included) has at least three goals. First, they want to understand the dynamics of the epidemic in terms of background conditions of population and environment. Thus, the first goal is to find a causal-mechanical explanation of why and how the infection spreads in populations. Second, modelers want to create an algorithm that allows them to predict how the epidemic will evolve over time. Third, modelers want to explore changes in model outcomes in response to parameter changes. In an iterative fashion, the algorithm can be modified to get closer and closer to predictions that can be confirmed or rejected by real-life data as time goes by.

I have mentioned above that one of the motivations to create ABMs is that they are considered superior to EBMs in terms of being more realistic (Hunter et al., 2017). Equation-based models are simple, static, and deterministic, because they are built like a mathematical formula such as a regression equation that gives a result on a dependent variable based on the value of one or more independent variables. Once the regression equation is derived from an observational study in a certain population, any new observation can be plugged into the regression formula and a predicted value for the dependent variable can be obtained. They are static in the sense of being non-dynamic. This means that once a regression equation is created, its result doesn't change if the covariates don't change. If one wants to look at other combinations of variables, different starting conditions, or changes over time, one needs to create new equations. And they are deterministic because the value of the dependent variable is fixed once the values of the independent variables are fixed. There is not much room for "natural variation" in equation-based modelling. Consider the following excerpt from an outline of ABMs on the website of one of the major schools of public health in the United States:

> *Agent-based models are computer simulations used to study the interactions between people, things, places, and time. They are stochastic models built from the bottom up meaning individual agents (often people in epidemiology) are assigned certain attributes. The agents are programmed to behave and interact with other agents and the environment in certain ways. These interactions pro-*

duce emergent effects that may differ from effects of individual agents. Agent-based modeling differs from traditional, regression-based methods in that, like systems dynamics modeling, it allows for the exploration of complex systems that display non-independence of individuals and feedback loops in causal mechanisms. It is not limited to observed data and can be used to model the counterfactual or experiments that may be impossible or unethical to conduct in the real world.[4]

Let me henceforth refer to this account as the *Columbia account of ABM* and rephrase its elements as three epistemological statements we can use as a guideline for the remainder of this chapter.

Agent-based models are epistemologically helpful because they

1. enable the exploration of complex systems characterized by (among other things) non-independence of individuals and feedback loops in causal *mechanisms*, i.e., the sequential processes of changes in agent "behavior" that connect the initial states among agents and outcomes established at the population level;
2. support the study of interactions at the levels of people, things, places, and time between programmed behaviors of and *interactions* between agents that produce *emergent effects*;
3. can explore mechanisms in ways that are *impossible* in observational and experimental research.

I will now turn to each one of these three epistemological benefits of ABMs in the next three subsections.

Mechanisms

In the basic biosciences, mechanistic views of biological processes appear to include the notions of *action* and *behavior* when it comes to the observation of changes among the mechanism's components and those that occur as part of the result of the process. For example, Olaf Wolkenhauer writes that systems biologists are interested in finding out "how biological function emerges from the interactions between the components of living systems and how these emergent properties enable and constrain the behavior of those components" (Wolkenhauer, 2014). First, note that Wolkenhauer says that biological function "emerges" from the interactions of components. We will come back to emergence in the next subsection. Second, consider this account of systems biology in light of one of the more frequently cited definitions of a mechanism in philosophy of science: "Mechanisms are entities and activities organized such that they are productive of regular changes from start or set-up to finish or termination conditions" (Machamer et al., 2000). Taken together, the two accounts suggest that at least some systems biologists see their work as identifying biological *mechanisms*. Wolkenhauer confirms this by saying that "[t]he iterative cycle of data-driven modeling and model-driven experimentation [...] helps in identifying new mechanistic details of cell-biological processes and previously unidentified regulatory *interactions* in the system" (italics mine). Thus, another important similarity between Wolkenhauer's account of computational systems biology and Machamer, Darden, and Craver's account of mechanism is that both refer to some sort of *action*, as in "interactions" and "activities", suggesting that at least some bioscientists think that biological mechanisms are characterized by interactions and activities among the element of those mechanisms.

Let us now move from biological to population mechanics. It seems that population health scientists have a similarly mechanistic view of population health as biologists view biological processes as mechanisms. Consider, for example, this quote from the book *The Future of the Public's Health in the Twenty-First Century* published by the Institute of Medicine (U.S.) Committee on Assuring the Health of the Public in the Twenty-First Century (Medicine, 2003): "(a)spects of discrimination might influence health through any number of mechanisms, including (socio-economic status)" (61) and "[t]here are several plausible mechanisms by which social cohesion might influence health through contextual effects" (71).

These quotes raise the question how social mechanisms are conceptualized. Let us first consider who or what the elements of social mechanisms are. Stinchcombe suggests that "[m]echanisms in a theory are defined here as bits of theory about entities at a different level (e.g., individuals) than the main entities being theorized about (e.g., groups), which serve to make the higher-level theory more supple, more accurate, or more general" (Stinchcombe, 1991). For our present discussion of epidemic ABMs as models of social mechanisms, the agent would be a representation of an individual person and the entirety of agents would be a representation of a social group or population. From this perspective, individuals (the A in ABMs) would be the actors. In what might be the most frequently cited text on social mechanisms *as explanations*, Hedström and Swedberg (1998) confirm this when they state that their concept of social mechanism is based on four core principles, i.e., action, precision, abstraction, and reduction (Hedström & Swedberg, 1998). They write that

> [t]he first of these principles—explanations based on actions—means, among other things, that it is actors and not variables who do the acting. A mechanism-based explanation is not built upon mere associations between variables but always refers directly to causes and consequences of individual action oriented to the behavior of others. (ibid.)

Are ABMs, therefore, models of social mechanisms? The following quote seems to answer in the affirmative. Conte and Paolucci write that

> [a] generative explanation of an observed social phenomenon consists of describing it in terms of the external (environmental and social) and internal (behavioral) mechanisms that generate them, rather than by inferring causes from observed co-variations. This is a vital property of explanation, which cannot easily be realized otherwise. When describing agent behavior by means of other formalisms (logic-based or numeric), we describe behavior from the outside, as perceived by an observer, but do not describe the way it is generated. ABM explains (sic) behavior from within, in terms of the mechanisms that are supposed to have generated it, that is, the mechanisms that operate in the agent when s/he behaves one way or another. (Conte & Paolucci, 2014)

However, note that Conte and Paolucci carefully distinguish between mechanisms as *natural constituents* of the real processes the ABM is supposed to be a model of, and the *structural and functional blueprint* for agents' interactions coded into the model algorithm. They appear to see social phenomena as generated (produced) by mechanisms (external and internal) and the advantage of ABMs over other kinds of models as their capability to offer a mechanistic explanation of system behavior. Topping and colleagues make it eminently clear that the mechanisms are *built into the model*. They begin their article about their ecological ABM model of the European brown hare (I am not joking) as follows:

> Agent-based models (ABMs) are gaining popularity in most scientific fields due to their ability to describe complex systems from first principles. Yet, they are also criticised for being 'black boxes' and impossible to fully understand. This is mainly due to the difficulty of testing, documenting and communicating the wealth of mechanisms built into such models. (Topping et al., 2010)

This view is confirmed by a group of researchers who designed an ABM on social distancing, testing, contact tracing, and quarantine on the occurrence of SARS-CoV-19 infections. Referring to multiple scenarios they modeled they write that "[t]he above scenarios are mechanistically simulated on the multi-layer network [...] by allowing different interactions (between effective contacts) according to the simulated strategy" (Aleta et al., 2020). Clearly, this team stresses the point that the *simulation* is mechanistic. They do *not* say that they think that the real-life phenomena they model are mechanistic as well. However, what other reason could they have creating mechanistic models than being convinced that the modeled social and behavioral processes are mechanistic as well? Perhaps, we can paraphrase Nancy Cartwright's "no causes in, no causes out" here as "no mechanisms in, no mechanisms out", meaning that only if we already have mechanistic background information can we see ABMs as representing such mechanisms. If ABMs are considered mechanistic explanations of a certain phenomenon, they explain the occurrence of the phenomenon as resulting from a mechanism by demonstrating that the phenomenon does indeed occur because of the mechanism modeled by the ABM. However, this does not yet allow for the inference that the phenomenon must be due to this mechanism. To do that, other potential mechanisms and the possibility of chance need to be ruled out, and of course, the existence of the mechanism needs to be demonstrated by real-world data.

Until now, I have tried to avoid the topic of causality because I wanted my focus to be on the role of ABMs as explaining mechanisms without reference to causation. However, some modelers talk about *causal mechanisms* when they talk about the relation between how they see causality in the world and in their models. Consider the Columbia account of ABM above: "exploration of complex systems that display non-independence of individuals and feedback loops in *causal mechanisms*" (italics mine). This notion resonates with Tracy and coworkers' view that

> ABMs are well suited to the exploration of causal mechanisms given their ability to incorporate multiple interacting causes and to test competing theories about causation, thus further elucidating what we do and do not know about how a given outcome arises. (Tracy et al., 2018, p. 85)

It seems as if knowledge about mechanisms is considered crucial because it can provide knowledge about causation. As much as I agree that causes and mechanisms have a very close working relationship, they are two very different things. Indeed, I have argued in the previous chapter for a distinction between causes and mechanisms in the context of illness occurrence as separate but closely related components of the causation process that represents the initial phase of illness etiology. In other words, I think that while mechanisms are not causes but rather the link between causes and their effects, there are nonetheless a component of the causation process that culminates in disease. They are also part of the disease process, which includes the mechanisms and the biological and clinical components of disease (see Fig. 8.1 in Chap. 8). However, this does not necessarily imply that all mechanisms must be causal. If non-causal mechanisms exist, and if ABMs can model any kind of mechanism, then not all mechanisms that can be represented in ABMs are causal. Therefore, any method that is supposed to extract information about causal mechanisms from ABMs would need to distinguish between causal and non-causal mechanisms in ABMs. On the other hand, it could be that all mechanisms are causal. We would not need to distinguish between causal and non-causal mechanisms because the latter would not exist. If all mechanisms are causal, and ABMs can model any mechanism, ABMs could be used in the exercise of generating causal-mechanical (etiological) explanations. If not, we would, again, need criteria for separating causal from non-causal mechanisms.

What could non-causal mechanisms look like apart from, say, non-functional mechanisms such as repetitive loops in which model parameters do not change? I am referring back to Machamer, Darden, and Craver's definition of mechanism as "entities and activities organized such that they are productive of regular changes". I take this to mean that according to their view mechanisms *produce* change. Mechanisms are the way by which causes make a difference. This perspective would mean that all mechanisms are causal. Therefore, if ABMs represent mechanisms, and if all mechanisms are causal, then ABMs are representations of causal mechanisms. Does this mean that ABMs can be used as tools in causal inference?

Let us assume that ABMs include causal interactions *by definition*. They are programmed to reflect a causal relationship between variables whenever one is coded to change in response to another. Indeed, this is a representation of a common causal intuition: X causes Y if Y changes whenever X changes. This could be called, somewhat informally, the light switch intuition. It is based on traditional philosophical accounts of causation such as regularity, difference-making, dependence, and so forth. However,

I see the argument that ABMs are helpful in causal inference as being based on circular reasoning: causality in, causality out (Cartwright, again). ABMs cannot help with causal inference because inference is the bottom-up support of a proposition by observed data. ABMs cannot provide such data because the data they provide are top-down, generated computationally by algorithms. Yes, the *model of the algorithm* itself, e.g., the assumptions and almost 200 parameters used by Hoertel et al. in our COVID-19 epidemic example above, may be based on observed data (such as disease incidence, contact frequency among agents, etc.), but the algorithm is designed to produce a result. Thus, the result is caused by the algorithm, and that causal fact does not support the notion that the underlying observed data are reflective of a causal scenario, but only the notion that the algorithm functions as a causal mechanism, and that an algorithmic causal mechanism can be interpreted as a depiction of an envisioned causal mechanism in real life, but not as evidence supporting the inference that the modeled real-life scenario is causal or that a real-life causal relationship even exists. An algorithmic causal mechanism only shows that such mechanism has the potential to yield the modeled phenomenon. The epistemic gain is demonstrative in a theoretical way (in silico) but not in a practical way as in experimentation with animal models (in vivo). Both in silico and in vivo demonstrations confirm the possibility of a role for the mechanism in the purported etiological process, but they do not confirm that it does indeed play that role in real-life scenarios.[5]

Another caveat comes from the observation that those who argue for or against methods for causal inference via some method or another usually do so while depending on their own, implicit and often unstated intuitions about the nature of causality (Casini & Manzo, 2016). What are epidemiologists' definitions of "causation"? Susser simply states that "a cause is what makes a difference" (Susser, 1991). A classic paper on the counterfactual definition of *causal effect* in epidemiology includes my favorite statement "in ideal randomized experiments, association *is* causation" (Hernán, 2004). My problem with this paper is, however, that it contrasts the term *causal effect* with the term *effect* because the latter is, according to the author, commonly used to mean "simply statistical association". I think the term causal effect introduces confusion, because there is simply no such thing as a non-causal effect. All effects are results of causal mechanisms *by definition*, although the exact mechanism itself is not always known. The more important issue here is, however, that Hernán sees the (population) definition of causal effect simply as tied to a probability differential of developing an outcome under two different exposure conditions (yes or no):

> We define the probability $Pr[\Upsilon_a = 1]$ as the proportion of subjects that would have developed the outcome Υ had all subjects in the population of interest received exposure value a. We also refer to $Pr[\Upsilon_a = 1]$ as the risk of Υ_a. The exposure has a causal effect in the population if $Pr[\Upsilon_{a=1} = 1] \neq Pr[\Upsilon_{a=0} = 1]$. (Hernán, 2004)

This definition strikes me as applicable to "statistical association", but by no means would I subscribe to the view that it defines "causal effect" without further explication of what Hernán *means* by "causal effect". Unless he intends to suggest that his definition *defines* causal effect. This would mean that causal effects are what epidemiologists tell us they are, in a sort of metaphysically unsatisfying and somewhat patronizing way.

Let me refer briefly to an exchange from the epidemiological literature about the capability of ABMs to contribute to causal inference. Marshall and Galea have argued that ABMs "represent a promising novel approach to identify and evaluate complex causal effects" (Marshall & Galea, 2015). Although they refer to causal inference in this quote and in the title of their paper, the authors seem to avoid this notion in the body of their paper and refer instead to the exploration, elucidation, and interrogation of the causal relationships modeled in an ABM. Their argument rests on the capability of ABMs to represent multiple causal interrelations (their view of a complex system):

> We argue that agent-based modeling offers an alternative and complementary approach to elucidate complex causal interdependencies that are of interest in epidemiology. Specifically, the forms of the relationships among causes (which are broadly defined here and can include agent traits as well as environments) are operationalized by the rules Z. The rule set consisting of functions $f()$, $g()$, and $h()$ can include nonlinear components, including feedback loops, such that linear independence need not be assumed. By altering the rule set Z and running the simulation under different assumed causal relationships and processes, the effect(s) of interdependent (i.e., joint) exposures can be explored and interrogated. (Marshall & Galea, 2015, p. 96)

Marshall and Galea call the causal interrelationships they are interested in "complex". I take it as implicit that by this they refer to *complex* systems, not just *complicated* ones. They stress the possibility to model nonlinear relationships—a characteristic of complex systems. Thus, their view seems to be in keeping with the notion discussed below that the sheer complexity of interactions of agents in ABMs may give rise to emergent phenomena. More importantly, it is the intervention by the modeler (altering the rule set under different causal assumptions) that renders the ABM a helpful tool in causal exploration and interrogation, to use Marshall and Galea's terms. This view grants epistemological value to ABMs based on the possibility to *manipulate* them and explore the consequences, which resonates with interventionist accounts of causation.

One invited commentator, Ana Diez-Roux, disagrees with the notion that ABMs can help with causal inference in epidemiology (Diez Roux, 2014). The following excerpt from her abstract puts her position in a nutshell, which I see as one point of departure for my proposal further below that ABMs provide etio-prognostic explanations:

> As discussed by Marshall and Galea [...], systems approaches are appealing because they allow explicit recognition of feedback, interference, adaptation over time, and nonlinearities. However, they differ fundamentally from the traditional approaches to causal inference used in epidemiology in that they involve creation of a virtual world. Systems modeling can help us understand the plausible implications of the knowledge that we have and how pieces can act together in ways that we might not have predicted. [...] However, the validity of any causal conclusions derived from systems models hinges on the extent to which the models represent the fundamental dynamics relevant to the process in the real world. For this reason, systems modeling will never replace causal inference based on empirical observation. Causal inference based on empirical observation and simulation modeling serve interrelated but different purposes. (Diez Roux, 2014, p. 100)

Of note, Diez-Roux does not say that ABMs are incapable of helping with causal inference in principle. She only says that ABM-generated models are not like epidemiological approaches to causal inference based on observed data. However, I agree with her notion that simulated data from ABMs are epistemologically inferior to observational epidemiological data simply because the underlying data are not real-world data but generated in silico.

Interaction and Emergence

Let us now move on to the question whether the system behavior of ABMs can be reduced to the interactions among agents' characteristics and behaviors or if it is an *emergent* phenomenon. The question I am interested in is about the relationship between mechanistic explanation and emergence. In brief, if ABMs are a non-deterministic black box and the system behavior they exhibit is truly emergent, what remains of the notion that ABMs represent causal-mechanistic explanations? What kind of causal mechanism would be explained by an ABMs whose inner workings remain in the dark and whose results are *by definition* unpredictable and surprising?[6] On the other hand, if ABMs really provide causal-mechanistic explanations we should be able to predict the phenomena they generate, which would render them non-emergent.

The classic reference on emergence, published by Jeffrey Goldstein in the first issue of the journal of the same name, defines emergence as

> *the arising of novel and coherent structures, patterns, and properties during the process of self-organization in complex systems. Emergent phenomena are conceptualized as occurring on the macro level, in contrast to the micro-level components and processes out of which they arise.* (Goldstein, 1999, p. 49)

Think of a complex system as having a micro-level (components) and a macro-level (surface). Goldstein defines emergent phenomena as (1) radically novel, (2) coherent, (3) macro-level, (4) dynamic, and (5) ostensive. *Radical novelty* refers to the fact that emergent phenomena appear at the macro-level without having previously been present in the complex system under study and cannot be derived from or predicted based on knowledge about what is going on at the micro-level. *Coherence* means that emergent properties maintain "some sense of identity over time" (ibid.); *macro-level* means that emergence is observable at the surface level of the observed system, not the micro-level constituted by its components; *dynamic* refers to emergent phenomena as not preformed but as developing over time; and *ostensive* as being recognized by "showing themselves".

Most important for our present discussion, however, is that Goldstein sees one of the main roles of emergence in science as explanatory:

> *In respect to its use in scientific explanation, the construct of emergence is appealed to when the dynamics of a system seem better understood by focusing on*

across-system organization rather than on the parts or properties of parts alone.
(Goldstein, 1999, p. 50)

Thus, in keeping with Goldstein's characterization of emergent phenomena, although their occurrence on the macro-level is *produced* by what is going on at the micro-level, they come "out of the blue" because they do not *depend* on the behavior of individual micro-level variables (agents in ABMs) but on the overarching function of the whole system. Thus, if ABMs are truly complex (non-deterministic, nonlinear) systems, they would produce emergent effects at the output level that are not predicted, or even predict*able*, by means of applying knowledge about the agents and their interactions. In contrast, these results would be ostensive occurrences that rely on the function of all interacting parts. The point here is that ABMs yield models of mechanisms that do not necessarily represent any real-world mechanism, be it biological or social mechanisms. They represent only themselves, based on input conditions and probabilistic rules for agent interactions and status changes. If an ABM yields an outcome, be it emergent or expected, the occurrence of that outcome can be explained by analyzing the workings of the modeled mechanism in silico.

What kind of mechanism consists of interactions between parts over time but is not "productive of regular changes" (per Machamer et al.'s definition) but instead to radically novel, dynamic, and ostensive phenomena? Can ABMs explain mechanisms or emergence, or both? The question whether ABMs can explain emergent phenomena is what Weisberg considers "the most controversial claim about IBMs [...] Not everyone is convinced" (Weisberg, 2014, p. 788). (Again, IBM and ABM refer to the same kind of model.) He quotes ecologist Joan Roughgarden as saying that she doesn't "think it's easy to discern the causation being revealed by an IBM simulation. And if we don't learn something about causation we don't learn anything scientifically important" (personal communication quoted in (Weisberg, 2014)).

Weisberg suggests to distinguish between explanations of emergent phenomena (mechanistic explanations) and explanations of the emergence of phenomena (emergence explanations). On his view, mechanistic explanations provide a "generalized mechanistic understanding of the dependence of higher-level properties and patterns on lower-level mechanistic factors" (Weisberg, 2014, p. 789). I take this to mean an explanation that is based on the description of the elements of a mechanism and their interactions as being what *somehow* leads to an emergent phenomenon. He shows how certain causal graphs (relational depictions of phenomena in boxes with causal arrows between them) can depict the relationships among micro-level factors that can help generate mechanistic explanations. Interestingly, the kind of causal graph he chooses suggests that on his view ABMs can model biological mechanisms because the causal mechanism depicted in his example permits feedback loops, an important characteristic of mechanisms in biological explanations (Bechtel, 2011). In contrast, the directed acyclic graphs (DAGs) that are frequently used in epidemiological causal reasoning (such as those in Fig. 7.1, Chap. 7) do *not* allow feedback loops, a feature preferred in causal reasoning because the vertices can be ordered, simplifying causal argumentation immensely. No such topological order is possible in cyclic graphs (Dasgupta et al., 2008, p. 96).

Emergence explanations, on the other hand, would require us to provide "reductive explanations that show how emergent phenomena arise from lower-level interactions" (Weisberg, 2014, p. 792).[7] They would require us to clarify what exactly it is that generates an emergent phenomenon. But one main problem with both cyclic and acyclic graphs is that it is unclear *what exactly the arrows represent*. If it is true that causation is "one word, many things" and that "there are different kinds of causal relations imbedded in different kinds of systems" (Cartwright, 2004), the edges between different vertices (characteristics of agents in ABMs) would potentially represent different sub-mechanisms. I read Weisberg as saying that we cannot use ABMs to provide emergence explanations unless we can specify exactly what is in each of these arrows, and I agree with him on that. On the other hand, he seems to say that ABMs can provide mechanistic explanations. Let me add that if all mechanisms are causal, I assume that Weisberg would conclude that ABMs can provide causal-mechanical explanations and I would agree with him on that as well. I also think that his usage of non-DAGs to depict what ABMs model not only fits biological but also social mechanisms. Note that the Columbia account of ABMs above explicitly mentions feedback loops. Indeed, some research on COVID-19 has revealed interesting feedback loops even across scales of representation (micro-level, macro-level). For example, one computational study suggests that macro-level dynamics such as social distancing can result in micro-level changes all the way down in the genetic makeup of SARS-CoV-2 (Barrett et al., 2021).

But perhaps, at least in the context of ABMs, we shouldn't ask too much of the arrow semantics in causal graphs, for in ABMs the relationship between all agents and all their characteristics is simply a mathematical relationship, not a biological one. This brings us to the third notion reflected in the Columbia account of ABM, impossible interactions.

Impossible Interactions

A major motivation to use ABMs comes from their flexibility to be manipulated in ways no observational or interventional epidemiological study could be manipulated. In essence, ABMs can be used to model the impossible because the characteristics of agents are variables created *for* the model and *by* the model. Furthermore, there is only one kind of relationship between and among variables in ABMs, a mathematical relationship represented by stochastic functions.

Based on the findings in the systems biology and population health/ sociological/ecological literature discussed in the previous sections, we can safely assume that ABMs are considered models of social mechanisms. Such mechanisms are modeled in ABMs by creating *interactions* between agent's characteristics among each other and between agents' and their environment's characteristics. How does this look like *inside* an ABM?

The term *interaction* is most often used in ABMs to denote the narrowing of virtual physical space between two agents to a level at which a status change occurs in at least one of them (Winkelmann et al., 2021). Based on certain parameters, each individual agent will move through virtual space until a pre-programmed fit between a set of characteristics of two agents leads to contact and infection with a certain prespecified likelihood. At this point the status of the heretofore "uninfected" agent switches to "infected". Because such status changes are dependent on certain constellations of variables at certain timepoints, and because these constellations are derived from a whole set of characteristics assigned to agents in a stochastic fashion, these interactions and associated status changes are *not* pre-determined. In this sense, ABMs are non-deterministic, and each run of the model will yield a slightly different result. Many runs need to be performed to narrow down the probability distribution of results at the macro-level, where population wide parameters such as "infection prevalence" change from starting conditions to a different value over the duration of model run time, depending on how many individuals will be newly infected (incidence) while the model is running. Such result is sometimes considered "emergent" since it is not fully determined by model parameters in an equation-like fashion.

In the above scenario, the interaction is between two agents. Interactions can also occur between agents and the spatial environment. For example, certain areas in the virtual space can be designated as different in terms of social characteristics (e.g., high-crime, low-crime, no-crime regions), and the likelihood of a status change of an agent (e.g., becoming the victim in a street mugging) would be different in these different regions. Moreover, agent-agent interactions could be modeled as representing just such a mugging (or not) and differ by section of the virtual space.

These considerations highlight one of the oft-praised advantages of ABMs, the possibility to design interactions *in any way* the modeler desires, even impossible or unethical ones. In essence, the functions of ABMs are completely devoid of the need for plausibility and ethical considerations. Nothing prevents the design of an ABM of a randomized-controlled trial of the effect of COVID-19 infection on survival. Obviously, although such trial would be possible in principle, it would (luckily) never be approved by an institutional review board.

But aside from being a potential tool for modeling the unethical, another important possibility is to model mechanistic relationships across levels along the bio-psycho-social spectrum. Agent-based models can evaluate interactions among and between agents and their environments regardless of a known mechanism between, say, agents' socioeconomic background, their immune status, and their risk of SARS-CoV-2 infection. The flip side of ABMs' *inability* to provide Weisbergian emergence explanations is the benefit for the modeler to simply ignore the *somehow* expected from such explanations without sacrificing the capability of their model to provide causal-mechanical explanations.

In epidemiological research, *multilevel modeling* that integrates variables across the individual, household, and community level is a common approach. Such models are called *multi-scale* or *nested* models and have become common in infectious disease modeling (Hart et al., 2020). Multi-scale models have traditionally been based on integro-differential equations (IDEs), but the usage of ABMs has recently become more frequent. Such models can easily integrate the interaction between biological and behavioral processes at the level of the individual and social processes at the population level.

At least some philosophers seem to feel comfortable with the idea of trans-level interaction and state that "our health is not just a metabolic response to toxins; it is about a complex social and biological interaction— a relational process or mechanism" (Parkkinen et al., 2018). Indeed, I believe that agent-based multi-scale models can provide the proposed integration of biological, behavioral, and social mechanism in a concept that Kelly, Kelly, and Russo have advocated for and called *mixed mechanisms* (Kelly et al., 2014). However, I think that they can do even more: they can explore comprehensive etio-prognostic explanations of illness occurrence, development, and prognosis. Indeed, ABMs can simulate not only the joint activities of determinants of illness occurrence (causes and mechanisms) in etiological explanations (Dammann, 2020) but also the joint activities of the determinants of the clinical course (disease development) and its outcomes (cure, death, or anything in between). They can even include the potential impact of etiological contributors such as *conditions* that may be different from causes in non-trivial ways (Broadbent, 2008), in ways that I regret not being able to rehearse here in detail. In the next and final section of this chapter, I propose that while ABMs' role in causal inference might be limited, they can provide etio-prognostic explanations by integrating determinants of illness occurrence (etiology) as well as determinants of disease development and outcome (prognosis).

ABMS AS ETIO-PROGNOSTIC EXPLANATIONS

Above, I have rejected the idea that ABMs can help with causal inference but offered support for the notion that ABMs can be helpful as explanations of causal-mechanical (etiological) processes of illness occurrence. Moreover, I propose that they can help even further by simulating the trajectory of illness development and outcome. Although I am aware that I am running the risk of repeating myself, let me first return to *etiological explanations* and how they are constructed, such as the one given in the previous chapter for ROP occurrence, and then explicate what I mean by *etio-prognostic explanation*.

In epidemiology, an obsession with causal inference abounds. The main idea seems to be that epidemiological methods can provide an apparatus that allows for causal inference based on observational epidemiological data. The underlying assumptions appear to be that observed statistical associations are not to be considered reflective of a causal relationship unless they come from ideal randomized experiments (Hernán, 2004). A simple and straightforward rejection of this proposal would need to show that ideal randomized experiments do not exist. Indeed, some philosophers have offered this argument as well as other considerations that should reduce our confidence in causal inference from randomized clinical trials, the gold standard of the randomized experiment in clinical epidemiology (Cartwright, 2007, 2010; Deaton & Cartwright, 2016; Worrall, 2007). If these arguments, which I cannot fully discuss here for reasons of space, carry any weight, there may just not be any way to reliably infer causality from epidemiological data that goes beyond the existing quasi-causometers introduced in Chap. 7. Instead of making causal inference of the holy grail of epidemiological research, a gentler, less exclusive perspective can be taken according to which epidemiology contributes to the generation of etiological explanations, which refer to purported causes of illness, the mechanisms they initiate, and the disease (illness) that occurs. This theoretical model of illness occurrence is a process model, with causation process and overlapping and jointly representing the etiological process (see Fig. 8.1 in Chap. 8). Providing such etiological explanation means providing a coherent set of hypotheses that support the observed data, explaining the occurrence of the disease and its clinical outcome.[8]

Comprehensive etiological explanations may include reference to initiators (causes), mediators, and modifiers. Causes (e.g., Sars-CoV-2 infection) are factors that initiate the mediating patho-mechanism (e.g., severe inflammation in the lung) which leads to pulmonary disease, sometimes respiratory failure, and death (outcome). Modifiers in this explanation are factors that change the impact of causes and mechanisms (e.g., vaccination or social distancing), while facilitators are any biological, behavioral, or societal conditions that have an impact on the remainder of the etiological process (such as age, race, access to healthcare, and so forth). Modeling such comprehensive etiological explanation is exactly what I see multi-scale ABMs as capable of doing. They can simulate what might happen in a population given a certain constellation of characteristics that describe the interactions between initiators/causes, mediators/mechanisms, and intrinsic as well as extrinsic modifiers of the causation process.

Etiological explanations are explanations that tell a cogent story of illness occurrence that is justified by reference to coherent causal and mechanistic evidence. Giving an etiological explanation means to provide a list of causes (even if the list has only one item) and mechanisms that, taken together, suffice to change the beliefs of the hitherto unconvinced about why and how the illness occurred. I think that this characterization of etiological explanations should work in both medical (single patient) settings as well as in epidemiological (population) contexts. Agent-based models that provide etiological explanations would be models of the entire etiological process from cause via mechanism to clinical disease (as depicted in

Fig. 8.1, Chap. 8). Any ABM that models COVID-19 infection incidence would provide an etiological explanation.

However, many ABMs that have been developed to model population-wide aspects of the pandemic do more: they also include estimates of hospitalizations based on estimates of illness severity, admission to intensive care, and mortality, as in the example provided above. These kinds of ABM not just explain illness occurrence but also what happens afterward, the *prognosis* of illness. Let me offer Table 9.1 to make some potentially helpful distinctions. Of note, the

> intended explicandum [of scientific explanations] is, very roughly, explanations of why things happen, where the 'things' in question can be either particular events or something more general—e.g., regularities or repeatable patterns in nature. (Woodward, 2017)

I am aware that explaining *why* something happens is a very different thing than explaining its *consequences*. Indeed, such an explanation would probably not be considered *scientific*. However, a slight change of perspective might allow us to reintroduce science through the backdoor. We could say that what happens after the initial occurrence of illness is just the *occurrence* of aspects of disease development and outcome. Thus, the

Table 9.1 Characteristics of causal, mechanical, clinical, and prognostic explanations

	Explanation			
	Causal	*Mechanical*	*Clinical*	*Prognostic*
Explanans	Cause (risk factors)	Pathogenesis (biology)	Signs and symptoms, clinical course	Outcome (cure, death, or anything in between)
Explanandum	Why? (roots)	How?	Clinical presentation	Prognosis
Source of evidence	Epidemiology, Causometry	Biosciences	Clinical medicine	Follow-up (medicine, epidemiology)
	Etiological explanation			
			Prognostic explanation	
	Etio-prognostic explanation			

prognostic part of etio-prognostic explanations can be viewed as providing a plain-old etiological explanation. This way, one could see prognostic explanations as scientific, i.e., by recognizing them as etiological explanations of a different, future target entity.

However, I am interested in the mere *practical* utility of explanations of illness occurrence and outcome for the purpose of uncertainty reduction. I prefer looking at ABMs as providing a pragmatic kind of explanation, which is simply helpful by illuminating both the *etiology and prognosis* of illness. This is exactly what we expect from ABMs in the context of the COVID-pandemic: explanations why and how illness occurrence patterns arise at the population level, how they evolve, and what their consequences are.

* * *

In this chapter, I have discussed the epistemological characteristics of ABMs, one type of simulation model used in the context of the COVID-19 pandemic. In contrast to equation-based models, ABMs are algorithms that use individual agents and attribute changing characteristics to each one, multiple times during multiple iterations over time. Based on my discussion, I conclude that ABMs can explain causal mechanisms but cannot provide emergence explanations, because they cannot provide information about exactly why low-level phenomena give rise to those emergent phenomena. This is also one reason why I believe that ABMs cannot help with causal inference. Another reason is that ABMs do not reflect real-world processes but the causal-mechanical intuitions of the modeler. On the other hand, ABMs can integrate "impossible" multi-scale interactions between initiators, mediators, moderators, and conditions, and may be useful as generators of comprehensive etio-prognostic explanations of illness occurrence and outcome, which in turn can go a long way reducing the uncertainty in medicine about disease etiology and prognosis.

Obviously, ABMs are not the only way to design etio-prognostic explanations. While they can be offered by simulation in silico, they can also be generated by mounting evidence in an explanatory-coherentist framework such as the one provided in the next chapter.

NOTES

1. This part of the chapter is a revised version of (Dammann, 2021a).
2. For a comparison of ABMs and EBMs, see (Van Dyke Parunak et al., 1998).
3. Quote from online material available at https://www.nature.com/articles/s41591-020-1001-6#Sec2 (accessed 06/13/2021).
4. https://www.publichealth.columbia.edu/research/population-health-methods/agent-based-modeling (accessed 06-04-2021).
5. See above, in Chap. 8, the remark that having an oxygen-induced retinopathy model of ROP that yields ROP-like abnormalities does not necessarily entail that all (or even any) ROP is induced by oxygen.
6. I see a similarity here to the current discussion about the transparency, explainability, and interpretability of machine learning algorithms (Roscher et al., 2020).
7. It would be fascinating to explore the potential impact of the purported distinction between weak and strong emergence in this context. See, e.g., (Bedau, 1997; Chalmers, 2006; O'Connor, 1994).
8. For a philosophical-ish take on explanatory coherence in epidemiology, see (Dammann, 2018).

REFERENCES

Aleta, A., Martin-Corral, D., Pastore, Y. Piontti A., Ajelli, M., Litvinova, M., Chinazzi, M., Dean, N. E., Halloran, M. E., Longini, I. M., Jr., Merler, S., Pentland, A., Vespignani, A., Moro, E., & Moreno, Y. (2020). Modelling the impact of testing, contact tracing and household quarantine on second waves of COVID-19. *Nature Human Behaviour, 4*(9), 964–971.

Barrett, C., Bura, A. C., He, Q., Huang, F. W., Li, T. J. X., Waterman, M. S., & Reidys, C. M. (2021). Multiscale feedback loops in SARS-CoV-2 viral evolution. *Journal of Computational Biology, 28*(3), 248–256.

Bechtel, W. (2011). Mechanism and biological explanation. *Philosophy of Science, 78*, 533–557.

Bedau, M. A. (1997). Weak emergence. *Philosophical Perspectives, 11*, 375–399.

Broadbent, A. (2008). The difference between cause and condition. *Proceedings of the Aristotelian Society, 108*(1pt3), 355–364.

Campaner, R., & Cerri, M. (2020). Manipulative evidence and medical interventions: some qualifications. *History and Philosophy of the Life Sciences, 42*, 15.

Cartwright, N. (2004). Causation: One word, many things. *Philosophy of Science, 71*, 805–819.

Cartwright, N. (2007). Are RCTs the gold standard? *BioSocieties, 1*, 11–20.

Cartwright, N. (2010). What are randomised controlled trials good for? *Philosophical Studies: An International Journal for Philosophy in the Analytic Tradition, 147*(1), 59–70.

Casini, L., & Manzo, G. (2016). Agent-based models and causality - a methodological appraisal. *The IAS Working Paper Series, 2016*(7). Linköping: University.

Chalmers, D. J. (2006). Strong and weak emergence. In P. Clayton & P. Davies (Eds.), *The re-emergence of emergence: The emergentist hypothesis from science to religion.* Oxford University Press.

Conte, R., & Paolucci, M. (2014). On agent-based modeling and computational social science. *Frontiers in Psychology, 5,* 668.

Cuevas, E. (2020). An agent-based model to evaluate the COVID-19 transmission risks in facilities. *Computers in Biology and Medicine, 121,* 103827.

Dammann, O. (2018). Hill's heuristics and explanatory coherentism in epidemiology. *American Journal of Epidemiology, 187*(1), 1–6.

Dammann, O. (2020). *Etiological explanations: Illness causation theory.* CRC Press.

Dammann, O. (2021a). Agent-based models as etio-prognostic explanations. *Argumenta, 1,* 19–38.

Dammann, O. (2021b). Evidence mapping to justify health interventions. *Perspectives in Biology and Medicine, 64*(2), 155–172.

Dasgupta, S., Papadimitriou, C. H., & Vazirani, U. V. (2008). *Algorithms.* McGraw-Hill Higher Education.

Deaton, A., & Cartwright, N. (2016). Understanding and misunderstanding randomized controlled trials. *National Bureau of Economic Research Working Paper Series, No. 22595.*

Diez Roux, A. V. (2014). Invited commentary: The virtual epidemiologist--promise and peril. *American Journal of Epidemiology, 181*(2), 100–102.

Douglas, H. E. (2009). Reintroducing prediction to explanation. *Philosophy of Science, 76*(4), 444–463.

Gillies, D. (2019). *Causality, probability, and medicine (1st edn).* Routledge.

Goldstein, J. (1999). Emergence as a construct: History and issues. *Emergence, 1*(1), 49–72.

Hart, W. S., Maini, P. K., Yates, C. A., & Thompson, R. N. (2020). A theoretical framework for transitioning from patient-level to population-scale epidemiological dynamics: Influenza A as a case study. *Journal of the Royal Society Interface, 17*(166), 20200230.

Hedström, P., & Swedberg, R. (1998). *Social mechanisms: An analytical approach to social theory.* Cambridge University Press.

Hempel, C. G., & Oppenheim, P. (1948). Studies in the logic of explanation. *Philosophy of Science, 15,* 135–175.

Hernán, M. A. (2004). A definition of causal effect for epidemiological research. *Journal of Epidemiology and Community Health, 58*(4), 265–271.

Hill, A. B. (1965). The environment and disease: Association or causation? *Proceedings of the Royal Society of Medicine, 58,* 295–300.

Hoertel, N., Blachier, M., Blanco, C., Olfson, M., Massetti, M., Rico, M. S., Limosin, F., & Leleu, H. (2020). A stochastic agent-based model of the SARS-CoV-2 epidemic in France. *Nature Medicine, 26*(9), 1417–1421.

Howick, J., Glasziou, P., & Aronson, J. K. (2009). The evolution of evidence hierarchies: What can Bradford Hill's 'guidelines for causation' contribute? *Journal of the Royal Society of Medicine, 102*(5), 186–194.

Hunter, E., Mac Namee, B., & Kelleher, J. D. (2017). A taxonomy for agent-based models in human infectious disease epidemiology. *Journal of Artificial Societies and Social Simulation, 20*(3), 2.

Kelly, M. P., Kelly, R. S., & Russo, F. (2014). The integration of social, behavioral, and biological mechanisms in models of pathogenesis. *Perspectives in Biology and Medicine, 57*(3), 308–328.

Kerr, C. C., Stuart, R. M., Mistry, D., Abeysuriya, R. G., Rosenfeld, K., Hart, G. R., Núñez, R. C., Cohen, J. A., Selvaraj, P., Hagedorn, B., George, L., Jastrzębski, M., Izzo, A., Fowler, G., Palmer, A., Delport, D., Scott, N., Kelly, S. B., Caroline, S., Wagner, B., Chang, S., Oron, A. P., Wenger, E., Panovska-Griffiths, J., Famulare, M., & Klein, D. J. (2021). Covasim: An agent-based model of COVID-19 dynamics and interventions. *PLoS Computational Biology, 17*(7), e1009149.

Machamer, P. K., Darden, L., & Craver, C. F. (2000). Thinking about mechanisms. *Philosophy in Science, 67*, 1–25.

Marshall, B. D., & Galea, S. (2015). Formalizing the role of agent-based modeling in causal inference and epidemiology. *American Journal of Epidemiology, 181*(2), 92–99.

Medicine, I., & o. (2003). *The future of the public's health in the 21st century.* National Academies Press.

O'Connor, T. (1994). Emergent properties. *American Philosophical Quarterly, 31*, 91–104.

Parkkinen, V.-P., Wallmann, C., Wilde, M., Clarke, B., Illari, P., Kelly, M. P., Norell, C., Russo, F., Shaw, B., & Williamson, J. (2018). *Evaluating evidence of mechanisms in medicine.* Springer.

Roscher, R., Bohn, B., Duarte, M. F., & Garcke, J. (2020). Explainable machine learning for scientific insights and discoveries. *IEEE Access, 8*, 42200–42216.

Shamil, M. S., Farheen, F., Ibtehaz, N., Khan, I. M., & Rahman, M. S. (2021). An agent-based modeling of COVID-19: Validation, analysis, and recommendations. *Cognitive Computation*, (2024) *16*, 1723–1734.

Silva, P. C. L., Batista, P. V. C., Lima, H. S., Alves, M. A., Guimarães, F. G., & Silva, R. C. P. (2020). COVID-ABS: An agent-based model of COVID-19 epidemic to simulate health and economic effects of social distancing interventions. *Chaos, Solitons & Fractals, 139*, 110088.

Staffini, A., Svensson, A. K., Chung, U.-I., & Svensson, T. (2021). An agent-based model of the local spread of SARS-CoV-2: Modeling study. *JMIR Medical Informatics, 9*(4), e24192.

Stinchcombe, A. L. (1991). The conditions of fruitfulness of theorizing about mechanisms in social science. *Philosophy of the Social Sciences, 21*(3), 367–388.

Susser, M. (1991). What is a cause and how do we know one? A grammar for pragmatic epidemiology. *American Journal of Epidemiology, 133*, 635–648.

Topping, C. J., Høye, T. T., & Olesen, C. R. (2010). Opening the black box—Development, testing and documentation of a mechanistically rich agent-based model. *Ecological Modelling, 221*(2), 245–255.

Tracy, M., Cerdá, M., & Keyes, K. M. (2018). Agent-based modeling in public health: Current applications and future directions. *Annual Review of Public Health, 39*(1), 77–94.

Truszkowska, A., Behring, B., Hasanyan, J., Zino, L., Butail, S., Caroppo, E., Jiang, Z.-P., Rizzo, A., & Porfiri, M. (2021). High-resolution agent-based modeling of COVID-19 spreading in a small town. *Advanced Theory and Simulations, 4*(3), 2000277.

Van Dyke Parunak, H., Savit, R., & Riolo, R. L. (1998). Agent-based modeling vs. equation-based modeling: A case study and users' guide. In J. S. Sichman, R. Conte, & N. Gilbert (Eds.), *Multi-agent systems and agent-based simulation*. Berlin, Heidelberg.

Venkatramanan, S., Lewis, B., Chen, J., Higdon, D., Vullikanti, A., & Marathe, M. (2018). Using data-driven agent-based models for forecasting emerging infectious diseases. *Epidemics, 22*, 43–49.

Weisberg, M. (2014). Understanding the emergence of population behavior in individual-based models. *Philosophy of Science, 81*(5), 785–797.

Winkelmann, S., Zonker, J., Schütte, C., & Conrad, N. D. (2021). Mathematical modeling of spatio-temporal population dynamics and application to epidemic spreading. *Mathematical Biosciences, 336*, 108619.

Wolkenhauer, O. (2014). Why model? *Frontiers in Physiology, 5*, 21.

Woodward, J. (2017). Scientific explanation. In E. N. Zalta (Ed.), *The Stanford encyclopedia of philosophy*, by Metaphysics Research Lab, Philosophy Department, Stanford University, Stanford, CA 94305.

Worrall, J. (2007). Why there's no cause to randomize. *British Journal for the Philosophy of Science, 58*(3), 451–488.

CHAPTER 10

Evidence-Mapping

Introduction

To support health interventions, biomedical and population health researchers need to collect solid evidence. In this chapter, I ask what type of evidence should be considered in light of the abundant uncertainty in medicine and the health sciences. I expand on previous work that focused on etiological explanations, i.e., causal-mechanical explanations of why and how illness occurs. I propose to add predictive evidence to the explanatory evidence to form a joint evidence set JES = [A,B,C,D] which consists of four different types of evidence: of association [A], of biology [B], of confirmation [C], and of difference-making [D]. I will consider explanatory coherence as a theoretical backbone for this proposal, suggest criteria for each type of evidence, and offer a rubric for multi-evidence mapping.

Health interventions need to be well-justified and, arguably, helpfulness is a good justifier. In turn, good justifications need to be supported by solid evidence. While some of the process of generating such evidence is formalized in individual branches of the health sciences, an overarching

---

This chapter is a modified version of Dammann [*Perspectives in Biology and Medicine*, 64(2), 155–172 (2021)]. The paper offers more tables and detail about evidence mapping.

O. Dammann, *Uncertainty and Explanation in Medicine and the Health Sciences*, https://doi.org/10.1007/978-3-031-82271-1_10

framework for the integration of multiple *different* types of evidence is lacking.

In this chapter, I propose a semi-formal methodological framework, i.e., *multilevel evidence mapping*, that helps organize and interpret the available evidence in support of health interventions. In brief, I will outline the collection of evidence from multiple sources in support of health interventions as a two-step process (Table 10.1). The first step is to gather *explanatory* evidence from epidemiological observations and mechanistic laboratory experiments. The second step involves making predictions based on these explanations and gathering *predictive* evidence by checking whether these predictions are accurate. My main argument is to show that it is not necessarily the randomized intervention trial, but the explanatory-predictive coherence of the above evidence that justifies health interventions, even in the absence of randomized trials. This argument dovetails with, e.g., Paneth and Joyner's discussion of evidence supporting the use of convalescent serum in COVID-19 patients, which includes the warning that "we should not be paralyzed into inaction when [RCTs] are not available" (Paneth & Joyner, 2021).

The argument builds on the nine viewpoints offered by Bradford Hill in support of causal inference based on observational epidemiological data (Hill, 1965) and my previous interpretation of Hill's viewpoints as an explanatory coherentist framework (Dammann, 2018b). We have considered Hill's heuristics previously (see Chap. 8, p. 219–222), but it might be helpful to list again his proposed nine viewpoints to be considered before attaching causal meaning to an association identified in observational epidemiological studies: *strength* of the association, *consistency and specificity*

Table 10.1 Fourfold table of explanatory (top) and predictive (bottom) evidence, provided by observational (left) and interventional (right) research (modified from Dammann, 2021)

	Observation	*Intervention*
Step 1 Explanation	**A. Association** *"There is something"* Observational (non-interventional) Epidemiology	**B. Biology** *"It might work like this"* Experimental Laboratory Science
Step 2 Prediction	**C. Confirmation** *"It happens – as expected"* Successfully predicted observation	**D. Difference** *"We can make a difference"* Clinical and population trials

of findings, cause before effect (*temporality*), *biological gradient* (dose-response), *plausibility, coherence, experiment (intervention success)*, and *analogy* (pre-existing knowledge about similar associations). Some, but not all of these viewpoints are captured in one way or another by the framework I propose in this chapter.

Here is a brief overview of the sections to follow. I begin by outlining how clinical and epidemiological observations provide evidence that a certain health phenomenon occurs and which risk factors, if any, are statistically *associated* with its occurrence [A]. Laboratory experiments are then designed to clarify the pathogenetic (*biological*) process that connects risk factors and their consequences mechanistically [B]. Together, [A] and [B] represent the first, explanatory step, providing what I have called *etiological explanations* (EE), comprehensive descriptions of the causes of illness and the pathogenetic mechanisms that connect the two. One way to establish the "fit" of EE is explanatory coherence modeling. The second step consists of two kinds of predictions. The first are correct predictions of the phenomenon under study outside of research settings, i.e., *confirmatory*-prospective evidence [C], as they are to be expected based on knowledge about the distribution of risk factors. The second includes predictions of *difference-making* in terms of intervention success, which comes ideally, but not necessarily, from randomized trials [D]. [C] and [D] stand in a confirmatory relationship to [A] and [B]. However, they also play an explanatory role together with A and B as members of the joint evidence set *JES* = [A,B,C,D] (Table 10.1).

In the subsequent section, I argue that *JES* exhibits *explanatory-predictive coherence* if (1.) members do not contradict each other (non-contradiction), (2.) their joint explanatory force is stronger than that of individual members of *JES* or of combinations of its members (additive synergism), and if (3.) the evidence they provide turns out to be successful in research settings (practical efficacy). If interventions based on such explanatory-predictive coherence also turn out to be *helpful* by successfully improving population health *outside* the research setting (practical effectiveness), we would consider this a final confirmation of success for the entire endeavor.

In the last section I describe how one recently developed kind of research synthesis, *evidence mapping*, can help arrange the available evidence in the form of an explanatory-predictive coherence model. The goal is to provide a structured rubric to document the availability or absence of different types of evidence, collected to justify interventions in medicine.

ETIOLOGICAL EXPLANATIONS

Modern biomedicine is an orchestrated response to the challenge of illness. The main target is the reduction of suffering by targeting the etiology of illness. The arguably most useful definition of the term includes *causes* that occur before any bodily response and *mechanisms* that lead from the initial bodily response to the first manifestations of illness (MacMahon & Pugh, 1970). In other words, this view conceptualizes illness development as a process with three main components: causal initiators set biological mechanisms in motion, which result in clinical illness (see Fig. 8.1 in Chap. 8).

The cognitive entry point into the system is knowledge about the characteristics of diseases, disorders, or defects. While some kinds of illness have very general, non-specific features, e.g., fever, others have very specific (pathognomonic) characteristics, such as the strawberry tongue in Kawasaki disease. Whatever the constellation of symptoms, their initial occurrence in a person can be defined as the onset of clinical illness.

Asking the etiological question of illness occurrence is asking for an explanation of *why* a person has become ill and *how*. In response, causal and mechanistic explanations are given, alone or together. A causal explanation is a response to the *why question* and it is given by listing factors that are considered responsible for the illness to occur. For example, infection with a human immunodeficiency virus (HIV) is considered to be the cause of AIDS, needle sharing among drug users is considered to be one major cause of HIV infection, and drug addiction is what leads to needle sharing, and so on. To give a mechanistic explanation is to explain *how* exposure to the cause culminates in the onset of illness. This mechanism is also known as the pathogenesis of the illness under consideration. It is the biological cascade of events that connects exposure to causes with illness, the outcome of the pathogenetic process.

Taken together, causal and mechanistic explanations describe the story of illness occurrence in the form of an EE. A good, comprehensive EE should be useful in at least two ways. First, it specifies the causes of illness to define targets for interventions that prevent illness occurrence. This is the task at hand for epidemiologists. The idea is that if we eliminate or at least reduce the occurrence of the cause (the epidemiological "exposure"), we might eliminate or reduce the disease (the epidemiological "outcome"). Preventive measures that lead to fewer people being infected with HIV should lead to fewer cases of AIDS. Reducing the number of drug addicts that share needles should lead to fewer cases of HIV infection. Thus, some AIDS prevention programs focus on reducing the need for needle sharing among drug users. Second, the EE identifies target points for medical interventions designed to interfere with the pathogenesis of illness. This task is tackled mainly by laboratory scientists. Drugs have been identified that inhibit viral replication and/or viral spread. Thus, EEs are very helpful in the design of health interventions by virtue of explaining both causal and patho-mechanistic factors.

Providing useful EEs requires solid evidence that supports causal-mechanistic claims. Causal claims are supported by good evidence from modern epidemiological risk factor studies. A candidate risk factor is studied in relation to illness occurrence. If certain requirements are fulfilled, the association between risk factor and illness is considered causal. The two classic causometric techniques to arrive at a point where experts consider causation likely are the quantitative *potential outcomes approach* (POA) (Rubin, 1974) and the qualitative approach according to Hill (Hill, 1965) (see Chap. 7 for details). While the former involves judgements based on the results of randomized or quasi-randomized epidemiologic studies, the latter requires the consideration of qualitative viewpoints when checking observed associations against external heuristics (Glass et al., 2013).

Pathogenetic mechanisms are studied in the laboratory by means of biomechanistic controlled experimentation. Clever experimental setup and intervention design ensure that the results can be considered causal. The rationale here is the same as in the POA for observational epidemiologic studies: comparing two randomly generated groups of otherwise identical groups of individuals (animals, cell cultures, or other comparatively simple systems) after only one of the groups has been exposed to a specific intervention will reveal differences between groups that can be considered to be caused by that intervention. In sum, EEs provide information about what causes a specific disease *and* how. In its simplest form, an EE looks like this: "Cause C contributes to the occurrence of disease D by initiating mechanism M which contributes to the occurrence of disease D". For more detailed discussions of the concept, see Dammann (2017, 2020).

Constructing etiological explanations is desirable even when causation cannot be proven. We all know the *association is not causation* paradigm. Although one may have simplistic situations of the sort that someone jumping off a cliff will *always* land in the water, one can also always create more or less clever exceptions that have a boat located underneath or the jumper happens to operate a hang-glider and so on. Here, causation is inferred from what David Hume (1711–1776) called a "constant connexion".

But causal inference is not this simple in the context of complex systems such as those that dominate the health sciences today. As mentioned before, Hernán states that in a perfectly designed and conducted randomized trial, association *is* causation (Hernán, 2004), but note that nothing more than association is observed, even in a randomized trial, while causation is not. What makes this association causal is Hernán's belief in randomization as a causometer; his causal inference, not some extra ingredient in the data renders the observed association different from an observation of a similar association in similar data from a prospective (non-randomized) cohort study. Therefore, I do not share the belief that perfect randomization *guarantees* causal associations and that randomization is an infallible causometer, while I can agree to consider it a "quasi-causometer" in light of the paucity of alternative approaches to causometry, Hill's heuristics being one (see below). Indeed, I do not believe that perfect randomization is achievable even with the most heroic efforts. There is always the possibility that results of randomized trials are affected by chance events or residual bias.

Instead, I hold that EE can be based solely on observed associations, if we have a coherent set of error-independent pieces of evidence like Hill's heuristics. It is the coherence among pieces of evidence that provides explanatory vigor. Think of such explanation as comparable to the coherence of evidence in a criminal law suit. It is not just the absence of an alibi that led to the conviction of the gardener, but the additional evidence provided by an eyewitness, who saw the gardener close to the victim's home at around the time the murder was committed, plus the presence of her DNA on the murder weapon.

The second requirement, error-independence, ensures that if individual pieces of evidence turn out to be erroneous, the remainder of the evidence remains unaffected and valid (Stegenga, 2009). In other words, evidential error independence makes sure that invalidation of evidence of one type of evidence does not invalidate any evidence of the other types. All evidence I refer to comes from observations in non-interventional epidemiological studies or in randomized trials, or from observations in lab experiments. No causal attribution is required. The causal notion is based entirely on the   degree   to   which   it   is   possible   to   integrate   the   available error-independent evidence from observed associations in a coherent explanatory framework.

In the next section I argue that for EEs to serve as a proper justification for health interventions, they should be coherent systems of multiple types of evidence that are strong individual predictors, they should be mutually coherent in their predictions (i.e., offer successful prognostic explanations), and should not be jointly weaker in their predictive success than individual predictors are.

EXPLANATORY-PREDICTIVE COHERENCE

What kind of characteristic must scientific evidence have to get us from the *belief* that an intervention will be helpful to the *knowledge* that it will be helpful? What distinguishes the belief that the rebound tenderness in a child's lower right abdominal quadrant might indicate appendicitis and that surgery might be needed, from the *knowledge* that it is in fact appendicitis and that surgery is needed? According to the tripartite definition of knowledge as justified, true belief, knowledge is separated from belief by truth and justification. Thus, I simply suggest that an evidential system that integrates explanatory and predictive components, is likely to become a belief-justifier, hence knowledge-maker, if it is consistently coherent and jointly more successful than its components. In keeping with the tripartite definition of knowledge, said evidential system should also be true.

In essence, I think that an explanatory-predictive coherentist approach will render a *justified* intervention *well-justified*. Explanatory coherentism claims that a well-justified belief requires multiple items of evidence that cohere with each other. When the items cohere, they can be offered together in support of hypotheses (Poston, 2014).

There is no foundation upon which all parts of the explanatory system are built (as in foundationalism), but only mutual support by all its parts. I have argued elsewhere that Hill's qualitative approach to causal inference in epidemiology is an interesting example of an explanatory coherentist framework (Dammann, 2018b) that can help integrating causal, mechanistic, and other evidence into comprehensive EE. In this chapter, I am going one step further and argue that adding *predictive* evidence to the mix will yield explanatory-predictive explanations that justify interventions designed to improve health if all types of evidence considered in one such set are coherent. Coherence refers to situations in which information becomes evidence by comparison (see section on Transitional Inference in Chap. 5), when pieces of information are put into perspective by being viewed in light of each other and examined for mutual and reciprocal coherence. If new information appears to be aligned with previously accepted information, and if they reinforce each other, the transformation from information to evidence is supported (Dammann, 2018a).

I distinguish between explanatory evidence, i.e., data that help us *cogently explain*, and prospective evidence, i.e., evidence that comes from *successful prediction*. Explanatory evidence is a set of facts that we use to tell the story of why and how a phenomenon comes about. Prospective evidence is a set of facts that tells us we can forecast when, why, and how future instances of the phenomenon are likely to occur. Explanatory evidence is provided by causal and mechanistic research, which tell us why and how illness occurs, respectively. While explanatory evidence comes from epidemiological association measures (type A evidence) and laboratory data (type B), while prospective evidence comes from the accurate prediction of an association (type C) and intervention success (type D). In the former situation, it is the observed data that count as evidence; in the latter situation, it is the accurate prediction. Prospective evidence comes from research that provides information about successful predictions. Explaining a fact is telling an evidence-based, plausible story why and how such fact occurred. Offering a prediction is telling an evidence-based, plausible story about the conditions under which future instances of such fact will occur. I am aware that the construct of etio-prognostic explanations used in the previous chapter appears to blur the distinction, but I am currently unable to offer a clean-cut distinction.

Now, let's dissect *JES* in terms of the evidence needed to support its *component relations* [A], [B], [C], and [D] (Table 10.1):

A. Association (Beyond Chance)

It needs to be demonstrable that the target health phenomenon is real, and that we have an idea *why* it occurs by demonstrating a strong *association* between putative determinants (exposures) and the phenomenon (outcome). We need to demonstrate that "there is something to intervene on". A cause c is anything that contributes to the occurrence of disease d as an initiator of a mechanism m which in turn contributes to the occurrence of d as a patho-mechanism.

Thus, we need to demonstrate that

- c is associated with d
- c is associated with m
- m is associated with d

These associations need to be statistical (and ideally statistically significant) because we are interested in the co-occurrence of c and d, of c and m, and of m and d beyond what would be expected by chance.

B. Biology

It further needs to be demonstrable that we have an idea of *how* the phenomenon occurs and what the underlying *biology* might be ("it might work like this");

- c can biologically plausibly initiate m
- m can biologically plausibly be a patho-mechanism for d

C. Confirmation

We must demonstrate that the phenomenon "occurs as expected" in real life, not just in the research lab, based on our knowledge from [A] and [B]; this is initially a *confirmatory* step and later, after successful confirmation of knowledge from [A] and [B], becomes a prospective explanation. We must demonstrate that one can predict the presence of m based on knowledge about the presence of c. Moreover, we must show that we can predict the occurrence of d given c and m. Thus, we need to demonstrate that knowledge about the presence of c or m enables the prediction of d. We must demonstrate that

- m occurs more frequently in the presence of c than in its absence;
- d occurs more frequently in the presence of c than in its absence;
- d occurs more frequently in the presence of m than in its absence.

Of note, I am not proposing that the other types of evidence in the *JES* would not benefit from confirmation as well. Indeed, experiments need confirmation by similar experiments in another laboratory and RCT results require confirmation by similar RCTs in different and larger populations (replication). Even confirmatory type C evidence becomes stronger if confirmed independently. What is special about the confirmation of the initial explanatory type A evidence by secondary predictive type C evidence is that *the mere existence* of a potential association needs to be ascertained.

D. Difference

The litmus test for establishing the $c{\rightarrow}m{\rightarrow}d$ sequence is successful (correct) prediction of intervention results. We must demonstrate that we can make a *difference* by intervening in controlled human research environments, such as randomized clinical or population trials (showing efficacy). We need to demonstrate that eliminating or reducing the occurrence of c eliminates or reduces m, and thereby d. In other words, we must successfully (correctly) predict that an intervention will make a difference. Of note, I do not think that randomization of an intervention trial is the main justifier of the kind of justification the current discussion is about, while the explanatory-predictive coherence of the error-independent components of a *JES* is.

Thus, to establish type D evidence we need to demonstrate that

- eliminating or reducing c is associated with elimination or reduced occurrence of m;
- interfering with m is associated with elimination or reduced occurrence of d.

Effective manipulation is part of components [B] and [D] in *JES*. I think that most of us would agree that if the consistently coherent joint evidence provided by *JES* achieves the targeted goal of health improvement, then health interventions based on *JES* are reasonably justified. Only if high-quality evidence of all four types is provided, i.e., if each one of the four types of evidence is plausibly supported by the other three, and none of the four contradicts any one of the other three, is the explanatory-predictive evidence coherent and the initiation of population health interventions fully justified. Note that some interventions may be justified even if the *JES* is still incomplete, e.g., if an intervention is desperately needed and preliminary evidence seems to suffice.

Consider the following brief example. Showing that [A] coffee consumption in pregnancy (risk factor $r1$) is associated with low birthweight and that [B] caffeine exposure in pregnant laboratory animals reduces the birthweight of mouse pups (by mechanism $m1$) (type B evidence) is not yet sufficient to fully justify population campaigns of coffee consumption reduction in pregnancy. Why not? It could very well be that another risk factor ($r2$) for low birthweight such as smoking is strongly associated with coffee consumption *and* has a much stronger effect on birthweight via another mechanism ($m2$) than does caffeine (via $m1$). For example, if pregnant women tend to hide smoking behavior in pregnancy from health researchers, but tell the truth about their coffee intake, it will seem as if $m1$ explains a stronger effect of $r1$ on birthweight than it really has, because the strength of the association is really determined by both $m1$ and $m2$, not just by $m1$. In such case, we would expect to be able to predict low birthweight based on knowledge about $r1$ and $m1$, without even knowing about $r2$ and $m2$, whose effect is screened off by (hidden behind) $r1$ and $m1$. However, any prediction based solely on such explanatory evidence of what would happen if we intervened on $r1$ would necessarily be an exaggeration, because such intervention would affect only $m1$, but not $m2$ (unless intervening on $r1$ somehow also modifies exposure to $r2$). We would probably be able to make a correct prediction about the occurrence of low birthweight based on [A] and [B], but we would likely be disappointed at step [D] because our intervention on (weak) $r1$ might reduce the risk for low birthweight only minimally, while an intervention on (strong) $r2$ would be much more effective. In this scenario, predictions [C] and [D] would yield incoherent results. My argument is that only if they are coherent, i.e., only if [C] and [D] cohere with each other *and* with [A] and [B], do they fully justify an intervention.

Of note, explanatory and predictive evidence are not based on the same data. While both may be based on the same *kind of* data (observations data from epidemiological studies), they cannot be based on identical data, i.e., data from the same study. Still, the confirmatory nature of type C evidence does not result from how and when the data are collected, but from the confirmatory relationship in which it stands to the initial explanatory evidence. The difference lies not in the repetition of an observation (in what Hill called consistency), but in the success of a prediction: explanatory evidence is data such as risk ratios or odds ratios and their confidence intervals, while predictive evidence is a simple yes/no answer to the question "is our prediction accurate?"

Furthermore, the explanatory *power* (vigor, thrust, oomph) of type A evidence lies in its capability to generate a causal hypothesis that explains the observed data. The explanatory power of type C evidence as stand-alone evidence would be the same as type A evidence, but given previous type A evidence, type C evidence also has additional *confirmatory* power that type A doesn't have, which comes from the success of the prediction we made based on type A evidence. In this sense, type A and C evidence are very different in the way they can be interpreted: type A evidence as being explained by a causal hypothesis and type C evidence as both, being explained by a causal hypothesis and by a hypothesis of accurate prediction.

My point is that while explanatory evidence may be pointing in the right direction and may, in some cases, even yield success once implemented, it is the added predictive evidence and the resulting coherence of items [C] and [D] that strengthens the justification of health interventions. In other words, I hold that providing *both* explanatory and predictive evidence in support of a proposition to intervene offers better evidence than does a cogent explanation alone. But my argument goes one step further, proposing that successful prediction joins explanatory evidence in transforming merely cogent evidence into evidence that justifies interventions.

This point may seem a departure from previous approaches that tend to separate explanation from confirmation. By integrating the explanation and confirmation, the overall explanatory power of the joint explanatory system of evidence is strengthened. At the point where all members of *JES* cohere, the *predictive* power of [C,D] adds to the *explanatory* power of [A,B] to form *JES*, whose joint explanatory power is greater than that of [A,B]. What makes me think that the joint explanatory power of *JES* goes beyond that of [A,B]? Consider, again, the notion of *evidential error-independence*. As explained above, this notion holds that the joint evidential power of two pieces of evidence is greater if they are error-independent than if they are not. Error-independence means that if one of the two pieces of evidence turns out to be faulty, the other one does not automatically fail as well. For example, if one witness saw the gardener arrive at the house of the victim on the evening of the murder *and also* saw the gardener having a heated argument with the victim on the back porch of the victims house an hour later, the explanatory power of these two pieces of evidence can usually be considered jointly stronger than either one alone. However, they might not be error-independent, since anything that limits the credibility of the witness (her having been inebriated that night as confirmed by a local bartender, or her being mentally ill and often confused if she forgets to take her medication, or her being the disgruntled ex-wife of the gardener) will limit the credibility of both pieces of evidence offered by her, not just one.

The notion that [A], [B], [C], and [D] are defined by their explanatory versus predictive characteristics and by their being gathered by observation versus intervention (Table 10.1) makes the error independent, at least along these two dimensions. Thus, error independence increases the evidential vigor of *JES* = [A,B,C,D] beyond that provided by just [A,B].

In sum, I argue that in order to promote a successful health intervention one needs (1.) explanatory evidence [A,B], (2.) strong individually successful predictors [C] and [D], which are (3.) mutually coherent in their predictions and thus form a coherent jointly predictive set [C,D] that is (4.) better in its predictive success compared to individual predictors [C] and [D]. At this moment, the predictive evidential set [C,D] is deemed coherent with the explanatory evidential set [A,B] and the joint explanatory-predictive coherence of *JES* justifies the proposed intervention. The presence of *incoherent* evidence would suggest, first, that starting an intervention might not be a good idea and, second, that the validity of the available incoherent evidence should be scrutinized.

EVIDENCE MAPPING

Mapping available evidence supports explanatory-predictive coherence claims. The result is an evidence map that systematically summarizes research data (Miake-Lye et al., 2016). Table 10.2 provides a proposed rubric for evidence mapping to support the claim that a health intervention is justified. Specific selection criteria and quality control methods, as well as effective ways to visually represent the evidence, are still to be developed. The following description of what kind of documentation should be available in support of explanatory-predictive coherence claims may serve as a humble beginning, and I invite proposals how to improve the framework.

Section A. Association

The first prerequisite for an intervention is having an observable target problem. This is often the identification of a health condition we want to alter, prevent, treat, and so forth. In part A of the map, I suggest documenting observational evidence from human individuals and populations in support of the hypothesis that the problem at hand is real (A.1, *occurrence*). Simple prevalence and incidence data provide such information. In the context of the discovery of AIDS, it was the publication of a case series

Table 10.2 Proposed multi-evidence map for documentation of evidence needed to form joint evidential set *JES* = [A,B,C,D] in support of health interventions

Section	Evidence type	Hypothesis supported	Evidence
A.	**Observation**		
A.1	Occurrence	The problem occurs naturally in humans	
A.2	Association	One or more candidate causes have been identified in well-performed observational studies	
B.	**Experiment**		
B.1.a	In vitro, effect	An in vitro laboratory model using the candidate cause(s) from A.2 induces characteristics of the target condition	
B.1.b	In vitro, effect blocked	Blocking the candidate causal mechanisms in above model prevents characteristics of the target condition from occurring	
B.2.a	In vivo, effect	An in vivo laboratory model using the candidate cause(s) from A.2 induces characteristics of the target condition	
B.2.b	In vivo, effect blocked	Blocking the candidate causal mechanisms in above model prevents characteristics of the target condition from occurring	
C.	**Confirmation**		
C.1.a	Similar population/ scenario; same type of observation	The problem continues to occur as predicted based on knowledge from type A evidence	
C.1.b	Similar population/ scenario; different type of observation	(as above)	
C.2.a	Different population/ scenario; different type of observation	(as above)	
C.2.b	Different population/ scenario; same type of observation	(as above)	
D.	**Difference**		
D.1	Clinical trial	An intervention targeting X turns out to be efficacious in clinical trial(s), randomized or not	

(*continued*)

Table 10.2   (continued)

Section	Evidence type	Hypothesis supported	Evidence
D.2	Population trial	An intervention targeting X turns out to be effective in population/community trial(s), randomized or not	
	Additional evidence		
C*	Effectiveness	Population-level changes based on vital data	
C*	Effectiveness	Post-marketing research	
D*	Supportive meta-analyses	e.g., Cochrane analyses suggest solid and significant efficacy	

of homosexual men with Kaposi's sarcoma and a rare form of pneumonia that helped identify AIDS as a population health problem (Centers for Disease, 1982).

If we don't know *what* to change, it is very hard to come up with a good idea what to do to bring about change. We need something to intervene upon to reduce the burden posed by the problem. Thus, we need to have some idea of what might be the causes of the condition of interest, risk factors that we think of as initiators of the process that culminates in the condition. This is achieved by detailed epidemiological studies. In the history of AIDS research, scientists found not only a strong association between HIV infection and the subsequent development of AIDS, but acquired data "from prospective epidemiological studies that document an absolute requirement for HIV infection for the development of AIDS" (Blattner et al., 1988). Evidence that certain candidate causes have been identified is documented in part A.2 of Table 10.2, *association*.

Section B. Biology

The second section is to be populated by detailed information about the mechanics of the process that leads from cause to effect. For obvious reasons, patho-mechanisms cannot be studied directly in humans. Thus, targeted laboratory experiments must be designed and performed to provide type [B] evidence. Such experiments come with two prominent drawbacks. First, the phenomena observed in such experiments are not occurring naturally, but only after some specific manipulation of the system parameters. Part of this caveat is that precisely what makes experiments credible as evidence for biological mechanisms (design, manipulation, controlled environment, randomization) also renders them un-natural in the sense of not being a reflection of what happens to a person while she is getting sick. Second, the biological phenomena observed in the experimental setting are frequently from work done *in vitro* ("in glass", test tube research) or *in vivo* ("in life", animal research). Neither system is identical with the "human system" (see translational inference in Chap. 5).

The focus on animal models comes from the intent to render experimental models as relevant to the (human) target condition as possible but also introduces new layers of ethical and comparability concerns. One striking example is the wide-ranging incongruence between human and murine inflammatory responses that might have important consequences for the use of experimental mouse data to support claims about human inflammatory disease (Seok et al., 2013). References that elucidate the mechanism that explains the association between the purported cause(s) and the illness under investigation are documented in section B of our evidence map; type B.1 being evidence from *in vitro*, type B.2 from *in vivo* studies. Either type can come without or with evidence from blocking experiments, which always strengthens experimental evidence.

Note that for the prevention of illness, knowledge of mechanisms (type [B] evidence) is sometimes not necessary. In the history of AIDS research, this concept was alluded to by Blattner, Gallo, and Temin in 1988, when they wrote "Epidemiological data show that transmission of HIV results in AIDS and blocking HIV transmission prevents the occurrence of AIDS" (Blattner et al., 1988). By "blocking HIV transmission" the authors refer to public health interventions that interrupt HIV transmission via blood transfusion, which resulted in an elimination of the occurrence of AIDS among individuals who had received transfusions containing HIV (type [D] evidence).

Section C. Confirmation

Repeated observation of the occurrence of the phenomenon under investigation, both in terms of incidence and prevalence of the illness and in terms of observed recurrent association between purported causes and the illness, serves as confirmation that we have a potential target for intervention (documented in section C). The term "confirmation" here refers to the confirmation of the natural occurrence of the illness, not the confirmation of research studies or experiments as is standard operating procedure in science (replication). The strength of the confirmatory evidence increases if we have such confirmation from multiple *different* populations and from multiple studies with *different designs*.

Section D. Difference

As discussed above, the scientific experiment is considered the litmus test for causal claims. What the lab experiment is for the explanatory axis, the intervention trial is for the predictive axis. Again, by *prediction* I do not refer to the simple forecasting of events, but the *accurate* prediction of intervention success. Results from a *successful* intervention would be entered in section D.1 of the evidence map, results from a successful population trial in section D.2.

As previously discussed, at least three conditions should be fulfilled by the evidence collected in the evidence map to justify interventions: High-quality evidence of all four types is provided, each one of the four types of evidence is plausibly supported by the other three, and none of the four types of evidence contradicts any of the other three.

The first requirement asks for high-quality evidence in all four areas. Here, the current scientific standard should guide judgement. In sections A and C, sufficient study size as well as control for confounding and other biases will be important. In section B, experiments should be controlled, blinded, statistical procedures should be appropriate, and in section D, published guidelines to rate the quality of the available evidence should be used, for example those from the GRADE initiative (Balshem et al., 2011).

Second, the evidence from all four sections should be mutually supportive in logical and biological ways. For example,

- the initial observational evidence that HIV is associated with AIDS (Laurence et al., 1984) (section A) was supported by
- confirmation (section C) of an association between HIV and AIDS in multiple or even many different populations (Quinn et al., 1989)
- by laboratory findings (section B) that a "virus-like infectious agent" transfected with DNA of an AIDS patient caused fatal wasting disease in monkeys and that zidovudine is an effective anti-HIV agent (Mitsuya et al., 1985), and
- by subsequent evidence that such intervention is effective in humans (section D) (Fischl et al., 1990)

Finally, any contradiction between the four types of evidence would reduce the coherence of the system. Of course, the absence of evidence of a different type is not directly contradictive. For example, an observed association between a purported cause and some disease [A] would not be contradicted by the mere absence of supporting experimental evidence [B], but by the failure to cause the illness in the lab using the purported cause as the experimental intervention.

* * *

In this chapter, I have attempted to bring together the concepts of etiological explanation and explanatory-predictive coherence by offering a proposed outline for a multi-evidence map, in which evidence of association, biology, confirmation, and difference can be documented with the goal to reduce interventional uncertainty. Moreover, I have proposed that high-quality evidence that is mutually supportive and non-contradictory might be a good starting point for judging the degree of explanatory-predictive coherence. More work is needed to outline formal ways to extract evidence from the literature and organize it using evidence mapping to curb interventional uncertainty and justify interventions in medicine.

REFERENCES

Balshem, H., Helfand, M., Schunemann, H. J., Oxman, A. D., Kunz, R., Brozek, J., et al. (2011). GRADE guidelines: 3. Rating the quality of evidence. *Journal of Clinical Epidemiology, 64*(4), 401–406.

Blattner, W., Gallo, R. C., & Temin, H. M. (1988). HIV causes AIDS. *Science, 241*(4865), 515–516.

Centers for Disease, C. (1982). A cluster of Kaposi's sarcoma and Pneumocystis carinii pneumonia among homosexual male residents of Los Angeles and orange counties, California. *MMWR. Morbidity and Mortality Weekly Report, 31*(23), 305–307.

Dammann, O. (2017). The etiological stance: Explaining illness occurrence. *Perspectives in Biology and Medicine, 60*(2), 151–165.

Dammann, O. (2018a). Data, information, evidence, and knowledge: A proposal for health informatics and data science. *Online Journal of Public Health Informatics, 10*(3), e224.

Dammann, O. (2018b). Hill's heuristics and explanatory coherentism in epidemiology. *American Journal of Epidemiology, 187*(1), 1–6.

Dammann, O. (2020). *Etiological explanations: Illness causation theory.* CRC Press.

Dammann, O. (2021). Evidence mapping to justify health interventions. *Perspectives in Biology and Medicine, 64*(2), 155–172.

Fischl, M. A., Richman, D. D., Hansen, N., Collier, A. C., Carey, J. T., Para, M. F., et al. (1990). The safety and efficacy of zidovudine (AZT) in the treatment of subjects with mildly symptomatic human immunodeficiency virus type 1 (HIV) infection. A double-blind, placebo-controlled trial. The AIDS Clinical Trials Group. *Annals of Internal Medicine, 112*(10), 727–737.

Glass, T. A., Goodman, S. N., Hernan, M. A., & Samet, J. M. (2013). Causal inference in public health. *Annual Review of Public Health, 34*, 61–75.

Hernán, M. A. (2004). A definition of causal effect for epidemiological research. *Journal of Epidemiology and Community Health, 58*(4), 265–271.

Hill, A. B. (1965). The environment and disease: Association or causation? *Proceedings of the Royal Society of Medicine, 58*, 295–300.

Laurence, J., Brun-Vezinet, F., Schutzer, S. E., Rouzioux, C., Klatzmann, D., Barre-Sinoussi, F., et al. (1984). Lymphadenopathy-associated viral antibody in AIDS. Immune correlations and definition of a carrier state. *The New England Journal of Medicine, 311*(20), 1269–1273.

MacMahon, B., & Pugh, T. F. (1970). *Epidemiology; principles and methods* (1st ed.). Little.

Miake-Lye, I. M., Hempel, S., Shanman, R., & Shekelle, P. G. (2016). What is an evidence map? A systematic review of published evidence maps and their definitions, methods, and products. *Systematic Reviews, 5*, 28.

Mitsuya, H., Weinhold, K. J., Furman, P. A., St Clair, M. H., Lehrman, S. N., Gallo, R. C., et al. (1985). 3'-Azido-3'-deoxythymidine (BW A509U): An antiviral agent that inhibits the infectivity and cytopathic effect of human T-lymphotropic virus type III/lymphadenopathy-associated virus in vitro. *Proceedings of the National Academy of Sciences of the United States of America, 82*(20), 7096–7100.

Paneth, N., & Joyner, M. (2021). The use of observational research to inform clinical practice. *The Journal of Clinical Investigation, 131*(2), e146392.

Poston, T. (2014). *Reason and explanation: A defense of explanatory coherentism* [text]. Palgrave Macmillan.

Quinn, T. C., Zacarias, F. R., & St John, R. K. (1989). HIV and HTLV-I infections in the Americas: A regional perspective. *Medicine (Baltimore), 68*(4), 189–209.

Rubin, D. B. (1974). Estimating causal effects of treatments in randomized and nonrandomized studies. *Journal of Educational Psychology, 66*(5), 688–701.

Seok, J., Warren, H. S., Cuenca, A. G., Mindrinos, M. N., Baker, H. V., Xu, W., et al. (2013). Genomic responses in mouse models poorly mimic human inflammatory diseases. *Proceedings of the National Academy of Sciences of the United States of America, 110*(9), 3507–3512.

Stegenga, J. (2009). Robustness, discordance, and relevance. *Philosophy of Science, 76*, 650–661.

CONCLUSION

I began this book by outlining Broadbent's puzzle of medical ineffectiveness and Stegenga's medical nihilism as a point of departure for my argument that medicine is less ineffective as these authors would like to make us believe. Instead, I offer an explanation why medicine might look as ineffective as it does: because of the inherent uncertainty in medicine, biology, and—indeed—the world. I subscribe to the view that such uncertainty is inherent in all processes that are central to medicine (aleatoric or A-uncertainty) and that our cognitive state vis-à-vis such wobbliness of data that reflect the uncertainty "out there" is one of epistemic or E-uncertainty "in here".

Above, and in the book, I have used the word *wobbly* as the adverb pointing to the tongue-in-cheek concept WOBBLY, an acronym for "We Better Be Looking Yonder". I have invented this concept to confer the essence of uncertainty, which includes the hard facts that the world is indeterministic, that its workings cannot be predicted with certainty, and that thinking of the world as predictable is futile. Looking beyond these facts means to acknowledge uncertainty as what it is—a natural variability of physical and biological processes that *via* their wobbliness can give rise to novelty, the emergence of phenomena not predictable with certainty based on their causes and mechanisms. It is erroneous to conceive of such wobbliness as random *error*. Yes, it may be random, but it isn't error. It is a

© The Author(s), under exclusive license to Springer Nature   291
Switzerland AG 2025
O. Dammann, *Uncertainty and Explanation in Medicine and the*
Health Sciences, https://doi.org/10.1007/978-3-031-82271-1

natural expression of what *can* happen based on the physical and biological constraints of the system at hand, with multiple different possible outcomes; which one *will* occur is estimable only with reference to probability distributions of repeatedly observable events.

Still, I believe it is possible to get a handle on uncertainty by organizing data, information, and evidence in ways that can yield reliable medical knowledge and, I think, those who work in the health sciences, such as epidemiology and the laboratory sciences, do just that when they *generate* data, information, and evidence. Similarly, I think that medics, such as doctors, nurses, and other clinicians, do just that when they *apply* such data, information, and evidence. The tools they use for this generation and usage are inferences, explanations, and causometry, among others that I have not discussed in this book. I have explored the first two, inference and explanation, from a very inclusive and pluralist vantage point. In fact, my interpretation of these terms and the underlying concepts is probably closer to their everyday meaning than to their philosophical definitions. I have granted myself this leeway not to evade difficulty but to gain space, needed to grasp the multiple different aspects of these concepts in medicine and the health sciences.

In this way, I have proposed to look at inference as transitional and translational—the former to describe the inferential transition from data to information to evidence and knowledge, and the latter to describe the inferential "leaps" that we make when we infer from association to causation, from animal to human, from population to individual, and from simple to complex. Moreover, I have looked at explanation in a rather mosaic-like fashion, not just as explaining *why* and *how* events occur, but also as explanations that do not represent responses to *why*- and *how*-questions, i.e., epistemic, justificatory, methodological, and anticipatory explanations. Taken together, these four types of explanation can have eight explanatory functions (in my model for medicine and public health), but I am certain that more types and functions can be defined in other contexts. Indeed, this is exactly what I intended: to open a door for more and more useful concepts of explanation for medicine and the health sciences, and the philosophy thereof.

Perhaps the most provocative proposal in this book is that, taken together, the epidemiological approaches to causal inference, i.e., randomization, POA, and Hill's heuristics, can be viewed as a causometric approach, a way to measure causal relationships. While it is possible that an association finds support from causometric analysis and still is not causal, I think this is highly unlikely. Although not necessarily watertight, associations that are vetted by causometric evaluation are "causal enough". It will still be up to decision-makers in medicine and public health to decide when they are satisfied that what they look at is causation, not just association—*those* decisions cannot be made by a causometer.

The last part of the book offers three pertinent examples how methods and concepts discussed in the previous chapters can be applied to generate etiological explanations, etio-prognostic explanations, and evidence maps to justify health interventions. None of the methods, concepts, and applications described in these pages are to be understood as hard-and-fast prescriptions. To the contrary, all I have said is open for discussion and revision. It would be an honor and privilege to receive feedback from my colleagues in the philosophy of medicine community how to amend and improve my views.

REFERENCES

Ackoff, R. L. (1989). From data to wisdom. *Journal of Applied Systems Analysis, 16,* 3–9.

Adler, N. E., & Rehkopf, D. H. (2008). U.S. disparities in health: Descriptions, causes, and mechanisms. *Annual Review of Public Health, 29*(1), 235–252.

Admon, A. J., Donnelly, J. P., Casey, J. D., Janz, D. R., Russell, D. W., Joffe, A. M., et al. (2019). Emulating a novel clinical trial using existing observational data. Predicting results of the prevent study. *Annals of the American Thoracic Society, 16*(8), 998–1007.

Aleta, A., Martin-Corral, D., Pastore, Y. Piontti, A., Ajelli, M., Litvinova, M., Chinazzi, M., Dean, N. E., Halloran, M. E., Longini, I. M., Jr., Merler, S., Pentland, A., Vespignani, A., Moro, E., & Moreno, Y. (2020). Modelling the impact of testing, contact tracing and household quarantine on second waves of COVID-19. *Nature Human Behaviour, 4*(9), 964–971.

Alshaikh, B., Yusuf, K., & Sauve, R. (2013). Neurodevelopmental outcomes of very low birth weight infants with neonatal sepsis: Systematic review and meta-analysis. *Journal of Perinatology, 33*(7), 558–564.

Amann, J., Blasimme, A., Vayena, E., Frey, D., & Madai, V. I. (2020). Explainability for artificial intelligence in healthcare: A multidisciplinary perspective. *BMC Medical Informatics and Decision Making, 20*(1), 310.

Amrhein, V., Greenland, S., & McShane, B. (2019). Scientists rise up against statistical significance. *Nature, 567*(7748), 305–307.

Anscombe, G. E. M. (1993). Causality and determination. In E. Sosa & M. Tooley (Eds.), *Causation* (pp. 88–104). OUP.

Appiah, A. (2006). *Cosmopolitanism: Ethics in a world of strangers* (1st ed.). W.W. Norton & Co..

© The Author(s), under exclusive license to Springer Nature 295
Switzerland AG 2025
O. Dammann, *Uncertainty and Explanation in Medicine and the Health Sciences,* https://doi.org/10.1007/978-3-031-82271-1

Apweiler, R., Beissbarth, T., Berthold, M. R., Bluthgen, N., Burmeister, Y., Dammann, O., et al. (2018). Whither systems medicine? *Experimental & Molecular Medicine, 50*(3), e453.

Aralikatti, A. K., Mitra, A., Denniston, A. K., Haque, M. S., Ewer, A. K., & Butler, L. (2010). Is ethnicity a risk factor for severe retinopathy of prematurity? *Archives of Disease in Childhood. Fetal and Neonatal Edition, 95*(3), F174–F176.

Arnauld, A., & Nicole, P. (1964). *The Art of Thinking; Port-Royal Logic.* Indianapolis: Bobbs-Merrill.

Ashton, N. (1954). Pathological basis of retrolental fibroplasia. *The British Journal of Ophthalmology, 38*(7), 385–396.

Ashton, N., Ward, B., & Serpell, G. (1954). Effect of oxygen on developing retinal vessels with particular reference to the problem of retrolental fibroplasia. *The British Journal of Ophthalmology, 38*(7), 397–432.

Audi, R. (1999). *The Cambridge dictionary of philosophy* (2nd ed.). Cambridge University Press.

Awadh, A., Chughtai, A. A., Dyda, A., Sheikh, M., Heslop, D. J., & MacIntyre, C. R. (2017). Does Zika virus cause microcephaly - Applying the Bradford Hill viewpoints. *PLoS Currents, 9.*

Azad, R., Gilbert, C., Gangwe, A. B., Zhao, P., Wu, W.-C., Sarbajna, P., et al. (2020). Retinopathy of prematurity: How to prevent the third epidemics in developing countries. *Asia-Pacific Journal of Ophthalmology, 9*(5), 440–448.

Baker, M. (2016). 1,500 scientists lift the lid on reproducibility. *Nature, 533*(7604), 452–454.

Balshem, H., Helfand, M., Schunemann, H. J., Oxman, A. D., Kunz, R., Brozek, J., et al. (2011). GRADE guidelines: 3. Rating the quality of evidence. *Journal of Clinical Epidemiology, 64*(4), 401–406.

Banker, B. Q., & Larroche, J. C. (1962). Periventricular leukomalacia of infancy. *Archives of Neurology, 7,* 386–410.

Barker, C. F., & Markmann, J. F. (2013). Historical overview of transplantation. *Cold Spring Harbor Perspectives in Medicine, 3*(4), a014977.

Baron, J. H. (2009). Sailors' scurvy before and after James Lind - a reassessment. *Nutrition Reviews, 67*(6), 315–332.

Barrett, C., Bura, A. C., He, Q., Huang, F. W., Li, T. J. X., Waterman, M. S., & Reidys, C. M. (2021). Multiscale feedback loops in SARS-CoV-2 viral evolution. *Journal of Computational Biology, 28*(3), 248–256.

Bechtel, W. (2011). Mechanism and biological explanation. *Philosophy of Science, 78,* 533–557.

Bedau, M. A. (1997). Weak emergence. *Philosophical Perspectives, 11,* 375–399.

Berzuini, C., Dawid, P., & Bernardinelli, L. (2012). *Causality: Statistical perspectives and applications.* Wiley.

Bharwani, S. K., & Dhanireddy, R. (2008). Systemic fungal infection is associated with the development of retinopathy of prematurity in very low birth weight infants: A meta-review. *Journal of Perinatology: Official Journal of the California Perinatal Association, 28,* 61–66.

Bird, A. (1998). *Philosophy of science.* Routledge.

Blattner, W., Gallo, R. C., & Temin, H. M. (1988). HIV causes AIDS. *Science, 241*(4865), 515–516.

Blodi, F. C., & Parke, P. C. (1953). Retrolental fibroplasia. *The American Journal of Nursing, 53*(6), 718–720.

Bombelli, L., Lee, J., Meyer, D., & Sorkin, R. D. (1987). Space-time as a causal set. *Physical Review Letters, 59*(5), 521–524.

Bonafiglia, E., Gusson, E., Longo, R., Ficial, B., Tisato, M. G., Rossignoli, S., et al. (2022). Early and late onset sepsis and retinopathy of prematurity in a cohort of preterm infants. *Scientific Reports, 12*(1), 11675.

Borger, T., Nel, E. J., Kok, L. M., Marinelli, F. E., & Woldendorp, K. H. (2021). Risk factors for musculoskeletal complaints in female musicians: A systematic review and exploration for future studies. *Medical Problems of Performing Artists, 36*(4), 279–296.

Bottomley, M. J., Brook, M. O., Shankar, S., Hester, J., & Issa, F. (2022). Towards regulatory cellular therapies in solid organ transplantation. *Trends in Immunology, 43*(1), 8–21.

Broadbent, A. (2008). The difference between cause and condition. *Proceedings of the Aristotelian Society, 108*(1pt3), 355–364.

Broadbent, A. (2018a). *Philosophy of medicine.* Oxford University Press.

Broadbent, A. (2018b). Prediction, understanding, and medicine. *The Journal of Medicine and Philosophy, 43,* 289–305.

Broadbent, A. (2019). *Philosophy of medicine* (p. 1). Oxford University Press.

Broadbent, A. (Ed.). (Forthcoming). *Oxford handbook of philosophy of medicine.*

Broadbent, A., & Smart, B. (2020). Kinds of explanation in public health policy. In J. Sholl & S. Rattan (Eds.), *Explaining health across the sciences* (pp. 405–415). Springer.

Brownson, R. C., Fielding, J. E., & Maylahn, C. M. (2009). Evidence-based public health: A fundamental concept for public health practice. *Annual Review of Public Health, 30,* 175–201.

Bryan, C. S., & Podolsky, S. H. (2009). Dr. Holmes at 200 — The spirit of skepticism. *New England Journal of Medicine, 361*(9), 846–847.

Cai, S., Thompson, D. K., Anderson, P. J., & Yang, J. Y.-M. (2019). Short- and long-term neurodevelopmental outcomes of very preterm infants with neonatal sepsis: A systematic review and meta-analysis. *Children, 6*(12), 131.

Cai, Z., Pan, Z. L., Pang, Y., Evans, O. B., & Rhodes, P. G. (2000). Cytokine induction in fetal rat brains and brain injury in neonatal rats after maternal lipopolysaccharide administration. *Pediatric Research, 47*(1), 64–72.

Campaner, R. (2019). *Varieties of causal explanations in medical contexts.* Mimesis International.

Campaner, R. (2022). *Explaining disease: Philosophical reflections on medical research and clinical practice.* Springer.

Campaner, R., & Cerri, M. (2020). Manipulative evidence and medical interventions: some qualifications. *History and Philosophy of the Life Sciences, 42,* 15.

Campbell, K. (1951). Intensive oxygen therapy as a possible cause of retrolental fibroplasias: A clinical approach. *The Medical Journal of Australia, 2,* 48–50.

Carel, H. (2016). *Phenomenology of illness* (1st ed.). Oxford University Press.

Cartwright, N. (1989). *Nature's capacities and their measurement.* Oxford University Press.

Cartwright, N. (1994). No causes in, no causes out. In *Nature's capacities and their measurement* (pp. 39–90). Oxford University Press.

Cartwright, N. (2004). Causation: One word, many things. *Philosophy of Science, 71,* 805–819.

Cartwright, N. (2007a). Are RCTs the gold standard? *BioSocieties, 1,* 11–20.

Cartwright, N. (2007b). *Hunting causes and using them: Approaches in philosophy and economics.* Cambridge University Press.

Cartwright, N. (2010). What are randomised controlled trials good for? *Philosophical Studies: An International Journal for Philosophy in the Analytic Tradition, 147*(1), 59–70.

Cartwright, N. (2011). A philosopher's view of the long road from RCTs to effectiveness. *The Lancet, 377*(9775), 1400–1401.

Cartwright, N. (2012). Will this policy work for you? predicting effectiveness better: How philosophy helps. *Philosophy of Science, 79*(5), 973–989.

Casini, L., & Manzo, G. (2016). Agent-based models and causality - a methodological appraisal. *The IAS Working Paper Series, 2016*(7). Linköping: University.

Cassidy, D. C. (1992). *Uncertainty: The life and science of Werner Heisenberg.* W.H. Freeman.

Cassidy, D. C. (2009). *Beyond uncertainty: Heisenberg, quantum physics, and the bomb.* Bellevue Literary Press.

Cats, B. P., & Tan, K. E. (1985). Retinopathy of prematurity: Review of a four-year period. *British Journal of Ophthalmology, 69*(7), 500–503.

CDC. (2012). *Public health surveillance: Preparing for the future.*

Centers for Disease, C. (1982). A cluster of Kaposi's sarcoma and Pneumocystis carinii pneumonia among homosexual male residents of Los Angeles and orange counties, California. *MMWR. Morbidity and Mortality Weekly Report, 31*(23), 305–307.

Chalmers, D. J. (2006). Strong and weak emergence. In P. Clayton & P. Davies (Eds.), *The re-emergence of emergence: The emergentist hypothesis from science to religion.* Oxford University Press.

Chalmers, J., Zhu, Z., Hua, X., Yu, Y., Zhu, P., Hong, K., et al. (2020). Effect of red blood cell transfusion on the development of retinopathy of prematurity: A systematic review and meta-analysis. *PLoS One, 15*(6), e0234266.

Chemtob, S., Hardy, P., Abran, D., Li, D. Y., Peri, K., Cuzzani, O., et al. (1995). Peroxide-cyclooxygenase interactions in postasphyxial changes in retinal and choroidal hemodynamics. *Journal of Applied Physiology, 78*(6), 2039–2046.

Chen, J., & Smith, L. E. (2007). Retinopathy of prematurity. *Angiogenesis, 10*(2), 133–140.

Chen, J. S., Anderson, J. E., Coyner, A. S., Ostmo, S., Sonmez, K., Erdogmus, D., et al. (2021). Quantification of early neonatal oxygen exposure as a risk factor for retinopathy of prematurity requiring treatment. *Ophthalmology Science, 1*(4), 100070.

Chen, M. L., Allred, E. N., Hecht, J. L., Onderdonk, A., Vanderveen, D. K., Wallace, D. K., et al. (2011). Placenta microbiology and histology and the risk for severe retinopathy of prematurity. *Investigative Ophthalmology & Visual Science, 52*, 7052–7058.

Chen, M. L., Citil, A., McCabe, F., Leicht, K. M., Fiascone, J., Dammann, C. E. L., et al. (2011). Infection, oxygen, and immaturity: Interacting risk factors for retinopathy of prematurity. *Neonatology, 99*, 125–132.

Chen, M. L., Guo, L., Smith, L. E., Dammann, C. E., & Dammann, O. (2010). High or low oxygen saturation and severe retinopathy of prematurity: A meta-analysis. *Pediatrics, 125*(6), e1483–e1492.

Cheng, P. W. (1997). From covariation to causation: A causal power theory. *Psychological Review, 104*(2), 367–405.

Cheung, B. M. Y. (2014). Behind the rosiglitazone controversy. *Expert Review of Clinical Pharmacology, 3*, 723–725.

Chu, A., Dhindsa, Y., Sim, M. S., Altendahl, M., & Tsui, I. (2020). Prenatal intrauterine growth restriction and risk of retinopathy of prematurity. *Scientific Reports, 10*(1), 17591.

Clark, S., & Weale, A. (2012). Social values in health priority setting: A conceptual framework. *Journal of Health Organization and Management, 26*(3), 293–316.

Claxton, S., & Fruttiger, M. (2003). Role of arteries in oxygen induced vaso-obliteration. *Experimental Eye Research, 77*(3), 305–311.

Coggins, S. A., & Glaser, K. (2022). Updates in Late-Onset Sepsis: Risk Assessment, Therapy, and Outcomes. *NeoReviews, 23*(11), 738–755.

Conee, E. B., & Feldman, R. (2004). *Evidentialism: Essays in epistemology.* Oxford University Press.

Conte, R., & Paolucci, M. (2014). On agent-based modeling and computational social science. *Frontiers in Psychology, 5*, 668.

Corradini, A., & O'Connor, T. (2010). *Emergence in science and philosophy.* Routledge.

Cortes, J., Rugo, H. S., Cescon, D. W., Im, S.-A., Yusof, M. M., Gallardo, C., et al. (2022). Pembrolizumab plus chemotherapy in advanced triple-negative breast cancer. *New England Journal of Medicine, 387*(3), 217–226.

Cox, D. R. (2012). Statistical causality: Some historical remarks. In C. Berzuini, P. Dawid, & L. Bernardinelli (Eds.), *Causality* (pp. 1–5). John Wiley & Sons.

Cuevas, E. (2020). An agent-based model to evaluate the COVID-19 transmission risks in facilities. *Computers in Biology and Medicine, 121,* 103827.

Dai, A. I., Demiryurek, S., Aksoy, S. N., Perk, P., Saygili, O., & Gungor, K. (2015). Maternal iron deficiency anemia as a risk factor for the development of retinopathy of prematurity. *Pediatric Neurology, 53*(2), 146–150.

Dammann, O. (2010). Inflammation and retinopathy of prematurity. *Acta Paediatrica, 99*(7), 975–977.

Dammann, O. (2017). The etiological stance: Explaining illness occurrence. *Perspectives in Biology and Medicine, 60*(2), 151–165.

Dammann, O. (2018a). Data, information, evidence, and knowledge: A proposal for health informatics and data science. *Online Journal of Public Health Informatics, 10*(3), e224.

Dammann, O. (2018b). Hill's heuristics and explanatory coherentism in epidemiology. *American Journal of Epidemiology, 187*(1), 1–6.

Dammann, O. (2020a). *Etiological explanations: Illness causation theory.* CRC Press.

Dammann, O. (2020b). Toward epistemic, intersectoral, and disciplinary humility for population health science. *American Journal of Public Health, 110*(4), 425–426.

Dammann, O. (2021a). Agent-based models as etio-prognostic explanations. *Argumenta, 1,* 19–38.

Dammann, O. (2021b). Evidence mapping to justify health interventions. *Perspectives in Biology and Medicine, 64*(2), 155–172.

Dammann, O. (2022). Explanation in Public Health. In S. Venkatapuram & A. Broadbent (Eds.), *Routledge handbook of the philosophy of public health.* Routledge.

Dammann, O. (2023). Does prematurity "per se" cause visual deficits in preterm infants without retinopathy of prematurity? *Eye (London, England), 37,* 2587–2589.

Dammann, O. (Forthcoming). Epidemiological inferences. In A. Broadbent (Ed.), *Oxford handbook of philosophy of medicine.* Oxford University Press.

Dammann, O., Brinkhaus, M. J., Bartels, D. B., Dordelmann, M., Dressler, F., Kerk, J., et al. (2009). Immaturity, perinatal inflammation, and retinopathy of prematurity: A multi-hit hypothesis. *Early Human Development, 85,* 325–329.

Dammann, O., Hartnett, M. E., & Stahl, A. (2022). Retinopathy of prematurity. *Developmental Medicine & Child Neurology, 65*(5), 625–631.

Dammann, O., & Leviton, A. (1997). Maternal intrauterine infection, cytokines, and brain damage in the preterm newborn. *Pediatric Research, 42*(1), 1–8.

Dammann, O., & Leviton, A. (1998). Infection remote from the brain, neonatal white matter damage, and cerebral palsy in the preterm infant. *Seminars in Pediatric Neurology, 5*(3), 190–201.

Dammann, O., & Leviton, A. (2006). Inflammation, brain damage and visual dysfunction in preterm infants. *Seminars in Fetal & Neonatal Medicine, 11*(5), 363–368.

Dammann, O., & Leviton, A. (2014). Intermittent or sustained systemic inflammation and the preterm brain. *Pediatric Research, 75*(3), 376–380.

Dammann, O., Leviton, A., O'Shea, T. M., & Paneth, N. (Eds.). (2021). *Extremely preterm birth and its consequences*. Mac Keith Press.

Dammann, O., Mezinska, S., & Gefenas, E. (2022). Health humanities in medicina: The auxiliary stance. *Medicina (Kaunas, Lithuania), 58*(3), 411.

Dammann, O., Poston, T., & Thagard, P. (2020). How do medical researchers make causal inferences? In K. McCain & K. Kampourakis (Eds.), *What is scientific knowledge? An introduction to contemporary epistemology of science* (pp. 33–51). Routledge.

Dammann, O., Rivera, J. C., & Chemtob, S. (2021). The prenatal phase of retinopathy of prematurity. *Acta Paediatrica, 110*(9), 2521–2528.

Dammann, O., & Smart, B. (2019). *Causation in population health informatics and data science*. Springer.

Dasgupta, S., Papadimitriou, C. H., & Vazirani, U. V. (2008). *Algorithms*. McGraw-Hill Higher Education.

Davis, C. S. (2021). The purdue pharma opioid settlement - accountability, or just the cost of doing business? *The New England Journal of Medicine, 384*(2), 97–99.

De Regt, H. (2017). *Understanding Scientific Understanding*. Oxford University Press.

Deaton, A., & Cartwright, N. (2016). Understanding and misunderstanding randomized controlled trials. *National Bureau of Economic Research Working Paper Series, No. 22595*.

Debillon, T., Gras-Leguen, C., Verielle, V., Winer, N., Caillon, J., Roze, J. C., et al. (2000). Intrauterine infection induces programmed cell death in rabbit periventricular white matter. *Pediatric Research, 47*, 736–742.

Degelman, M. L., & Herman, K. M. (2017). Smoking and multiple sclerosis: A systematic review and meta-analysis using the Bradford Hill criteria for causation. *Multiple Sclerosis and Related Disorders, 17*, 207–216.

Dekkers, O. M., Elm, E. v., Algra, A., Romijn, J. A., & Vandenbroucke, J. P. (2009). How to assess the external validity of therapeutic trials: A conceptual approach. *International Journal of Epidemiology, 39*(1), 89–94.

Dellsén, F. (2016). There may yet be non-causal explanations. *Journal for General Philosophy of Science, 47*(2), 377–384.

Devanesan, A. (2020). Medical nihilism: The limits of a decontextualised critique of medicine. *Studies in History and Philosophy of Biological and Biomedical Sciences, 79*, 101189.

Diez Roux, A. V. (2014). Invited commentary: The virtual epidemiologist--promise and peril. *American Journal of Epidemiology, 181*(2), 100–102.

Doll, R., & Hill, A. B. (1950). Smoking and carcinoma of the lung. *BMJ, 2*(4682), 739–748.

Douglas, H. E. (2009). Reintroducing prediction to explanation. *Philosophy of Science, 76*(4), 444–463.

Edwards, R. T., Charles, J. M., & Lloyd-Williams, H. (2013). Public health economics: A systematic review of guidance for the economic evaluation of public health interventions and discussion of key methodological issues. *BMC Public Health, 13*, 1001.

Erdal, H., Demirtas, M. S., Kılıcbay, F., & Tunc, G. (2023). Evaluation of oxidative stress levels and dynamic thiol-disulfide balance in patients with retinopathy of prematurity. *Current Eye Research 48*(11), 1026–1033.

Erdei, C., & Dammann, O. (2014). The perfect storm: Preterm birth, neurodevelopmental mechanisms, and autism causation. *Perspectives in Biology and Medicine, 57*(4), 470–481.

Erdil, D., Koku Aksu, A. E., Falay Gur, T., & Gurel, M. S. (2020). Hand eczema treatment: Change behaviour with text messaging, a randomized trial. *Contact Dermatitis, 82*(3), 153–160.

Estrada, M. M., Tomlinson, L. A., Yu, Y., Ying, G.-S., & Binenbaum, G. (2022). Daily oxygen supplementation and risk of retinopathy of prematurity. *Ophthalmic Epidemiology, 30*, 1–9.

Faden, R. R., & Shebaya, S. (2019). Public health programs and policies: Ethical justifications. In A. C. Mastroianni, J. P. Kahn, & N. E. Kass (Eds.), *The Oxford handbook of public health ethics* (pp. 20–32). Oxford University Press.

Fedak, K. M., Bernal, A., Capshaw, Z. A., & Gross, S. (2015). Applying the Bradford Hill criteria in the 21st century: How data integration has changed causal inference in molecular epidemiology. *Emerging Themes in Epidemiology, 12*(1), 14.

Fevereiro-Martins, M., Guimarães, H., Marques-Neves, C., & Bicho, M. (2022). Retinopathy of prematurity: Contribution of inflammatory and genetic factors. *Molecular and Cellular Biochemistry, 477*(6), 1739–1763.

Fevereiro-Martins, M., Marques-Neves, C., Guimarães, H., & Bicho, M. (2023). Retinopathy of prematurity: A review of pathophysiology and signaling pathways. *Survey of Ophthalmology, 68*(2), 175–210.

Finkelstein, L., & Leaning, M. S. (1984). A review of the fundamental concepts of measurement. *Measurement, 2*(1), 25–34.

Fischl, M. A., Richman, D. D., Hansen, N., Collier, A. C., Carey, J. T., Para, M. F., et al. (1990). The safety and efficacy of zidovudine (AZT) in the treatment of subjects with mildly symptomatic human immunodeficiency virus type 1 (HIV) infection. A double-blind, placebo-controlled trial. The AIDS Clinical Trials Group. *Annals of Internal Medicine, 112*(10), 727–737.

Fleischmann, C., Reichert, F., Cassini, A., Horner, R., Harder, T., Markwart, R., et al. (2021). Global incidence and mortality of neonatal sepsis: A systematic review and meta-analysis. *Archives of Disease in Childhood, 106*(8), 745–752.

Fortes Filho, J. B., Valiatti, F. B., Eckert, G. U., Costa, M. C., Silveira, R. C., & Procianoy, R. S. (2009). Is being small for gestational age a risk factor for retinopathy of prematurity? A study with 345 very low birth weight preterm infants. *Jornal de Pediatria, 85*(1), 48–54.

Fox, C. R., & Ülkümen, G. (2011). Distinguishing two dimensions of uncertainty. In W. Brun, G. Keren, G. Kirkebøen, & H. Montgomery (Eds.), *Perspectives on thinking, judging, and decision making.* Universitetsforlaget.

Frank, C., Faber, M., & Stark, K. (2016). Causal or not: Applying the Bradford Hill aspects of evidence to the association between Zika virus and microcephaly. *EMBO Molecular Medicine, 8*(4), 305–307.

Friedman, M. (1974). Explanation and scientific understanding. *Journal of Philosophy, 71*(1), 5–19.

Friedman-Kien, A. E. (1981). Disseminated Kaposi's sarcoma syndrome in young homosexual men. *Journal of the American Academy of Dermatology, 5*(4), 468–471.

Fuller, J. (2020). Medical Nihilism by Jacob Stegenga: What is the right dose? *Studies in History and Philosophy of Science Part C: Studies in History and Philosophy of Biological and Biomedical Sciences, 81*, 101270.

Fuller, J. (2022). Epidemiological evidence: Use at your 'own risk'? *Philosophy of Science, 87*(5), 1119–1129.

Fuller, J., & Flores, L. J. (2015). The Risk GP Model: The standard model of prediction in medicine. *Studies in History and Philosophy of Biological and Biomedical Sciences, 54*, 49–61.

Gauvreau, K., & Pagano, M. (1994). Why 5%? *Nutrition, 10*(1), 93–94.

Gebharter, A. (2017). *Causal nets, interventionism, and mechanisms: Philosophical foundations and applications, synthese library, studies in epistemology, logic, methodology, and philosophy of science* (1st edn, p. 1). Springer International Publishing (VII, 184 pages 155 illustrations). https://doi.org/10.1007/978-3-319-49908-6

Gerwin, M. E. (1985). Bas van Fraassen, the scientific image. *Canadian Journal of Philosophy, 15*(2), 363–378.

Giannantonio, C., Papacci, P., Cota, F., Vento, G., Tesfagabir, M. G., Purcaro, V., et al. (2012). Analysis of risk factors for progression to treatment-requiring ROP in a single neonatal intensive care unit: Is the exposure time relevant? *The Journal of Maternal-Fetal & Neonatal Medicine, 25*(5), 471–477.

Gibian, P. (2001). *Oliver Wendell Holmes and the culture of conversation.* Cambridge University Press.

Gilles, F. H., Leviton, A., & Kerr, C. S. (1976). Endotoxin leucoencephalopathy in the telencephalon of the newborn kitten. *Journal of the Neurological Sciences,* 27(2), 183–191.

Gillies, D. (2000). *Philosophical theories of probability.* Routledge.

Gillies, D. (2019). *Causality, probability, and medicine (1st edn).* Routledge.

Glaser, K., Hartel, C., Klingenberg, C., Herting, E., Fortmann, M. I., Speer, C. P., Stensvold, H. J., Huncikova, Z., Ronnestad, A. E., Nentwich, M. M., Stahl, A., Dammann, O., Gopel, W., German Neonatal Network, t.N.N.N.I., the Infection, I.I., Immunisation section of the European Society for Paediatric, R. (2024). Neonatal Sepsis Episodes and Retinopathy of Prematurity in Very Preterm Infants. JAMA Netw Open 7, e2423933.

Glass, T. A., Goodman, S. N., Hernan, M. A., & Samet, J. M. (2013). Causal inference in public health. *Annual Review of Public Health, 34,* 61–75.

Glymour, C., Zhang, K., & Spirtes, P. (2019). Review of causal discovery methods based on graphical models. *Frontiers in Genetics, 10,* 524.

Godfrey, E. L., & Rana, A. (2019). Outcomes in solid-organ transplantation: Success and stagnation. *Texas Heart Institute Journal, 46*(1), 75–76.

Goldenberg, M. (2021). *Vaccine hesitancy.* University of Pittsburg Press.

Goldstein, G. P., Leonard, S. A., Kan, P., Koo, E. B., Lee, H. C., & Carmichael, S. L. (2019). Prenatal and postnatal inflammation-related risk factors for retinopathy of prematurity. *Journal of Perinatology, 39*(7), 964–973.

Goldstein, J. (1999). Emergence as a construct: History and issues. *Emergence, 1*(1), 49–72.

Gottlieb, M. S., Schroff, R., Schanker, H. M., Weisman, J. D., Fan, P. T., Wolf, R. A., et al. (1981). Pneumocystis carinii pneumonia and mucosal candidiasis in previously healthy homosexual men: Evidence of a new acquired cellular immunodeficiency. *The New England Journal of Medicine, 305*(24), 1425–1431.

Graunt, J. (1665). *Natural and political observations mentioned in a following index, and made upon the bills of mortality* (3rd edn). Printed by John Martyn, and James Allestry.

Groopman, J. E. (1984). Causation of AIDS revealed. *Nature, 308*(5962), 769.

Gunn, T. R., Easdown, J., Outerbridge, E. W., & Aranda, J. V. (1980). Risk factors in retrolental fibroplasia. *Pediatrics, 65*(6), 1096–1100.

Gyllensten, L. J., & Hellström, B. E. (1952). Retrolental fibroplasia - animal experiments - the effect of the eyes of fullterm mice. a preliminary report. *Acta Paediatrica, 41*(6), 577–582.

Hacking, I. (2001). *An introduction to probability and inductive logic.* Cambridge University Press.

Haefeli, M., & Elfering, A. (2005). Pain assessment. *European Spine Journal, 15*(S1), S17–S24.

Hall, H. I., Correa, A., Yoon, P. W., Braden, C. R., & Centers for Disease, C., & Prevention. (2012). Lexicon, definitions, and conceptual framework for public health surveillance. *MMWR Surveillance Summaries, 61*, 10–14.

Hall, N. S. (2007). R. A. Fisher and his advocacy of randomization. *Journal of the History of Biology, 40*(2), 295–325.

Halliday, S. (2016). William Farr: Campaigning statistician. *Journal of Medical Biography, 8*(4), 220–227.

Han, P. K. J. (2021). *Uncertainty in medicine: A framework for tolerance*. Oxford University Press.

Hardy, P., Abran, D., Li, D. Y., Fernandez, H., Varma, D. R., & Chemtob, S. (1994). Free radicals in retinal and choroidal blood flow autoregulation in the piglet: Interaction with prostaglandins. *Investigative Ophthalmology & Visual Science, 35*(2), 580–591.

Hariton, E., & Locascio, J. J. (2018). Randomised controlled trials - the gold standard for effectiveness research. *BJOG: An International Journal of Obstetrics & Gynaecology, 125*(13), 1716–1716.

Haroon Parupia, M. F., & Dhanireddy, R. (2001). Association of postnatal dexamethasone use and fungal sepsis in the development of severe retinopathy of prematurity and progression to laser therapy in extremely low-birth-weight infants. *Journal of Perinatology, 21*(4), 242–247.

Hart, W. S., Maini, P. K., Yates, C. A., & Thompson, R. N. (2020). A theoretical framework for transitioning from patient-level to population-scale epidemiological dynamics: Influenza A as a case study. *Journal of the Royal Society Interface, 17*(166), 20200230.

Hartnett, M. E. (2015). Pathophysiology and mechanisms of severe retinopathy of prematurity. *Ophthalmology, 122*(1), 200–210.

Hartnett, M. E. (2020). Retinopathy of prematurity: Evolving treatment with anti–vascular endothelial growth factor. *American Journal of Ophthalmology, 218*, 208–213.

Hartnett, M. E., & Lane, R. H. (2013). Effects of oxygen on the development and severity of retinopathy of prematurity. *Journal of AAPOS, 17*(3), 229–234.

Hartnett, M. E., & Penn, J. S. (2012). Mechanisms and management of retinopathy of prematurity. *The New England Journal of Medicine, 367*(26), 2515–2526.

Havmose, M., Thyssen, J. P., Zachariae, C., & Johansen, J. D. (2022). Long-term follow-up of hand eczema in hairdressers: A prospective cohort study of Danish hairdressers graduating from 1985 to 2007. *Journal of the European Academy of Dermatology and Venereology, 36*(2), 263–270.

Hayes, R., Hartnett, J., Semova, G., Murray, C., Murphy, K., Carroll, L., et al. (2021). Neonatal sepsis definitions from randomised clinical trials. *Pediatric Research, 93*(5), 1141–1148.

Hedström, P., & Swedberg, R. (1998). *Social mechanisms: An analytical approach to social theory*. Cambridge University Press.

Heisenberg, W. (1927). Über den anschaulichen Inhalt der quantentheoretischen Kinematik und Mechanik. *Zeitschrift für Physik, 43*(3–4), 172–198.

Hellstrom, A., Smith, L. E., & Dammann, O. (2013). Retinopathy of prematurity. *Lancet, 382*(9902), 1445–1457.

Hempel, C. G. (1962). Deductive-nomological versus statistical explanation. In H. Feigl & G. Maxwell (Eds.), *Scientific explanation, space, and time* (Vol. III, pp. 98–169). University of Minnesota Press.

Hempel, C. G., & Oppenheim, P. (1948). Studies in the logic of explanation. *Philosophy of Science, 15*, 135–175.

Hernán, M. A. (2004). A definition of causal effect for epidemiological research. *Journal of Epidemiology and Community Health, 58*(4), 265–271.

Hernán, M. A. (2021). Methods of public health research — Strengthening causal inference from observational data. *New England Journal of Medicine, 385*(15), 1345–1348.

Hernán, M. A., & Robins, J. M. (2006). Estimating causal effects from epidemiologic data. *Journal of Epidemiology and Community Health, 60*, 578–586.

Hernán, M. A., & Robins, J. M. (2016). Using big data to emulate a target trial when a randomized trial is not available. *American Journal of Epidemiology, 183*(8), 758–764.

Hernán, M. A., & Robins, J. M. (2020). *Causal inference: What if? In.* Chapman & Hall/CRC.

Hernandez, R., Teruel, T., & Lorenzo, M. (2003). Rosiglitazone produces insulin sensitisation by increasing expression of the insulin receptor and its tyrosine kinase activity in brown adipocytes. *Diabetologia, 46*, 1618–1628.

Hess, K., & Philipp, W. (2001). Bell's theorem and the problem of decidability between the views of Einstein and Bohr. *Proceedings of the National Academy of Sciences, 98*(25), 14228–14233.

Higgins, R. D. (2019). Oxygen saturation and retinopathy of prematurity. *Clinics in Perinatology, 46*(3), 593–599.

Hill, A. B. (1965). The environment and disease: Association or causation? *Proceedings of the Royal Society of Medicine, 58*, 295–300.

Hill, B., Lagerlund, H., & Psillos, S. (2021). *Reconsidering causal powers: Historical and conceptual perspectives.* Oxford University Press.

Hill, E. R., O'Connor, L. E., Wang, Y., Clark, C. M., McGowan, B. S., Forman, M. R., et al. (2022). Red and processed meat intakes and cardiovascular disease and type 2 diabetes mellitus: An umbrella systematic review and assessment of causal relations using Bradford Hill's criteria. *Critical Reviews in Food Science and Nutrition, 64*, 1–18.

Hingorani, A. D., Kuan, V., Finan, C., Kruger, F. A., Gaulton, A., Chopade, S., et al. (2019). Improving the odds of drug development success through human genomics: Modelling study. *Scientific Reports, 9*(1), 18911.

Hittner, H. M., Godio, L. B., Rudolph, A. J., Adams, J. M., Garcia-Prats, J. A., Friedman, Z., et al. (1981). Retrolental fibroplasia: Efficacy of vitamin E in a double-blind clinical study of preterm infants. *New England Journal of Medicine, 305*(23), 1365–1371.

Hoertel, N., Blachier, M., Blanco, C., Olfson, M., Massetti, M., Rico, M. S., Limosin, F., & Leleu, H. (2020). A stochastic agent-based model of the SARS-CoV-2 epidemic in France. *Nature Medicine, 26*(9), 1417–1421.

Höfler, M. (2005). Causal inference based on counterfactuals. *BMC Medical Research Methodology, 5*(1), 28.

Holm, M., Morken, T. S., Fichorova, R., VanderVeen, D., Allred, E. N., Dammann, O., et al. (2017). Systemic inflammation-associated proteins and retinopathy of prematurity in infants born before the 28th week of gestation. *Investigative Ophthalmology & Visual Science, 58*, 6419–6428.

Holmes, O. W. (1860). *Currents and counter-currents in medical science. An address delivered before the Massachusetts medical society, at the annual meeting, May 30, 1860.* Ticknor and Fields.

Home, P. D., Pocock, S. J., Beck-Nielsen, H., Gomis, R., Hanefeld, M., Dargie, H., Komajda, M., Gubb, J., Biswas, N., & Jones, N. P. (2005). Rosiglitazone Evaluated for Cardiac Outcomes and Regulation of Glycaemia in Diabetes (RECORD): Study design and protocol. *Diabetologia, 48*, 1726–1735.

Home, P. D., Pocock, S. J., Beck-Nielsen, H., Curtis, P. S., Gomis, R., Hanefeld, M., Jones, N. P., Komajda, M., McMurray, J. J. V., & RECORD Study Team. (2009). Rosiglitazone evaluated for cardiovascular outcomes in oral agent combination therapy for type 2 diabetes (RECORD): A multicentre, randomised, open-label trial. *Lancet, 373*, 2125–2135.

Home, P. D., Pocock, S. J., Beck-Nielsen, H., Gomis, R., Hanefeld, M., Jones, N. P., Komajda, M., McMurray, J. J. V., & RECORD Study Group. (2007). Rosiglitazone evaluated for cardiovascular outcomes--an interim analysis. *The New England Journal of Medicine, 357*, 28–38.

Hong, E. H., Shin, Y. U., Bae, G. H., Choi, Y. J., Ahn, S. J., Sobrin, L., et al. (2021). Nationwide incidence and treatment pattern of retinopathy of prematurity in South Korea using the 2007–2018 national health insurance claims data. *Scientific Reports, 11*(1), 1451.

Hong, H. K., Lee, H. J., Ko, J. H., Park, J. H., Park, J. Y., Choi, C. W., et al. (2014). Neonatal systemic inflammation in rats alters retinal vessel development and simulates pathologic features of retinopathy of prematurity. *Journal of Neuroinflammation, 11*, 87.

Howick, J. (2011). *The philosophy of evidence-based medicine.* Wiley-Blackwell, BMJ Books.

Howick, J., Glasziou, P., & Aronson, J. K. (2009). The evolution of evidence hierarchies: What can Bradford Hill's 'guidelines for causation' contribute? *Journal of the Royal Society of Medicine, 102*(5), 186–194.

Huang, J., Tang, Y., Zhu, T., Li, Y., Chun, H., Qu, Y., et al. (2019). Cumulative evidence for association of sepsis and retinopathy of prematurity. *Medicine (Baltimore)*, *98*(42), e17512.

Huang, Y.-H., Kuo, C.-H., Peng, I. C., Chang, Y.-S., Tseng, S.-H., Conway, E. M., et al. (2021). Recombinant thrombomodulin domain 1 rescues pathological angiogenesis by inhibition of HIF-1α-VEGF pathway. *Cellular and Molecular Life Sciences*, *78*(23), 7681–7692.

Hudalla, H., Bruckner, T., Poschl, J., Strowitzki, T., & Kuon, R. J. (2021). Maternal smoking as an independent risk factor for the development of severe retinopathy of prematurity in very preterm infants. *Eye (London, England)*, *35*(3), 799–804.

Huncikova, Z., Vatne, A., Stensvold, H. J., Lang, A. M., Stoen, R., Brigtsen, A. K., et al. (2023). Late-onset sepsis in very preterm infants in Norway in 2009–2018: A population-based study. *Archives of Disease in Childhood. Fetal and Neonatal Edition*, *108*(5), 478–484.

Hunter, E., Mac Namee, B., & Kelleher, J. D. (2017). A taxonomy for agent-based models in human infectious disease epidemiology. *Journal of Artificial Societies and Social Simulation*, *20*(3), 2.

Illari, P. M., & Russo, F. (2014). *Causality: Philosophical theory meets scientific practice* (1st ed.). Oxford University Press.

Imbens, G., & Rubin, D. B. (2015). *Causal inference for statistics, social, and biomedical sciences - an introduction*. CUP.

Ingvaldsen, S. H., Morken, T. S., Austeng, D., & Dammann, O. (2021). Visuopathy of prematurity: Is retinopathy just the tip of the iceberg? *Pediatric Research*, *91*(5), 1043–1048.

Ioannidis, J. P. (2005). Why most published research findings are false. *PLoS Medicine*, *2*(8), e124.

Ioannidis, J. P. (2015). Exposure-wide epidemiology: Revisiting Bradford Hill. *Statistics in Medicine*, *35*(11), 1749–1762.

Isaacs, D., & Fitzgerald, D. (1999). Seven alternatives to evidence based medicine. *BMJ*, *319*(7225), 1618–1618.

Jaffiol, C. (2009). Current management of type 2 diabetes in France. *Bulletin de l'Académie Nationale de Médecine*, *193*(7), 1645–1661.

James, S. L., Abate, D., Abate, K. H., Abay, S. M., Abbafati, C., Abbasi, N., et al. (2018). Global, regional, and national incidence, prevalence, and years lived with disability for 354 diseases and injuries for 195 countries and territories, 1990–2017: A systematic analysis for the Global Burden of Disease Study 2017. *The Lancet*, *392*(10159), 1789–1858.

Jamil, W., Svensson, A., Josefson, A., Lindberg, M., & Von Kobyletzki, L. (2022). Incidence rate of hand eczema in different occupations: A systematic review and meta-analysis. *Acta Dermato-Venereologica*, *102*, adv00681.

Joussen, A. M., Poulaki, V., Le, M. L., Koizumi, K., Esser, C., Janicki, H., et al. (2004). A central role for inflammation in the pathogenesis of diabetic retinopathy. *The FASEB Journal, 18*(12), 1450–1452.

Justice, M. J., & Dhillon, P. (2016). Using the mouse to model human disease: Increasing validity and reproducibility. *Disease Models & Mechanisms, 9*(2), 101–103.

Karlowicz, M. G., Giannone, P. J., Pestian, J., Morrow, A. L., & Shults, J. (2000). Does candidemia predict threshold retinopathy of prematurity in extremely low birth weight (</=1000 g) neonates? *Pediatrics, 105*(5), 1036–1040.

Kathpalia, A., & Nagaraj, N. (2021). Measuring causality. *Resonance, 26*(2), 191–210.

Keller, L. O., Strohschein, S., Lia-Hoagberg, B., & Schaffer, M. (1998). Population-based public health nursing interventions: A model from practice. *Public Health Nursing, 15*(3), 207–215.

Keller, L. O., Strohschein, S., Lia-Hoagberg, B., & Schaffer, M. A. (2004). Population-based public health interventions: Practice-based and evidence-supported. Part I. *Public Health Nursing, 21*(5), 453–468.

Kelly, M. P., Kelly, R. S., & Russo, F. (2014). The integration of social, behavioral, and biological mechanisms in models of pathogenesis. *Perspectives in Biology and Medicine, 57*(3), 308–328.

Kerr, C. C., Stuart, R. M., Mistry, D., Abeysuriya, R. G., Rosenfeld, K., Hart, G. R., Núñez, R. C., Cohen, J. A., Selvaraj, P., Hagedorn, B., George, L., Jastrzębski, M., Izzo, A., Fowler, G., Palmer, A., Delport, D., Scott, N., Kelly, S. B., Caroline, S., Wagner, B., Chang, S., Oron, A. P., Wenger, E., Panovska-Griffiths, J., Famulare, M., Klein, D. J. (2021). Covasim: An agent-based model of COVID-19 dynamics and interventions. *PLoS Computational Biology, 17*(7), e1009149.

Keyes, K. M., & Galea, S. (2016). *Population health science*. Oxford University Press.

Khoury, M. J., Bowen, M. S., Clyne, M., Dotson, W. D., Gwinn, M. L., Green, R. F., et al. (2018). From public health genomics to precision public health: A 20-year journey. *Genetics in Medicine, 20*(6), 574–582.

Kieffer, C. M., & Robertson, A. S. (2020). Impact of FDA-required cardiovascular outcome trials on type 2 diabetes clinical study initiation from 2008 to 2017. *Therapeutic Innovation & Regulatory Science, 54*, 640–644.

Kim, S. J., Port, A. D., Swan, R., Campbell, J. P., Chan, R. V. P., & Chiang, M. F. (2018). Retinopathy of prematurity: A review of risk factors and their clinical significance. *Survey of Ophthalmology, 63*(5), 618–637.

Kitcher, P. (1981). Explanatory unification. *Philosophy of Science, 48*(4), 507–531.

Kitcher, P. (1989). Explanatory unification and the causal structure of the world. In P. Kitcher & W. Salmon (Eds.), *Scientific explanation* (Vol. 8, pp. 410–505). University of Minnesota Press.

Klaic, M., Kapp, S., Hudson, P., Chapman, W., Denehy, L., Story, D., et al. (2022). Implementability of healthcare interventions: An overview of reviews and development of a conceptual framework. *Implementation Science, 17*(1), 10.

Kleinbaum, D. G., Kupper, L. L., & Morgenstern, H. (1982). *Epidemiologic research: Principles and quantitative methods.* Lifetime Learning Publications.

Kleinberg, S. (2013). *Causality, probability, and time.* Cambridge University Press.

Kolata, G. B. (2015). *The New York Times book of medicine.* Sterling Publishing Co..

Koller, D., & Friedman, N. (2009). *Probabilistic graphical models: Principles and techniques.* MIT Press.

Kremer, I., Naor, N., Davidson, S., Arbizo, M., & Nissenkorn, I. (1992). Systemic candidiasis in babies with retinopathy of prematurity. *Graefe's Archive for Clinical and Experimental Ophthalmology, 230*(6), 592–594.

Krieger, N. (2001). Theories for social epidemiology in the 21st century: An eco-social perspective. *International Journal of Epidemiology, 30*(4), 668–677.

Krieger, N. (2011). *Epidemiology and the people's health: Theory and context.* Oxford University Press.

Kronik, A. (2018). *How young are you? Understanding psychological age, time, causometry, to create meaningful, harmonious, productive lives.* New Academia Pub.

Kruskal, W., & Mosteller, F. (1979a). Representative sampling, I: Non-scientific literature. *International Statistical Review/Revue Internationale de Statistique, 47*(1), 13–24.

Kruskal, W., & Mosteller, F. (1979b). Representative sampling, II: Scientific literature, excluding statistics. *International Statistical Review/Revue Internationale de Statistique, 47*(2), 111–127.

Kruskal, W., & Mosteller, F. (1979c). Representative sampling, III: The current statistical literature. *International Statistical Review/Revue Internationale de Statistique, 47*(3), 245–265.

Lafreniere, J. D., Toguri, J. T., Gupta, R. R., Samad, A., O'Brien, D. M., Dickinson, J., et al. (2019). Effects of intravitreal bevacizumab in Gram-positive and Gram-negative models of ocular inflammation. *Clinical & Experimental Ophthalmology, 47*(5), 638–645.

Lam, D., Lively, S., & Schlichter, L. C. (2017). Responses of rat and mouse primary microglia to pro- and anti-inflammatory stimuli: Molecular profiles, K+ channels and migration. *Journal of Neuroinflammation, 14*(1), 166.

Lange, M. (2017). *Because without cause: Non-causal explanation in science and mathematics.* Oxford University Press.

Laurence, J., Brun-Vezinet, F., Schutzer, S. E., Rouzioux, C., Klatzmann, D., Barre-Sinoussi, F., et al. (1984). Lymphadenopathy-associated viral antibody in AIDS. Immune correlations and definition of a carrier state. *The New England Journal of Medicine, 311*(20), 1269–1273.

Lee, J., & Dammann, O. (2012). Perinatal infection, inflammation, and retinopathy of prematurity. *Seminars in Fetal & Neonatal Medicine, 17*(1), 26–29.

Lee, J. W., McElrath, T., Chen, M., Wallace, D. K., Allred, E. N., Leviton, A., et al. (2013). Pregnancy disorders appear to modify the risk for retinopathy of prematurity associated with neonatal hyperoxemia and bacteremia. *The Journal of Maternal-Fetal & Neonatal Medicine, 26*(8), 811–818.

Lemoine, M. (2017). Explanation in medicine. In M. Solomon, J. R. Simon, & H. Kincaid (Eds.), *The Routledge companion to philosophy of medicine* (pp. 296–309). Routledge.

Leong, A. (2019). The struggle over parcel C: How Boston's Chinatown won a victory in the fight against institutional expansion and environmental racism. *Amerasia Journal, 21*(3), 99–120.

Leviton, A. (1993). Preterm birth and cerebral palsy: Is tumor necrosis factor the missing link? *Developmental Medicine and Child Neurology, 35*(6), 553–558.

Leviton, A., & Gilles, F. H. (1973). An epidemiologic study of perinatal telencephalic leucoencephalopathy in an autopsy population. *Journal of the Neurological Sciences, 18*(1), 53–66.

Lewis, D. (1980). A subjectivist's guide to objective chance. In R. C. Jeffrey (Ed.), *Studies in inductive logic and probability* (Vol. II, pp. 263–293). University of California Press.

Lewis, D. (1986). Causal explanation. In *Philosophical papers* (Vol. II, pp. 214–240). Oxford University Press.

Lim, R. R., Hainsworth, D. P., Mohan, R. R., & Chaurasia, S. S. (2019). Characterization of a functionally active primary microglial cell culture from the pig retina. *Experimental Eye Research, 185*, 107670.

Lipton, P. (1991). *Inference to the best explanation.* Routledge.

Liu, T., Tomlinson, L. A., Yu, Y., Ying, G. S., Quinn, G. E., Binenbaum, G., et al. (2022). Changes in institutional oxygen saturation targets are associated with an increased rate of severe retinopathy of prematurity. *Journal of AAPOS, 26*(1), 18.

Loeliger, M. M., Mackintosh, A., De Matteo, R., Harding, R., & Rees, S. M. (2011). Erythropoietin protects the developing retina in an ovine model of endotoxin-induced retinal injury. *Investigative Opthalmology & Visual Science, 52*(5), 2656–2661.

Lou, J., Liu, X., Fan, X., Xu, X., Wang, Z., & Wang, L. (2023). Lncrna FEZfl–as1 negatively regulates ETNK1 to promote malignant progression of renal cell carcinoma. *Journal Of Medical Biochemistry, 42*(2), 232–238.

Loudon, I. (2013). Ignaz Phillip Semmelweis' studies of death in childbirth. *Journal of the Royal Society of Medicine, 106*(11), 461–463.

Lundgren, P., Kistner, A., Andersson, E. M., Hansen Pupp, I., Holmstrom, G., Ley, D., et al. (2014). Low birth weight is a risk factor for severe retinopathy of prematurity depending on gestational age. *PLoS One, 9*(10), e109460.

Machamer, P. K., Darden, L., & Craver, C. F. (2000). Thinking about mechanisms. *Philosophy in Science, 67*, 1–25.

Mackie, J. L. (1974). *The cement of the universe; a study of causation*. Clarendon Press.

MacMahon, B., & Pugh, T. F. (1970). *Epidemiology; principles and methods* (1st ed.). Little.

Mahaffey, K. W., Hafley, G., Dickerson, S., Burns, S., Tourt-Uhlig, S., White, J., Newby, L. K., Komajda, M., McMurray, J., Bigelow, R., Home, P. D., & Lopes, R. D. (2013). Results of a reevaluation of cardiovascular outcomes in the RECORD trial. *American Heart Journal, 166*(240–249), e241.

Mahipal, V., & Alam, M. A. U. (2022). Estimating heterogeneous causal effect of polysubstance usage on drug overdose from large-scale electronic health record. In *2022 44th Annual International Conference of the IEEE Engineering in Medicine & Biology Society (EMBC)*.

Mahmood, S. S., Levy, D., Vasan, R. S., & Wang, T. J. (2014). The Framingham Heart Study and the epidemiology of cardiovascular disease: A historical perspective. *Lancet, 383*(9921), 999–1008.

Malkov, M. I., Lee, C. T., & Taylor, C. T. (2021). Regulation of the Hypoxia-Inducible Factor (HIF) by pro-inflammatory cytokines. *Cells, 10*(9), 2340.

Manchikanti, L., Helm, S., Fellows, B., Janata, J. W., Pampati, V., Grider, J. S., et al. (2012). Opioid epidemic in the United States. *Pain Physician, 15*(3 Suppl), ES9–E38.

Manschot, W. A. (1954). Etiology of retrolental fibroplasia. *Archives of Ophthalmology, 52*(6), 833–845.

Manzoni, P., Maestri, A., Leonessa, M., Mostert, M., Farina, D., & Gomirato, G. (2006). Fungal and bacterial sepsis and threshold ROP in preterm very low birth weight neonates. *Journal of Perinatology, 26*(1), 23–30.

Marcuse, H. (1964). *One-dimensional man; studies in the ideology of advanced industrial society*. Beacon Press.

Marshall, B. D., & Galea, S. (2015). Formalizing the role of agent-based modeling in causal inference and epidemiology. *American Journal of Epidemiology, 181*(2), 92–99.

McCain, K. (2014). *Evidentialism and epistemic justification* (1st ed.). Routledge, Taylor & Francis Group.

McColm, J. R., Cunningham, S., Wade, J., Sedowofia, K., Gellen, B., Sharma, T., et al. (2004). Hypoxic oxygen fluctuations produce less severe retinopathy than hyperoxic fluctuations in a rat model of retinopathy of prematurity. *Pediatric Research, 55*(1), 107–113.

McLeod, D. S., Brownstein, R., & Lutty, G. A. (1996). Vaso-obliteration in the canine model of oxygen-induced retinopathy. *Investigative Ophthalmology & Visual Science, 37*(2), 300–311.

Medicine, I., & o. (2003). *The future of the public's health in the 21st century*. National Academies Press.

Miake-Lye, I. M., Hempel, S., Shanman, R., & Shekelle, P. G. (2016). What is an evidence map? A systematic review of published evidence maps and their definitions, methods, and products. *Systematic Reviews, 5*, 28.

Miettinen, O. S. (1985). *Theoretical epidemiology.* John Wiley & Sons.

Mill, J. S. (1856). *A system of logic* (4th ed.). John W. Parker & Son.

Milstein, B., & Wetterhall, S. (2016). A framework featuring steps and standards for program evaluation. *Health Promotion Practice, 1*(3), 221–228.

Mises, R. v (1981 (1957)). *Probability, statistics, and truth.* Dover.

Mishel, M. H. (1981). The measurement of uncertainty in illness. *Nursing Research, 30*(5), 258–263.

Mitra, S., Aune, D., Speer, C. P., & Saugstad, O. D. (2014). Chorioamnionitis as a risk factor for retinopathy of prematurity: A systematic review and meta-analysis. *Neonatology, 105*(3), 189–199.

Mitsuya, H., Weinhold, K. J., Furman, P. A., St Clair, M. H., Lehrman, S. N., Gallo, R. C., et al. (1985). 3'-Azido-3'-deoxythymidine (BW A509U): An antiviral agent that inhibits the infectivity and cytopathic effect of human T-lymphotropic virus type III/lymphadenopathy-associated virus in vitro. *Proceedings of the National Academy of Sciences of the United States of America, 82*(20), 7096–7100.

Mittal, M., Dhanireddy, R., & Higgins, R. D. (1998). Candida sepsis and association with retinopathy of prematurity. *Pediatrics, 101*(4 Pt 1), 654–657.

Miyazaki, Y., He, H., Mandarino, L. J., & DeFronzo, R. A. (2003). Rosiglitazone improves downstream insulin receptor signaling in Type 2 diabetic patients. *Diabetes, 52,* 1943–1950.

Mohamed, S., Murray, J. C., Dagle, J. M., & Colaizy, T. (2013). Hyperglycemia as a risk factor for the development of retinopathy of prematurity. *BMC Pediatrics, 13,* 78.

Mohammad-Taheri, S., Zucker, J., Hoyt, C. T., Sachs, K., Tewari, V., Ness, R., et al. (2022). Do-calculus enables estimation of causal effects in partially observed biomolecular pathways. *Bioinformatics, 38*(Supplement_1), i350–i358.

Moore, M. S. (2009). *Causation and responsibility: An essay in law, morals, and metaphysics.* Oxford University Press.

Morabia, A. (1991). On the origin of Hill's causal criteria. *Epidemiology, 2*(5), 367–369.

Morabia, A. (2010). Janet Lane-Claypon--interphase epitome. *Epidemiology, 21*(4), 573–576.

Morabia, A. (2013). Hume, Mill, Hill, and the sui generis epidemiologic approach to causal inference. *American Journal of Epidemiology, 178*(10), 1526–1532.

Morken, T. S., Dammann, O., Skranes, J., & Austeng, D. (2019). Retinopathy of prematurity, visual and neurodevelopmental outcome, and imaging of the central nervous system. *Seminars in Perinatology, 43*(6), 381–389.

Mumford, S., & Anjum, R. L. (2011). *Getting causes from powers.* Oxford University Press.

Nissen, S. E. (2010). The rise and fall of rosiglitazone. *European Heart Journal, 31,* 773–776.

Nissen, S. E., & Wolski, K. (2007). Effect of rosiglitazone on the risk of myocardial infarction and death from cardiovascular causes. *The New England Journal of Medicine, 356,* 2457–2471.

Nissen, S. E., & Wolski, K. (2010). Rosiglitazone revisited: An updated meta-analysis of risk for myocardial infarction and cardiovascular mortality. *Archives of Internal Medicine, 170,* 1191–1201.

Northrop, R. B. (2011). *Introduction to complexity and complex systems.* Taylor & Francis.

Noyola, D. E., Bohra, L., Paysse, E. A., Fernandez, M., & Coats, D. K. (2002). Association of candidemia and retinopathy of prematurity in very low birthweight infants. *Ophthalmology, 109*(1), 80–84.

O'Connor, T. (1994). Emergent properties. *American Philosophical Quarterly, 31,* 91–104.

Opara, C. N., Akintorin, M., Byrd, A., Cirignani, N., Akintorin, S., & Soyemi, K. (2020). Maternal diabetes mellitus as an independent risk factor for clinically significant retinopathy of prematurity severity in neonates less than 1500g. *PLoS One, 15*(8), e0236639.

Organ Donation and Transplantation Activities 2019 Report. (2019).

Padhi, T. R., Rath, S., Jalali, S., Pradhan, L., Kesarwani, S., Nayak, M., et al. (2014). Larger and near-term baby retinopathy: A rare case series. *Eye, 29*(2), 286–289.

Paneth, N., & Joyner, M. (2021). The use of observational research to inform clinical practice. *The Journal of Clinical Investigation, 131*(2), e146392.

Park, S. Y., Staicu, A.-M., Xiao, L., & Crainiceanu, C. M. (2018). Simple fixed-effects inference for complex functional models. *Biostatistics, 19*(2), 137–152.

Parkkinen, V.-P., Wallmann, C., Wilde, M., Clarke, B., Illari, P., Kelly, M. P., Norell, C., Russo, F., Shaw, B., & Williamson, J. (2018). *Evaluating evidence of mechanisms in medicine.* Springer.

Pearce, N. (2012). Classification of epidemiological study designs. *International Journal of Epidemiology, 41*(2), 393–397.

Pearl, J. (2000). *Causality - models, reasoning and inference.* Cambridge University Press.

Pearl, J. (2009). *Causality: Models, reasoning, and inference.* Cambridge University Press.

Pearl, J., Glymour, M., & Jewell, N. P. (2016). *Causal inference in statistics: A primer.* Wiley.

Pearson, K. (1900). *The grammar of science* (2nd ed.). A. and C. Black.

Pellegrino, E. D., & Thomasma, D. C. (1981). *A philosophical basis of medical practice: Toward a philosophy and ethic of the healing professions.* Oxford University Press.

Penn, J. S., Madan, A., Caldwell, R. B., Bartoli, M., Caldwell, R. W., & Hartnett, M. E. (2008). Vascular endothelial growth factor in eye disease. *Progress in Retinal and Eye Research, 27*(4), 331–371.

Peters, J., Janzing, D., & Schölkopf, B. (2017). *Elements of causal inference: Foundations and learning algorithms.* The MIT Press.

Phillips, C. J., Fordham, R., Marsh, K., Bertranou, E., Davies, S., Hale, J., et al. (2011). Exploring the role of economics in prioritization in public health: What do stakeholders think? *European Journal of Public Health, 21*(5), 578–584.

Phillips, C. V., & Goodman, K. J. (2006). Causal criteria and counterfactuals; nothing more (or less) than scientific common sense. *Emerging Themes in Epidemiology, 3,* 5.

Pierce, E. A., Avery, R. L., Foley, E. D., Aiello, L. P., & Smith, L. E. (1995). Vascular endothelial growth factor/vascular permeability factor expression in a mouse model of retinal neovascularization. *Proceedings of the National Academy of Sciences of the United States of America, 92*(3), 905–909.

Porter, R. (1998). *The greatest benefit to mankind: A medical history of humanity* (1st American ed.). W. W. Norton.

Poston, T. (2014). *Reason and explanation: A defense of explanatory coherentism* [text]. Palgrave Macmillan.

Pound, P., Ebrahim, S., Sandercock, P., Bracken, M. B., Roberts, I., & Reviewing Animal Trials Systematically, G. (2004). Where is the evidence that animal research benefits humans? *BMJ, 328*(7438), 514–517.

Proctor, R. N. (2012). The history of the discovery of the cigarette-lung cancer link: Evidentiary traditions, corporate denial, global toll. *Tobacco Control, 21*(2), 87–91.

Purohit, D. M., Ellison, R. C., Zierler, S., Miettinen, O. S., & Nadas, A. S. (1985). Risk factors for retrolental fibroplasia: Experience with 3,025 premature infants. *Pediatrics, 76*(3), 339–344.

Quinn, G. (2016). Retinopathy of prematurity blindness worldwide: Phenotypes in the third epidemic. *Eye and Brain, 8,* 31–36.

Quinn, G. E., Ying, G.-s., Bell, E. F., Donohue, P. K., Morrison, D., Tomlinson, L. A., et al. (2018). Incidence and early course of retinopathy of prematurity. *JAMA Ophthalmol, 136*(12), 1383–1389.

Quinn, T. C., Zacarias, F. R., & St John, R. K. (1989). HIV and HTLV-I infections in the Americas: A regional perspective. *Medicine (Baltimore), 68*(4), 189–209.

Ramshekar, A., & Hartnett, M. E. (2021). Vascular endothelial growth factor signaling in models of oxygen-induced retinopathy: Insights into mechanisms of pathology in retinopathy of prematurity. *Frontiers in Pediatrics, 9,* 796143.

Range, M. M., Arbic, B. K., Johnson, B. C., Moore, T. C., Titov, V., Adcroft, A. J., et al. (2022). The Chicxulub impact produced a powerful global Tsunami. *AGU Advances, 3*(5). https://doi.org/10.1029/2021AV000627

Rasmussen, S. A., Jamieson, D. J., Honein, M. A., & Petersen, L. R. (2016). Zika virus and birth defects--reviewing the evidence for causality. *The New England Journal of Medicine, 374*(20), 1981–1987.

Ratra, D., Akhundova, L., & Das, M. (2017). Retinopathy of prematurity like reti-nopathy in full-term infants. *Oman Journal of Ophthalmology, 10*(3), 167–172.

Reiss, J. (2015). *Causation, evidence, and inference.* Routledge.

Reutlinger, A., & Saatsi, J. (2018). *Explanation beyond causation: Philosophical perspectives on non-causal explanations* (1st ed.). Oxford University Press.

Ricci, B. (1990). Oxygen-induced retinopathy in the rat model. *Documenta Ophthalmologica, 74*(3), 171–177.

Rice, J. E. d., Vannucci, R. C., & Brierley, J. B. (1981). The influence of immatu-rity on hypoxic-ischemic brain damage in the rat. *Annals of Neurology, 9*(2), 131–141.

Richards, C. L., Iademarco, M. F., & Anderson, T. C. (2014). A new strategy for public health surveillance at CDC: Improving national surveillance activities and outcomes. *Public Health Reports, 129*(6), 472–476.

Ridker, P. M., Cook, N. R., Lee, I. M., Gordon, D., Gaziano, J. M., Manson, J. E., et al. (2005). A randomized trial of low-dose aspirin in the primary pre-vention of cardiovascular disease in women. *The New England Journal of Medicine, 352*(13), 1293–1304.

Riley, D., Fischer, M., Singh, B., Haidvogl, M., & Heger, M. (2001). Homeopathy and conventional medicine: An outcomes study comparing effectiveness in a primary care setting. *Journal of Alternative and Complementary Medicine, 7*(2), 149–159.

Rivera, J. C., Holm, M., Austeng, D., Morken, T. S., Zhou, T. E., Beaudry-Richard, A., et al. (2017). Retinopathy of prematurity: Inflammation, choroi-dal degeneration, and novel promising therapeutic strategies. *Journal of Neuroinflammation, 14*(1), 165.

Robins, J., & Wasserman, L. (1999). On the impossibility of inferring causation from association without background knowledge. In C. Glymour & G. F. Cooper (Eds.), *Computation, causation, discovery* (pp. 305–321). AAAI/MIT Press.

Rocca, E., & Anjum, R. L. (2020). Causal evidence and dispositions in medicine and public health. *International Journal of Environmental Research and Public Health, 17*(6), 1813.

Rodriguez, S. H., Ells, A. L., Blair, M. P., Shah, P. K., Harper, C. A., Martinez-Castellanos, M. A., et al. (2023). Retinopathy of prematurity in the 21st cen-tury and the complex impact of supplemental oxygen. *Journal of Clinical Medicine, 12*(3), 1228.

Roscher, R., Bohn, B., Duarte, M. F., & Garcke, J. (2020). Explainable machine learning for scientific insights and discoveries. *IEEE Access, 8*, 42200–42216.

Ross, L. (2023). Explanation in contexts of causal complexity: Lessons from psychiatric genetics. In William C. Bausman, Janella K. Baxter & Oliver M. Lean (eds.), *From Biological Practice to Scientific Metaphysics.* Minneapolis: University of Minnesota Press.

Ross, L. N. (2018). The doctrine of specific etiology. *Biology and Philosophy, 33*, 37.

Rothman, B. K. (2021). *The biomedical empire: Lessons learned from the Covid-19 pandemic.* Stanford Briefs, an imprint of Stanford University Press.

Rothman, K. J. (1976). Causes. *American Journal of Epidemiology, 104*, 87–92.

Rothman, K. J. (1986). *Modern epidemiology.* Little, Brown & Company.

Rothman, K. J. (1996). Lessons from John Graunt. *Lancet, 347*(8993), 37–39.

Rothman, K. J., & Greenland, S. (1998). *Modern epidemiology* (2nd ed.). Lippincott-Raven.

Rothman, K. J., & Greenland, S. (2005a). Causation and causal inference in epidemiology. *American Journal of Public Health, 95*(*Suppl 1*), S144–S150.

Rothman, K. J., & Greenland, S. (2005b). *Hill's criteria for causality* (0470011815). (Encyclopedia of biostatistics), Online, Issue.

Rothman, K. J., Greenland, S., Poole, C., & Lash, T. L. (2008). Causation and causal inference. In K. J. Rothman, S. Greenland, & T. L. Lash (Eds.), *Modern epidemiology* (3rd ed., pp. 5–31). Lippincott Williams & Wilkins.

Rothman, K. J., Lash, T. L., VanderWeele, T. J., & Haneuse, S. (2021). *Modern epidemiology* (4th ed.). Wolters Kluwer.

Ruben, D. H. (1990). *Explaining explanation.* Routledge.

Rubin, D. B. (1974). Estimating causal effects of treatments in randomized and nonrandomized studies. *Journal of Educational Psychology, 66*(5), 688–701.

Salmon, W. C. (1984). *Scientific explanation and the causal structure of the world.* Princeton University Press.

Salmon, W. C. (1997). Causality and explanation: A reply to two critiques. *Philosophy of Science, 64*(3), 461–477.

Saugstad, O. D. (2006). Oxygen and retinopathy of prematurity. *Journal of Perinatology, 26* (Suppl 1), S46–50; discussion S63–44.

Schmid, P., Cortes, J., Dent, R., Pusztai, L., McArthur, H., Kümmel, S., et al. (2022). Event-free survival with pembrolizumab in early triple-negative breast cancer. *New England Journal of Medicine, 386*(6), 556–567.

Schmid, P., Cortes, J., Pusztai, L., McArthur, H., Kümmel, S., Bergh, J., et al. (2020). Pembrolizumab for early triple-negative breast cancer. *New England Journal of Medicine, 382*(9), 810–821.

Schouten, B., Cobben, F., & Bethlehem, J. (2009). Indicators for the representativeness of survey response. *Survey Methodology, 35*(1), 101–113.

Schramme, T., & Edwards, S. (Eds.). (2016). *Handbook of the philosophy of medicine.* Springer.

Schulman, J., Jampol, L. M., & Schwartz, H. (1980). Peripheral proliferative retinopathy without oxygen therapy in a full-term infant. *American Journal of Ophthalmology, 90*(4), 509–514.

Schulzke, S. M., Stoecklin, B., & von Ungern-Sternberg, B. (2021). Update on ventilatory management of extremely preterm infants—A Neonatal Intensive Care Unit perspective. *Pediatric Anesthesia, 32*(2), 363–371.

Secker-Walker, R. H., Flynn, B. S., Solomon, L. J., Skelly, J. M., Dorwaldt, A. L., & Ashikaga, T. (2000). Helping women quit smoking: Results of a community intervention program. *American Journal of Public Health, 90*(6), 940–946.

Seema, R. K., Mandal, R. N., Tandon, A., Randhawa, V. S., Mehta, G., et al. (1999). Serum TNF-alpha and free radical scavengers in neonatal septicemia. *The Indian Journal of Pediatrics, 66*(4), 511–516.

Sekhon, M., Cartwright, M., & Francis, J. J. (2017). Acceptability of healthcare interventions: An overview of reviews and development of a theoretical framework. *BMC Health Services Research, 17*(1), 88.

Seok, J., Warren, H. S., Cuenca, A. G., Mindrinos, M. N., Baker, H. V., Xu, W., et al. (2013). Genomic responses in mouse models poorly mimic human inflammatory diseases. *Proceedings of the National Academy of Sciences of the United States of America, 110*(9), 3507–3512.

Shah, P. K., Narendran, V., & Kalpana, N. (2012). Aggressive posterior retinopathy of prematurity in large preterm babies in South India. *Archives of Disease in Childhood - Fetal and Neonatal Edition, 97*(5), F371–F375.

Sham, P. C., & Cherny, S. S. (2011). Genetic architecture of complex diseases. In E. Zeggini & A. Morris (Eds.), *Analysis of complex disease association studies* (pp. 1–13). Academic Press.

Shamil, M. S., Farheen, F., Ibtehaz, N., Khan, I. M., & Rahman, M. S. (2021). An agent-based modeling of COVID-19: Validation, analysis, and recommendations. *Cognitive Computation,* (2024) *16*, 1723–1734.

Shang, A., Huwiler-Muntener, K., Nartey, L., Juni, P., Dorig, S., Sterne, J. A., et al. (2005). Are the clinical effects of homoeopathy placebo effects? Comparative study of placebo-controlled trials of homoeopathy and allopathy. *Lancet, 366*(9487), 726–732.

Shipley, B. (2000). *Cause and correlation in biology.* Cambridge University Press.

Shulman, J. P., Weng, C., Wilkes, J., Greene, T., & Hartnett, M. E. (2017). Association of maternal preeclampsia with infant risk of premature birth and retinopathy of prematurity. *JAMA Ophthalmol, 135*(9), 947–953.

Silva, P. C. L., Batista, P. V. C., Lima, H. S., Alves, M. A., Guimarães, F. G., & Silva, R. C. P. (2020). COVID-ABS: An agent-based model of COVID-19 epidemic to simulate health and economic effects of social distancing interventions. *Chaos, Solitons & Fractals, 139*, 110088.

Silveira, R. C., Fortes Filho, J. B., & Procianoy, R. S. (2011). Assessment of the contribution of cytokine plasma levels to detect retinopathy of prematurity in very low birth weight infants. *Investigative Ophthalmology & Visual Science, 52*, 1297–1301.

Silverman, W. A. (1977). The lesson of retrolental fibroplasia. *Scientific American, 236*(6), 100–107.

Silverman, W. A. (1982). Retinopathy of prematurity: Oxygen dogma challenged. *Archives of Disease in Childhood, 57*(10), 731–733.

Silverman, W. A. (1986). Epoche in retinopathy of prematurity. *Archives of Disease in Childhood, 61*(5), 522–525.

Singham, M. (2020). *The great paradox of science: Why its conclusions can be relied upon even though they cannot be proven.* Oxford University Press.

Sjoberg, E. A. (2017). Logical fallacies in animal model research. *Behavioral and Brain Functions, 13*(1), Article no. 3.

Skow, B. (2015). Scientific explanation. In P. Humphreys (Ed.), *The Oxford handbook of philosophy of science.* OUP.

Skow, B. (2016). *Reasons why,* First edition. ed. Oxford University Press, Oxford, United Kingdom; New York, NY.

Smart, B. (2016). *Concepts and causes in the philosophy of disease.* Palgrave Macmillan.

Smart, B. T. H. (2023). The core business of medicine: A defence of the best available intervention thesis. *Synthese, 201,* 194.

Smith, L. E., Wesolowski, E., McLellan, A., Kostyk, S. K., D'Amato, R., Sullivan, R., et al. (1994). Oxygen-induced retinopathy in the mouse. *Investigative Ophthalmology & Visual Science, 35*(1), 101–111.

Snowise, N. G. (2021). Memorials to John Snow - Pioneer in anaesthesia and epidemiology. *Journal of Medical Biography, 31*(1), 47–50. https://doi.org/10.1177/09677720211013807

Solomon, M. (2015). *Making medical knowledge* (1st ed.). Oxford University Press.

Solomon, M., Simon, J. R., & Kincaid, H. (2017). *The Routledge companion to philosophy of medicine.* Routledge, Taylor & Francis Group.

Sood, B. G., Madan, A., Saha, S., Schendel, D., Thorsen, P., Skogstrand, K., et al. (2010). Perinatal systemic inflammatory response syndrome and retinopathy of prematurity. *Pediatric Research, 67*(4), 394–400.

Spirtes, P., & Glymour, C. (1991). An algorithm for fast recovery of sparse causal graphs. *Social Science Computer Review, 9*(1), 62–72.

Spirtes, P., Glymour, C., & Scheines, R. (1991). From probability to causality. *Philosophical Studies: An International Journal for Philosophy in the Analytic Tradition, 64,* 1–36.

Spirtes, P., Glymour, C., & Scheines, R. (2000). *Causation, prediction, and search* (2nd ed.). MIT Press.

Spirtes, P., Glymour, C. N., & Scheines, R. (1993). *Causation, prediction, and search.* Springer-Verlag.

Staffini, A., Svensson, A. K., Chung, U.-I., & Svensson, T. (2021). An agent-based model of the local spread of SARS-CoV-2: Modeling study. *JMIR Medical Informatics, 9*(4), e24192.

Stegenga, J. (2009). Robustness, discordance, and relevance. *Philosophy of Science, 76,* 650–661.

Stegenga, J. (2018). *Medical nihilism.* Oxford University Press.

Stinchcombe, A. L. (1991). The conditions of fruitfulness of theorizing about mechanisms in social science. *Philosophy of the Social Sciences, 21*(3), 367–388.

Stockel, D., Schmidt, F., Trampert, P., & Lenhof, H. P. (2015). CausalTrail: Testing hypothesis using causal Bayesian networks. *F1000Res, 4*.

Stout, R. (1996). *Things that happen because they should.* Oxford University Press.

Sun, M., Wadehra, M., Casero, D., Lin, M.-C., Aguirre, B., Parikh, S., et al. (2020). Epithelial Membrane Protein 2 (EMP2) Promotes VEGF-induced pathological neovascularization in murine oxygen-induced retinopathy. *Investigative Opthalmology & Visual Science, 61*(2), 3.

Susser, M. (1991). What is a cause and how do we know one? A grammar for pragmatic epidemiology. *American Journal of Epidemiology, 133*, 635–648.

Tadesse, M., Dhanireddy, R., Mittal, M., & Higgins, R. D. (2002). Race, Candida sepsis, and retinopathy of prematurity. *Biology of the Neonate, 81*(2), 86–90.

Tamm, M. (2021). Is causality a necessary tool for understanding our universe, or is it a part of the problem? *Entropy, 23*(7), 886.

Termote, J. U., Schalij-Delfos, N. E., Wittebol-Post, D., Brouwers, H. A., Hoogervorst, B. R., & Cats, B. P. (1994). Surfactant replacement therapy: A new risk factor in developing retinopathy of prematurity? *European Journal of Pediatrics, 153*(2), 113–116.

Terry, T. L. (1942a). Extreme prematurity and fibroblastic overgrowth of persistent vascular sheath behind each crystalline lens. *American Journal of Ophthalmology, 25*, 203–204.

Terry, T. L. (1942b). Fibroblastic overgrowth of persistent tunica vasculosa lentis in infants born prematurely: II. Report of cases-clinical aspects. *Transactions of the American Ophthalmological Society, 40*, 262–284.

Terry, T. L. (1944). Retrolental fibroplasia in the premature infant: V. further studies on fibroplastic overgrowth of the persistent tunica vasculosa lentis. *Transactions of the American Ophthalmological Society, 42*, 383–396.

Tettamanti, G., Auvinen, A., Åkerstedt, T., Kojo, K., Ahlbom, A., Heinävaara, S., et al. (2020). Long-term effect of mobile phone use on sleep quality: Results from the cohort study of mobile phone use and health (COSMOS). *Environment International, 140*, 105687.

Thagard, P. (2006). Evaluating explanations in law, science, and everyday life. *Current Directions in Psychological Science, 15*(3), 141–145.

Thompson, R. P., & Upshur, R. (2018). *Philosophy of medicine: An introduction.* Routledge, Taylor & Francis Group.

Thygesen, L. C., Andersen, G. S., & Andersen, H. (2005). A philosophical analysis of the Hill criteria. *Journal of Epidemiology and Community Health, 59*(6), 512–516.

Tolsma, K. W., Allred, E. N., Chen, M. L., Duker, J., Leviton, A., & Dammann, O. (2011). Neonatal bacteremia and retinopathy of prematurity: The ELGAN study. *Archives of Ophthalmology, 129*(12), 1555–1563.

Topping, C. J., Høye, T. T., & Olesen, C. R. (2010). Opening the black box—Development, testing and documentation of a mechanistically rich agent-based model. *Ecological Modelling, 221*(2), 245–255.

Tracy, M., Cerdá, M., & Keyes, K. M. (2018). Agent-based modeling in public health: Current applications and future directions. *Annual Review of Public Health, 39*(1), 77–94.

Truszkowska, A., Behring, B., Hasanyan, J., Zino, L., Butail, S., Caroppo, E., Jiang, Z.-P., Rizzo, A., & Porfiri, M. (2021). High-resolution agent-based modeling of COVID-19 spreading in a small town. *Advanced Theory and Simulations, 4*(3), 2000277.

Tremblay, S., Miloudi, K., Chaychi, S., Favret, S., Binet, F., Polosa, A., et al. (2013). Systemic inflammation perturbs developmental retinal angiogenesis and neuroretinal function. *Investigative Ophthalmology & Visual Science, 54*(13), 8125–8139.

Trifonova, K., Slaveykov, K., Mumdzhiev, H., & Dzhelebov, D. (2018). Artificial reproductive technology - a risk factor for retinopathy of prematurity. *Open Access Macedonian Journal of Medical Sciences, 6*(11), 2245–2249.

Truszkowska, A., Behring, B., Hasanyan, J., Zino, L., Butail, S., Caroppo, E., et al. (2021). High-resolution agent-based modeling of COVID-19 spreading in a small town. *Advanced Theory and Simulations, 4*(3), 2000277.

Tsai, A. S., Chou, H. D., Ling, X. C., Al-Khaled, T., Valikodath, N., Cole, E., et al. (2022). Assessment and management of retinopathy of prematurity in the era of anti-vascular endothelial growth factor (VEGF). *Progress in Retinal and Eye Research, 88*, 101018.

Tulchinsky, T. H. (2018). John snow, cholera, the broad street pump; Waterborne diseases then and now. In *Case studies in public health* (pp. 77–99). Elsevier.

United States. Surgeon General's Advisory Committee on Smoking and Health. (1964). *Smoking and health; report of the advisory committee to the Surgeon General of the Public Health Service.* U., S. Dept. of Health, Education, and Welfare, Public Health Service; for sale by the Superintendent of Documents, U.S. Govt. Print. Off.

Upshur, R., & Goldenberg, M. J. (2020). Countering medical nihilism by reconnecting facts and values. *Studies in History and Philosophy of Science, 84*, 75–83.

Upshur, R. E. (2002). Principles for the justification of public health intervention. *Canadian Journal of Public Health, 93*(2), 101–103.

Ushio-Fukai, M. (2007). VEGF signaling through NADPH oxidase-derived ROS. *Antioxidants & Redox Signaling, 9*(6), 731–739.

Van Dyke Parunak, H., Savit, R., & Riolo, R. L. (1998). Agent-based modeling vs. equation-based modeling: A case study and users' guide. In J. S. Sichman, R. Conte, & N. Gilbert (Eds.), *Multi-agent systems and agent-based simulation.* Berlin, Heidelberg.

Vandenbroucke, J. P., Broadbent, A., & Pearce, N. (2016). Causality and causal inference in epidemiology: The need for a pluralistic approach. *International Journal of Epidemiology, 45*(6), 1776–1786.

VanderVeen, D. K., & Cataltepe, S. U. (2019). Anti-vascular endothelial growth factor intravitreal therapy for retinopathy of prematurity. *Seminars in Perinatology, 43*(6), 375–380.

VanderWeele, T. J. (2015). *Explanation in causal inference: Methods for mediation and interaction.* Oxford University Press.

Van Fraassen Bas, C. (1980). *The Scientific Image.* Oxford University Press.

Vannucci, S. J., & Back, S. A. (2022). The Vannucci model of hypoxic-ischemic injury in the neonatal rodent: 40 years later. *Developmental Neuroscience, 44*(4–5), 186–193.

Venkatramanan, S., Lewis, B., Chen, J., Higdon, D., Vullikanti, A., & Marathe, M. (2018). Using data-driven agent-based models for forecasting emerging infectious diseases. *Epidemics, 22,* 43–49.

Walker, W. E., Harremoës, P., Rotmans, J., van der Sluijs, J. P., van Asselt, M. B. A., Janssen, P., et al. (2003). Defining uncertainty: A conceptual basis for uncertainty management in model-based decision support. *Integrated Assessment, 4*(1), 5–17.

Wallace, D. K., Kylstra, J. A., Phillips, S. J., & Hall, J. G. (2000). Poor postnatal weight gain: A risk factor for severe retinopathy of prematurity. *Journal of AAPOS, 4*(6), 343–347.

Wang, X., Tang, K., Chen, L., Cheng, S., & Xu, H. (2019). Association between sepsis and retinopathy of prematurity: A systematic review and meta-analysis. *BMJ Open, 9*(5), e025440.

Weed, D. L. (2008). Truth, epidemiology, and general causation. *Brooklyn Law Review, 73*(3), 943–957.

Weinberger, B., Laskin, D. L., Heck, D. E., & Laskin, J. D. (2002). Oxygen toxicity in premature infants. *Toxicology and Applied Pharmacology, 181*(1), 60–67.

Weisberg, M. (2014). Understanding the emergence of population behavior in individual-based models. *Philosophy of Science, 81*(5), 785–797.

White, C. (1990). Research on smoking and lung cancer: A landmark in the history of chronic disease epidemiology. *The Yale Journal of Biology and Medicine, 63*(1), 29–46.

Williamson, J. (2005). *Bayesian nets and causality: Philosophical and computational foundations.* Oxford University Press.

Winkelmann, S., Zonker, J., Schütte, C., & Conrad, N. D. (2021). Mathematical modeling of spatio-temporal population dynamics and application to epidemic spreading. *Mathematical Biosciences, 336,* 108619.

Wolkenhauer, O. (2014). Why model? *Frontiers in Physiology, 5,* 21.

Woodcock, J., Sharfstein, J. M., & Hamburg, M. (2010). Regulatory action on rosiglitazone by the U.S. food and drug administration. *New England Journal of Medicine, 363,* 1489–1491.

Woodward, J. (2003). *Making things happen - A theory of causal explanation.* Oxford University Press.

Woodward, J. (2017). Scientific explanation. In E. N. Zalta (Ed.), *The Stanford encyclopedia of philosophy* (Fall edn). Metaphysics Research Lab, Stanford University.

Woodward, J., & Ross, L. (2021). Scientific explanation. In E. N. Zalta (Ed.), *The Stanford Encyclopedia of Philosophy* (Summer edn). Metaphysics Research Lab, Stanford University.

Worrall, J. (2007). Why there's no cause to randomize. *British Journal for the Philosophy of Science, 58*(3), 451–488.

Worrall, J. (2011). Causality in medicine: Getting back to the Hill top. *Preventive Medicine, 53*(4–5), 235–238.

Wright, L. (1976). *Teleological explanations: An etiological analysis of goals and functions.* University of California Press.

Wu, P. Y., Fu, Y. K., Lien, R. I., Chiang, M. C., Lee, C. C., Chen, H. C., et al. (2023). Systemic cytokines in retinopathy of prematurity. *Journal of Personalized Medicine, 13*(2), 291.

Xu, Y., Lu, X., Hu, Y., Yang, B., Tsui, C.-K., Yu, S., et al. (2018). Melatonin attenuated retinal neovascularization and neuroglial dysfunction by inhibition of HIF-1α-VEGF pathway in oxygen-induced retinopathy mice. *Journal of Pineal Research, 64*(4), e12473.

Yang, B., Xu, Y., Yu, S., Huang, Y., Lu, L., & Liang, X. (2016). Anti-angiogenic and anti-inflammatory effect of Magnolol in the oxygen-induced retinopathy model. *Inflammation Research, 65*(1), 81–93.

Yeravdekar, R. C., & Singh, A. (2022). Physician-scientists: Fixing the leaking pipeline — A scoping review. *Medical Science Educator, 32*(6), 1413–1424.

Young, R. H. (2005). A brief history of the pathology of the gonads. *Modern Pathology, 18*(Suppl 2), S3–S17.

Yu, C. W., Popovic, M. M., Dhoot, A. S., Arjmand, P., Muni, R. H., Tehrani, N. N., et al. (2022). Demographic risk factors of retinopathy of prematurity: A systematic review of population-based studies. *Neonatology, 119*, 1–13.

Yu, H., Yuan, L., Zou, Y., Peng, L., Wang, Y., Li, T., et al. (2014). Serum concentrations of cytokines in infants with retinopathy of prematurity. *APMIS, 122*(9), 818–823.

Zeggini, E., & Morris, A. P. (2011). *Analysis of complex disease association studies: A practical guide* (1st ed.). Academic Press/Elsevier.

Zhao, K., Jiang, Y., Zhang, J., Shi, J., Zheng, P., Yang, C., et al. (2022). Celastrol inhibits pathologic neovascularization in oxygen-induced retinopathy by targeting the miR-17-5p/HIF-1α/VEGF pathway. *Cell Cycle, 21*(19), 2091–2108.

Author Index[1]

B
Broadbent, Alex, viii, 3–6, 8, 9, 11,
  15n5, 19–29, 32n1, 32n2, 32n5,
  36, 42n1, 45, 65–67, 109n2,
  110n14, 153, 223n3, 262, 291

C
Campaner, Raffaella, 36, 40–42,
  42–43n1, 238
Cartwright, Nancy, 82, 83, 92, 93,
  110n11, 164, 173, 203, 252,
  254, 259, 263

H
Han, Paul, viii, 31, 47, 48, 52,
  61n1, 61n2
Heisenberg, Werner, 10, 48–50, 120

Hill, Austin Bradford, 13, 72, 85,
  93, 111n31, 165, 170, 173,
  180, 187, 189, 199,
  202–204, 218–223, 223n6,
  244, 272, 275–277,
  281, 292
Howick, Jeremy, 42n1, 180, 238

I
Ioannidis, John, 3, 6, 180

K
Kolata, Gina, 2, 3, 15n4, 20

R
Ross, Lauren, 107, 108, 130

---

[1] Note: Page numbers followed by 'n' refer to notes.

Subject Index[1]

[1] Note: Page numbers followed by 'n' refer to notes.

© The Author(s), under exclusive license to Springer Nature Switzerland AG 2025
O. Dammann, *Uncertainty and Explanation in Medicine and the Health Sciences*, https://doi.org/10.1007/978-3-031-82271-1